Endodontic Materials in Clinical Practice

Endodontic Materials in Clinical Practice

Edited by

Josette Camilleri
University of Birmingham
Birmingham, UK

WILEY Blackwell

Registered Offices
John Wiley & Sons, Inc., 111 River Street, Hoboken, NJ 07030, USA
John Wiley & Sons Ltd, The Atrium, Southern Gate, Chichester, West Sussex, PO19 8SQ, UK

Editorial Office
9600 Garsington Road, Oxford, OX4 2DQ, UK

For details of our global editorial offices, customer services, and more information about Wiley products visit us at www.wiley.com.

Wiley also publishes its books in a variety of electronic formats and by print-on-demand. Some content that appears in standard print versions of this book may not be available in other formats.

Library of Congress Cataloging-in-Publication Data

Names: Camilleri, Josette, editor.
Title: Endodontic materials in clinical practice / edited by Josette
    Camilleri.
Description: First edition. | Hoboken, NJ : Wiley-Blackwell, 2021. | Includes
    bibliographical references and index. | Description based on print version
    record and CIP data provided by publisher; resource not viewed.
Identifiers: LCCN 2020028477 (print) | LCCN 2020028478 (ebook) | ISBN
    9781119513612 (epub) | ISBN 9781119513605 (adobe pdf) | ISBN 9781119513520
    (hardback)
Subjects: | MESH: Dental Pulp Diseases–therapy | Root Canal Filling
    Materials–therapeutic use | Pulp Capping and Pulpectomy
    Agents–therapeutic use
Classification: LCC RK351 (ebook) | LCC RK351 (print) | NLM WU 230 | DDC
    617.6/342–dc23
LC record available at https://lccn.loc.gov/2020028477
LC record available at https://lccn.loc.gov/2020028478

Cover Design: Wiley
Cover Image: © Hal Duncan, © Josette Camilleri, © Nastaran Meschi, © Laurence Jordan

Set in 9.5/12.5pt STIXTwoText by SPi Global, Pondicherry, India

Printed in Singapore

M090196_120321

Contents

List of Contributors

Maria Teresa Arias-Moliz
Department of Microbiology
Faculty of Dentistry
University of Granada
Granada
Spain

Christos Boutsioukis
Department of Endodontology
Academic Centre for Dentistry
Amsterdam (ACTA)
University of Amsterdam and Vrije
Universiteit Amsterdam
Amsterdam
The Netherlands

Francois Bronnec
Private practice
Paris
France

Josette Camilleri
School of Dentistry
Institute of Clinical Sciences
College of Medical and Dental Sciences
University of Birmingham
Birmingham
UK

Nicholas Chandler
Sir John Walsh Research Institute
University of Otago
Dunedin
New Zealand

Bun San Chong
Institute of Dentistry
Barts and The London School of Medicine
and Dentistry
Queen Mary University of London
London, UK

Paul R. Cooper
Sir John Walsh Research Institute
Department of Oral Sciences
Faculty of Dentistry
University of Otago
Dunedin, New Zealand

Luiz Fernando D'Altoé
Department of Dentistry
University of the Extreme South of Santa
Catarina (UNESC)
Criciúma
Santa Catarina
Brazil

Brian W. Darvell
School of Dentistry
Institute of Clinical Sciences
College of Medical and Dental Sciences
University of Birmingham
Birmingham, UK

Henry F. Duncan
Division of Restorative Dentistry and
Periodontology
Dublin Dental University Hospital
Trinity College Dublin
Dublin, Ireland

Mostafa EzEldeen
Department of Oral Health Sciences
KU Leuven

Dentistry
University Hospitals Leuven
Leuven
Belgium

Kerstin M. Galler
Department of Conservative Dentistry and
Periodontology
University Hospital Regensburg
Regensburg
Germany

Laurence Jordan
Faculty of Dentistry
Paris University
Paris, France

Chimie ParisTech
PSL Research University
Paris, France

Rothschild Hospital AP-HP
Paris, France

Paul Lambrechts
Department of Oral Health Sciences
KU Leuven

Dentistry
University Hospitals Leuven
Leuven
Belgium

Pierre Machtou
UFR d'Odontologie
Paris Diderot University
Paris, France

Nastaran Meschi
Department of Oral Health Sciences
KU Leuven

Dentistry
University Hospitals Leuven
Leuven
Belgium

Mutlu Özcan
Division of Dental Biomaterials
Center for Dental and Oral Medicine
Clinic for Reconstructive Dentistry
University of Zürich
Zürich
Switzerland

Christof Pertl
Department of Dental Medicine and Oral
Health
Medical University of Graz
Austria

Harvard School of Dental Medicine
Boston
MA
USA

Phillip L. Tomson
School of Dentistry
Institute of Clinical Sciences
University of Birmingham
Birmingham
UK

Gertrude Van Gorp
Department of Oral Health Sciences
KU Leuven

Dentistry
University Hospitals Leuven
Leuven
Belgium

Claudia Angela Maziero Volpato
Department of Dentistry
Federal University of Santa Catarina (UFSC)
Florianópolis
Santa Catarina
Brazil

Matthias Widbiller
Department of Conservative Dentistry and
Periodontology
University Hospital Regensburg
Regensburg
Germany

1

Introduction

Materials Chemistry as a Means to an End(o) – The Invisible Foundation

Brian W. Darvell

School of Dentistry, Institute of Clinical Sciences, College of Medical and Dental Sciences, University of Birmingham, Birmingham, UK

1.1   Introduction

In the last 70 years or so, our understanding of dental materials has progressed from the more or less purely pragmatic to a more structure–function design-based science. This process is not yet complete. That is, despite the currency of 'evidence-based dentistry' – which has its own Wikipedia entry and an eponymous journal – there remains much work to be done to make everyone appreciate the value of the science of those materials. Inadequate teaching and dogmatic schools of thought are also manifest in endodontics to no lesser extent. It is my understanding that this book represents an attempt to begin the essential process of modernization in this field. Accordingly, I shall attempt to provide some foundations for the necessary insight.

Once the vitality of the dental pulp becomes compromised, endodontic intervention is necessary to preserve a functional natural dentition, with natural alveolar (as opposed to ankylosed) bone attachment, and thus the preservation of that very bone. More, perhaps, than in some other areas of dentistry, the materials used in endodontic work have an intimate relationship with tissues. Most obviously, the dentine is subject to exposure to a variety of more or less aggressive irrigants as well as fillers and (putative) sealers, often involving calcium hydroxide. Another possibility is of a strong oxidizing agent in the form of hypochlorite. Whilst the need for microbial elimination is not disputed, it is appropriate to be aware of the implications of such treatments: the chemistry demands that if a reaction is possible, it will occur, whether you like it or not, whether you meant it or not, and whether you are aware of it or not. Of course, apical extrusion of almost all materials can have very unfortunate consequences. Such intimacy is quite undesirable.

At the least, a foreign body reaction will be elicited; at the worst, destruction of periapical bone – but the risk of infection is always high, with potentially wider implications.

1.2 The Substrate

Dentine has a complex composite structure whose matrix is largely proteinaceous, but it also has an inorganic component, biological apatite. As such, it is vulnerable to hydrolysis (whether acid- or base-catalysed), even at pH 7 – although this may then be at a very low rate [1]. Since the mechanical properties of a composite structure are dependent on the integrity of the matrix, any such hydrolysis must be considered detrimental. In this light, the frequent finding that root fracture is associated with the use of calcium hydroxide, or materials containing it, is a predictable outcome for inevitable chemistry. The increased risk has to be treated as a necessary sequela of such a treatment, with the unhappy implication that the life of the remaining tooth may be limited (bearing in mind that the loads experienced by such teeth depend on a number of circumstances). Indeed, the use of oxidants such as sodium hypochlorite (which also deliberately has a high pH) must likewise contribute to such deterioration, because all organic material must be subject to oxidation, and indiscriminately. Add to this the penetration and diffusion of fluids and the effect can be seen to be not necessarily local. We therefore need to recognize that all such treatments involve compromise, a trade-off between immediate benefit and longer-term failure risk.

Disruption of the dentine matrix has further implications. As is discussed in Chapter 3, many biologically important molecules become bound within it during its development. Should these molecules be released through matrix breakdown, they may become once again biologically active and thus be important in reparative or regenerative processes. Such release through mechanical processes has little implication for that activity. Likewise, demineralization under mild conditions, such as with ethylene diamine tetra-acetic acid or 'EDTA' (what is used in dentistry is actually closer to the trisodium salt, in order to provide enough solubility at around pH 7–8), may be considered in the same context. Such demineralization can be presumed to offer an easier diffusive path through the now much more porous tissue, and so may release these molecules without detriment to them, although perhaps the larger ones – proteins, for example – may emerge more slowly. It is, however, worth considering whether the more aggressive media at high pH cause any destruction of such molecules: proteins of whatever kind are still subject to hydrolysis. Are any of the other important matrix components capable of reaction, and thus damage and inactivation, under those conditions? Naturally, this is not necessarily an all-or-nothing kind of event – the kinetics of the reaction determines how much survives. It would follow, though, given that these molecules are believed to be of value in the course of treatment, that finding more benign means of release than the presently documented range of products would be of value for a more reliable effect of full efficacy. It would be wrong to assume, again, that the chemical reaction that destroys the matrix and releases these substances is selective. For example, urea may solubilize (that is, make soluble, as opposed to merely releasing) the matrix protein, but at the risk of unfolding, and therefore inactivating, enzymes of interest. There will probably not be a perfect resolution of this problem, but the means may conceivably be designed or selected for specific targets. It should be apparent that oxidizing agents are liable to destroy any and all biologically active molecules more rapidly than high pH alone. What appear to be needed are assays of the sequestered substances for comparison with release rates and survival in an active form after the various possible treatments.

The use of demineralizing and matrix-destroying agents has an important implication. If bonding to collagen is intended, it must be left intact. If interaction with the calcium or phosphate of the mineral is contemplated, that must remain available. It is clearly illogical to use a treatment that removes an essential component of a subsequently intended process.

The preceding discussions are essentially of simple chemistry. It is curious then that in the historical focus on sterility and its maintenance in the present context, there has been little consideration of the inevitable effects of some of the agents used. Ignorance of the chemistry is no excuse, and to claim, for example, that a particular effect is not required is a chemical absurdity: as already stressed, if a reaction is possible, it will occur; if a pathway exists, it will be taken. The only debate is about relative rates. Materials science – and no less in endodontics than anywhere else – must recognize the chemistry of systems and design accordingly. The dogma mentioned must be designed out of dentistry. Again, though, compromise is inevitable; perfection is – at best – unlikely. Rational assessment is not optional, it is essential.

1.3 Nomenclatural Hype: 'Bioactivity', 'Bioceramics'

It is clear that substances released unaltered from the dentine matrix must retain their biological function and activity, although whether the balance that originally obtained during development in the many complex interacting pathways is effectively and usefully maintained remains a matter for investigation. Nevertheless, it is proper to argue that this is indeed biological activity – bioactivity, to use the current jargon – because these are natural substances involved in entirely normal biological processes. Unfortunately, the field of dentistry is heavily trampled and muddied by the indiscriminate use of the term in any

context where a biological response is elicited. That is, in the absence of those natural biological substances, any action, process, or material that provokes a response of any kind is automatically labelled 'bioactive'. Such responses fall for now into just two classes: simple chemical and challenge defence.

Simple chemical responses typically involve the provision of a species that perturbs a chemical equilibrium, such as by changing the local pH. To take an ordinary example, adding sufficient calcium ions to a tissue fluid (by dissolution of a component of a material, say) must locally drive the precipitation of a calcium phosphate, assuming nucleation can occur. Because this is inevitable simple chemistry, with no sign of the involvement of a biological process, there is no logic or sense in labelling the source material 'bioactive', yet this is commonplace. We may note in passing that a frequently-used test of 'bioactivity' involves immersing the test material in a metastable supersaturated solution of calcium and phosphate, the criterion being the appearance in due course of an apatitic precipitate on that material. The fact is that almost everything produces that effect, due to the ease with which apatitic material nucleates under those circumstances – there are many papers reporting such an outcome. It is worth remembering that tissue fluids are not, in general, supersaturated with respect to apatites. Simplistic calculations based on analytical values without taking into account speciation (and, especially, binding by many specialized protein systems) fail to give sensible results. Whilst hypercalcification (heterotopic ossification) is a real and distressing disease, we do not as a matter of course calcify promptly and locally in response to cuts and bruises, which effect would otherwise be expected. To make this point more clearly, highly supersaturated calcium phosphate solutions can be prepared that can stand for days without doing anything. Yet, merely shaking the flask can result in the prompt and massive precipitation of the excess: any seed is enough. There is no discernible chemical difference between such a system and the 'bioactivity' test. There is simply no biology involved.

Challenge defence responses are elicited by anything that represents a foreign body, toxicity, osmotic imbalance, boundary layer disturbance (*via* zeta potentials or surface chemistry), pH change, or merely an unusual ion – that is, a chemical challenge, an insult to the tissue. The body's natural reaction is to mount a defensive response such as encapsulation and immune reactions, if outright apoptosis and necrosis does not occur. When calcification (*e.g.* dentine formation) is involved, it is greeted with pleasure. But then, such an effect occurs with low-level challenges such as caries anyway. It does not seem to be sensible to label materials that provoke a defensive response, however natural or normal, as 'bioactive'. On that basis, formaldehyde is bioactive, zinc oxide-eugenol is bioactive, and calcium hydroxide is bioactive.

By extension, then, it is a puzzle how materials that cause disruption or degradation of the dentine matrix can be labelled 'bioactive' simply because in the course of that damage some truly biologically active substances happen to be released, and quite regardless of the fact that such substances may have local beneficial effects. What we see is a creeping inflation of titular importance that bears no relation to underlying processes. It is one of the worst examples of the hijacking of a term to make the products it is attached to seem more valuable and useful. There are many such in dentistry. The problem is that, in the absence of understanding by the general user of the products' actual chemistry, their use and effects are misunderstood. We do not serve patients' best interests by such exaggeration and misinformation.

All that said, there is a conceptual class of material that can truly be described as bioactive, and although there is nothing at present on the market, it has been demonstrated in principle. That is, the incorporation of a naturally occurring biological substance or substances that may stimulate or trigger a natural process that leads to a suitable outcome, such as bone growth or dentine deposition. By definition, this is a substance that is normally involved, but whose artificial provision enables, facilitates, or amplifies the pathway. One would expect that the vehicle for such a delivery would be otherwise benign, not representing a challenge in itself – for example, a resorbable, noninflammatory material.

We must be careful, though, not to stray into the realm of pharmaceutical products (which incidentally has all kinds of implications for marketing and promotion, never mind supply and use). That is, pharmaceuticals are intended to be biologically active in that they may, for example, modulate or trigger natural processes. The question is whether a material that is the vehicle for a substance not normally involved in the usual biochemistry of repair can be considered 'bioactive'. Imagine a material carrying, say, aspirin: it would be wrong to say this is bioactive. Thus, salicylate-based cements and liners are not. Whether the provision of a normal, human, biological substance in such a fashion is pharmaceutical is for others to debate and decide. Ponder the taking of vitamin D, or melatonin, for example. Antibiotics clearly cross the line.

Overall, then, the key is that we must inspect the chemistry to ascertain what is going on. If it is a simple chemical effect that does not involve any biology as such, or if it is a chemical challenge that results in a defensive (albeit normal) response, it is quite improper to apply the term 'bioactive': it is an advertising malfeasance. If – or, perhaps, when – materials are available that are the vehicles for any of the many biologically active substances that offer the possibility of true reparative or regenerative responses, the label will be fully justified and accurate. Until then, it is suggested that much more careful thought is required, which goes beyond the allure of advertising hype and wishful thinking. Mere repetition does not make it so. Believing one's own propaganda is not scientific.

A similar abuse occurs in the term 'bioceramic'. A ceramic material is, in simple chemical terms, anything that is not metallic or organic polymeric. The prefix 'bio' only seems to refer to the context in which it is used: in a medical or dental application. This is pretentiously misleading. It does not automatically confer special properties on the material in question, which has in any case been chosen (one hopes) on grounds of its general inertness and suitable mechanical properties. There are no classes of materials that in any sense earn the label, except possibly those of bone, dentine, and enamel – natural hard tissues – and even then, it serves no real purpose. Can it be applied to mollusc shells? Quite possibly. But how does that help us understand the value of marketing hype? Its extension to setting cements and sealers is incomprehensible [2].

Chemistry is frequently a weak point in other areas. Take 'MTA' as perhaps the most egregious example: this is the trade-name abbreviation for what is described as 'mineral trioxide aggregate'. Try as one might, this phrase makes no sense whatsoever: it does not inform in any way at all – it does not even describe the material itself – yet it is bandied about as if it were a meaningful label. It is inorganic, admittedly, but as the Oxford English Dictionary has it: 'Mineral: A naturally occurring substance of neither animal nor vegetable origin; an inorganic substance. (Not now in technical use.)'. MTA plainly does not qualify.[1] The only 'mineral' present as such is gypsum, possibly – but not originally. Then again, 'mineral aggregate' is a term for 'rock' that has fallen out of fashion. This kind of product is not a rock, nor derived as such from one. Otherwise, 'aggregate' ordinarily means the rough granular material used in concrete, for example, such as pebbles, crushed rock, slag, and so on – the first thing that springs to mind – but that is clearly not what is meant

(where it is in fact the core or filler in that composite material).

The first publication to refer to 'MTA' claims that one of the 'principle [sic] compounds present' is 'tricalcium oxide silicate oxide' [3]. This is not an identifiable substance; indeed, it is chemical nonsense. There are no details given whatsoever of provenance, processing, or analysis. The next paper says, 'The principle compounds present…tricalcium oxide, and silicate oxide', which speaks of a lack of understanding and an earlier failure to proof-read (and of very poor reviewing on both occasions), but quite simply neither compound exists, nor can the labels be parsed in a chemically meaningful fashion [4]. Later, we find: 'All MTA was divided into calcium oxide and calcium phosphate' – this was for the set material [5]. Calcium oxide cannot survive contact with water, and no calcium phosphate has been seen since. There is not a trioxide anywhere claimed, not does one exist in either the initial or the reacted powder. The word 'aggregate' seems merely to have been used as a synonym for 'mixture'. Can it be that 'MTA' simply stands for 'mixture of three solid oxides'? Even that is quite untrue. (The later-incorporated so-called 'bismuth trioxide' does not exist as such – the Bi(III) oxide actually used would better be called 'sesquioxide', which would be accurate if not currently the standard term). The point of all this is to say that accuracy and precision are required for science and proper communication – to understand what is being done and what might be expected to happen.

It is, of course, necessary to identify products fully and accurately in recording and reporting work, whether clinical or experimental. However – and especially given the number of products subsequently sold – it is clear that the continual use of the trade name as a generic is both wrong and misleading. Genericization, or 'trademark erosion', is commonly viewed as detrimental to (and by) the owners of trademarks, but in the contexts of teaching, research, insurance, and standardization, too, it plainly has severe drawbacks. It is proper

---

1 The irony of having to refer to the 'mineral' of tooth tissue is not lost on me.

then to use a label that conveys the essential information succinctly, for a class of materials. It was on the basis of this argument that the term 'hydraulic silicate cement' (HSC) was proposed [6]. The qualifying 'hydraulic' is necessary and sufficient to distinguish such materials from the now-obsolete silicate cements which relied on reaction with phosphoric acid (*i.e.* a type of acid–base system): water is the reactant for the setting of an HSC. The persistence of 'MTA' might reflect chemical ignorance, again, but certainly it represents an unthinking adherence to habit.

The term 'hydraulic' is also applied in another context: so-called 'hydraulic condensation', or the technique of forcing a fluid material to fill the space of a root canal by means of, say, a gutta-percha cone pushed into it. The relationship of the term to hydraulic machinery is obvious: transmission of pressure using a liquid. In that physical sense, it is legitimate [7] (but then a syringe is also 'hydraulic'). The difficulty seems to be in prevention of extrusion (*v.s.*) – simple hydrostatics says that this is likely, and promotional material seems to imply that it is expected. It is for others to decide whether the use of such techniques is appropriate.

1.4 Chemical Interactions and Irrigation

Another weakness is found in the use of irrigants. It is perhaps well known that chlorhexidine reacts with EDTA-containing products, precipitating material that will clog tubules and canals. But reaction also occurs between chlorhexidine and various other irrigants, producing with NaOCl various chlorinated substances and precipitates, which may be coloured [8]. Hydrolysis to produce 4-chloroaniline, a toxic substance, has also been suggested [9]. Essentially, the possible chemical interaction between all substances used in any sequential treatment should be considered for adverse effects as a matter of routine. Neither independence, nor complementarity, nor synergy may be assumed. It makes sense to ensure that some rinsing occurs between each irrigant used to minimize risks. Even so, since diffusion into tubules and accessory canals must occur, the efficiency of that rinsing cannot be very great. Reactions in the deeper tissue must be expected. In fact, that is how staining occurs in the first place. Indeed, even a mixture that is advocated (Chapter 5), HEDP-NaOCl, clearly has an oxidation reaction proceeding fairly rapidly, although the speculated details appear not yet to be verified [10].

A related issue arises in respect of the formulation of products. It is incumbent on researchers to know what they are working with, the composition of materials, and all setting, mechanical, and physical properties and subsequent degradations. Failure to do so can be considered a lapse. However, it is often singularly difficult to get such information: it does not appear in full in product literature, it does not appear in Material Safety Data Sheets because only known or expected hazardous materials need be declared, and it is often denied to enquirers by the manufacturer on grounds of trade secrets. We are owed full declaration of ingredients in manufactured foodstuffs, even if the wording is obfuscated by industry jargon, so that we can avoid adverse reactions or belief violations. We expect to know what is in cosmetics, perfumes, and anything else we put on our bodies, for similar reasons. Likewise with pharmaceuticals. So why, then, is it permissible to sell products that will be implanted in patients without a full list of ingredients and components? The possibility of direct adverse effects is certainly of great concern (especially because we differ widely in our sensitivities). Given that many materials are used in sequence or are contiguous on completion, that concern is raised to an imperative. It is surely inappropriate, if not arrogant, for a manufacturer tacitly to imply that we do not need to know because they have decided it is safe, and that no regulation is thereby contravened. The regulations must be addressed.

The word 'activation' is also frequently mis-applied in chemical contexts. Thus, so-called 'electrochemically activated water' is in fact a solution of various substances produced by electrolysis. The water as such is not 'activated' in any sense whatsoever. The word is used out-side dentistry in a variety of similar contexts, similarly vacuously. The most relevant mean-ing is the switching of a system into a new state or condition, as for example the electronic transition in a photosensitizer, making it capa-ble of the next step in a reaction. Simply raising temperature, for example, often has clear chemical rate effects – but that is not 'activa-tion' (such an approach of course ignores the detrimental effect on vital tissue of tempera-tures above 42 °C and cannot be recommended for that reason anyway). Likewise, (ultra)soni-cation cannot 'activate' anything in this switch-ing sense. Although it does have some remarkable effects in what is termed 'sono-chemistry', outcomes in the present context can be attributed simply to mechanical actions, including stirring through induced flow: no specific chemistry is known to have been dem-onstrated. Care must be taken, of course, when discussing the standard chemical term 'activa-tion energy': what is required to overcome an energy barrier to a process. Sonication may well provide that for some chemical processes by means of cavitation effects, but as far as can be ascertained, this does not apply here (cavi-tation is also mechanically destructive). Laser-based techniques also appear to be purely mechanical in effect. 'Activation' is likewise unhelpfully applied to mere agitation of a reac-tive solution by stirring or pumping, such as moving an irrigating solution with a gutta-per-cha point or the like. Whilst this may allow faster bulk reaction, overcoming the limitation of reliance on diffusive processes to some extent, the actual chemical kinetics of the reac-tion are totally unaffected. Such magic is not scientific.

Whilst on the subject of irrigation, it is often said that a solution is applied specifically to remove the smear layer resulting from instrumentation. That smear layer must, of course, be composed of the same proportions of matrix and mineral as the underlying tissue. It follows that no single solution can achieve such removal: mineral can be dissolved, and matrix oxidized, but not by the same agent. Likewise, there can be no selectivity on the part of the agents: chemically, smeared material is essentially indistinguishable from its source. Diffusion ensures that an acid or chelator, say, will reach underlying material in due course (and, of course, reach more remote areas than the canal being treated via accessory canals and so on). Very often, one sees references to so-called 'appropriate con-centrations', which supposedly avoid overex-tended reaction, without recognizing that both time and concentration – to say nothing of temperature – affect rate, whilst the extent of dissolution depends on the relative amounts of smeared material and reactant (volume × concentration), assuming that factors such as flow and streaming are not involved. Even then, one cannot assume uniformity of thick-ness or of any of the relevant factors over the entire space, most especially because it is tapered. Always, there is a compromise – in particular because the extent of the smeared material is unknown and progress cannot be monitored. Protocols based on the mean behaviour of a laboratory series cannot inform on the status of the individual case – an exam-ple of the fallacy of averages: sample means convey no information on distribution and thus on behaviour in the tails [11].

Following irrigation, it is necessary to dry the canal. This makes sense in that free liquid as such could interfere (mechanically) with subsequent processes, or even chemically via dilution or dissolution. However, it is wrong to imagine that water (as a substance) can be removed and then excluded from tooth tissue: desiccation is neither achievable not desirable. Dentine matrix, being proteinaceous, is hydrated. Removal of that water would be detrimental to its structure and properties. However, all tooth tissues are permeable, both grossly through patent canals and tubules and diffusively through soft and hard tissues, including enamel and cementum, and the vast majority of materials (solid ceramics and metals excluded). Water is therefore always available, everywhere, always. What matters, chemically, is its activity, not its concentration. That is, the equilibrium condition to be expected is that the activity of the water in all diffusively contiguous regions – that means everywhere in the mouth and surrounding structures – is the same. This is a thermodynamic condition that cannot be gainsaid. 'Humidity' is therefore 100%, always (although this really is not the proper term, except in a void, where it refers to the relative saturation of the vapour – 'wet' is preferable). How long it takes is a separate matter: diffusivity depends on the medium (we assume close enough to constant temperature). Even so, approach to equilibrium can be expected within a couple of weeks at most in the majority of materials and relevant circumstances [12, 13]. Any reactions that are possible (including absorption, and thus swelling) are therefore necessarily going to occur, but the extent in a given timeframe – the rate – depends on the availability of the water: gradients, diffusivity, and reaction kinetics. Avoidance of 'leakage', meaning actual liquid flow or diffusion through liquid pathways, may properly be the goal, but exclusion of water as a reactive substance is not possible.

In the context of leakage, there is clearly much interest in how well a material may be attached to tooth tissue. Commonly, this is referred to in terms of 'bond strength', yet it is acknowledged that for many materials this is ordinarily attributable only to a mechanical key – the result of the interlocking of the cast asperities of the material on those of the substrate [14]. It would seem preferable in such cases simply to refer to 'retention', as then it is accepted that there is nothing else going on. This thought raises an interesting point: on what is actual bond strength measured? Most systems of interest in dentistry involve a carefully prepared rough surface, whether through instrumentation, grit-blasting, or etching, seemingly acknowledging that this is the main source of interaction. Would it not be sensible to test the adhesive qualities of materials using a smoothly polished, unetched substrate? That way, the true bond strength could be ascertained; that is, the benefit of any chemical interactions could be measured directly, instead of being confounded by the mechanical key. Proper efforts could then be directed to improving the chemistry, even if the key was to be used to augment the retention in normal service.

In passing, we may note that there is no such thing as a meaningful shear test in dentistry, as has been shown several times. Its continued use – in numerous highly idiosyncratic and ill-controlled forms – is both pointless and bemusing: the results are uninterpretable, and certainly of no clinical relevance. Whilst that leaves axial tension as the only viable method, no material in any dental context is known to fail in that mode either: the service interpretability of all such results is problematic, therefore. A related problem occurs with 'push-out' tests. The assumed interfacial shear is confounded by parasitic stresses and distortions that vitiate intent and thus interpretation. The absence of appreciation of the mechanics of such systems is disappointing.

A distinction also needs to be drawn between adhesion and seal. The latter can arise from a coating that has no specific bonding beyond the van der Waals (*i.e.* simple wetting) or from a material that expands (for whatever reason) and is sufficiently plastic to conform to the surface. It might help to ponder the way in which an O-ring seal works: a purely elastic system that has no bond requirement of any kind. Quality of 'seal' is plainly not related to 'bond strength' in any fundamental fashion, although in a dental context its continued existence might be. There are evident dangers in expanding materials in what are unavoidably weakened roots, but thought must be given to what scale of gap might be considered appropriate: does it matter at the molecular scale, say of water (the answer has to be no, since this is probably unavoidable), or is it just that of bacteria that is required? Perhaps somewhere in between is acceptable. This needs thinking through.

Lack of thinking is also evident in the use of methods taken from dental International Standards (ISO) documents, showing both a misapprehension of their purpose and unfamiliarity with the subtleties – indeed, outright difficulties – of testing, especially for mechanical properties, which is an exacting field [15]. Such 'standardized' methods are to be understood as economically sensible means of ascertaining safety and efficacy; as quality-control (QC) methods. To call them quick and dirty is perhaps going too far, but they cannot necessarily represent the last word for scientific studies, because the manufacturer, for example, would not be prepared to pay for such accreditation testing, and they make their views known in the drafting committees and national bodies. It is essential to give a full appraisal of a proposed method, refining and elaborating it as necessary, to avoid pitfalls and increase the value of the results in terms of clinical relevance and interpretability. The fact that there are no universally recognized methods of unimpeachable protocol speaks of the difficulties of doing a good job, but also imposes severe requirements on those doing any testing. That severity is rarely even acknowledged, let alone honoured. Crude methods are taken from the literature simply because they have been used before (sometimes for many years), and that precedent is the only defence – there is no science. But on top of that, modifications are made without justification, seemingly for convenience. Comparability between papers evaporates.

1.5 Terminology

The history of the names of chemical substances is worth some study as it reveals the development of chemical thought from the earliest attempts to study the way the world works. Some old forms persist in literary contexts (*e.g.* brimstone), others are retained in common speech (*e.g.* acetic acid). The field of chemistry itself has endeavoured to standardize a systematic approach to a variety of areas on a number of occasions since the nineteenth century, culminating in the system of preferred names developed by the International Union of Pure and Applied Chemistry (IUPAC). The point of all this effort, of course, is to be able to communicate exactly, unambiguously, the substance involved. One can understand that the literature will show the progression over time as understanding and rigour develop, and it remains necessary to be able to decode old names. Yet, when perusing a list such as that for EDTA [16], several points emerge. Firstly, the use of trade names as if they were chemically meaningful (*v.s.* 'MTA'), when the cessation of the sale of the product would mean that decoding the reference might take some considerable effort in the future (and we have to assume and accept that trade products will at some point cease to be sold). Some products are the same but sold with different labels, such as the Endosequence, Totalfill, and iRoot ranges. Researchers can waste a lot of effort trying to compare these when it is not necessary. Secondly, the import of foreign-language versions without translation or checking can only confuse. Thirdly, the arcane terms used by manufacturers in their product information might seem intelligible, but you only have to read the ingredients of certain prepared foodstuffs or cosmetics to see how they would leave even a chemist stymied and bemused (part of the reason for the introduction of the E-number system by the European Food Safety Authority (EFSA)). Fourthly, there are several ways of being systematic. But then, looking at the dental literature, we can discern other problems. Manufacturers wish to obscure their formulations for commercial reasons, but the substance names used commonly convey very little to help understand their chemical, mechanical, or biological properties, such as interactions and allergies – points that have already been made. For these to be parroted uncritically as technically correct labels betrays many things. The fact that there are documented instances of advertising copy-writers (presumably not chemists) garbling text in the manner we are used to from the press, only for this to be propagated by 'research' papers, is at best disappointing. We have a duty to communicate accurately. It is incumbent on us to check. We are obliged to review material critically, and report accordingly. In many cases, a preferable approach would be to identify a substance and state its IUPAC name, then be consistent in using a proper chemical term: the appearance of several names for the same substance in the same text underlines the complete absence of understanding. Reviewers should insist on clarity.

As we should appreciate, all materials used in dentistry represent compromise. It is simply not possible to obtain all desirable attributes (chemical, physical, mechanical, biological, economic, practical) simultaneously. We routinely trade off one thing against another, and accept some deficiency for some other benefit. There are commonly strong grounds for believing that ideality is unapproachable: physics is a hard taskmaster, and thermodynamics ineluctable. Nevertheless, it is proper to enquire as to the amelioration or refinement that might be possible. This should be on rational grounds, not guesswork or wishful thinking. We have seen such awkward proposals before in a number of instances, such as 'resin-modified' glass ionomer cement (GIC). If GIC has some good properties but is weak and moisture-sensitive, whilst light-cured materials are strong and insensitive, surely we can do both? No. Firstly, the one function replaces the other: in a given volume, something has to go to make space for something else. All too often, 'additions' are made that are not recognized as the replacements they are. Given that, something must be diminished even if something is gained. Secondly, by including competing reactions that have no chemistry in common, the trade-off

depends on the relative rates and timings: it is a very fine balance, the probability of attaining which is low [17]. This is a complicated and messy system that falls between two stools. It is well recognized that 'compomers', where a GIC-type glass was used as the core in a resin matrix, failed to work as hoped [13, 18] – so why now do we see supposedly *light-cured hydraulic silicate* cement? Similar arguments apply, similar outcomes are to be expected. The triumph of advertising over substance? Wishful thinking is the bane of dentistry.

We see similar failures of appreciation in the seemingly random selections of additives regularly studied and proposed for many applications. For example, a material is too weak for a certain use, but a strong material is known that can be made as a powder – why not add this? Again, the replacement aspect of such a design is not recognized, but a key requirement of such composite structures is missing: bonding. Composite structures require a bond – that is, a chemical bond – between the matrix and the core (*alias* the 'filler', a term that betrays a less than honourable economic incentive in some contexts) for stress transfer to occur and the benefit to be realized. This is 'matrix constraint'. With it, there are remarkable improvements. Without it, the material behaves as if it were full of holes, with the obvious outcome. This was seen in the attempts to strengthen silver amalgam with (silver-plated!) sapphire whiskers, GIC with zirconia powder, and GIC with amalgam alloy powder ('miracle mix') to name but three egregious examples. Now we have 'microsilica' added to HSC. In fact, we should be careful to distinguish between materials that are included to do a job – such as reactants or bonded core – and those that have no other purpose than to dilute the system, which is all a true filler actually is. Of course, the inclusion of pharmaceutically active substances such as antimicrobials must also be treated rationally, because they are then part of the matrix (occupying volume) and therefore affect all its properties, always – poor discriminatory power experiments notwithstanding.

It is often the case that such an additive will be explored at a range of proportions (and, sadly, when it matters, not accounting for the consequent changes in other, more important, ratios). Then, through the sequential application of Student's *t*-test, the maximum amount that does not give a statistically significant result (*i.e.* a 'nonsignificant $P > 0.05$', 'N.S.') will be decided upon. This is fallacious in several respects. Firstly, anything that interferes with the setting reaction or the resulting structure must, by definition, cause a deterioration. Secondly, the 'failure to detect' is not the same as an assertion of no effect; it is the entirely expected consequence of the poor discriminatory power of testing with a small sample size, large scatter, and relatively weak effect. Whether it matters is not the focus of attention as it should be, but the claim is made that the addition is safe because 'nonsignificant' is enough. In fact, with a large enough sample size, you will always get a 'significant' result. In addition, the test is weak because it is piecemeal instead of looking for the covariance of the outcome with input, when the full power can be obtained. It is also wrong because it is trawling without multiple test protection. What is proper is to determine the size of the effect, then determine – from other considerations – how much is tolerable. If reviewers do not understand all this, what hope is there?

1.6 Classification of HSCs

As enthusiasm for this kind of material has grown, a range of variations has been produced, but many of them make reference to the original (nonsensical) labelling (*v.s.*). Consequently, there is a deal of confusion as to the nature of the various formulations and what behaviour might be expected from them. There are numerous products available now, and some systematic classification would be helpful to inform product selection. The chemistry is essential to understanding what

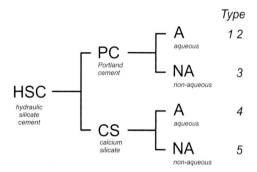

Figure 1.1 Fundamental classification of hydraulic silicate cements at the point of use. The types referred to for clinical purposes elsewhere in this book are shown. Type 1 is the original formulation of the class, without any additive. All others have one or more additives of various kinds, for various purposes [19].

is going on – how could it be otherwise? – and thus to enabling the statement of a simple, informative, and (most importantly) accurate classification. As already indicated, an HSC is defined by the reaction of a silicate system with water (a simple classification of HSCs based on their chemistry is shown in Figure 1.1). That silicate system might be a Portland cement-like (PC) complex mixture (regardless of its provenance, *i.e.* whether it is derived directly from a commercial PC or created in a similar fashion from less-contaminated feedstock) or a simpler calcium silicate (CS) or mixture of related compounds that has been synthesized for 'purity' (to avoid heavy metals) or for other reasons. We therefore have a very simple division into PC and CS. The main subdivision then is based on the water that is needed for the material hydration reaction. Some HSCs are to be mixed with water (*i.e.* they are an aqueous mixture at the point of application), and some are presented as a slurry or paste in a non-aqueous vehicle, which is subsequently lost entirely, diffusing away. In the latter case, setting is still specifically hydraulic, as it relies on water from the surroundings (*v.s.* re: drying) diffusing into the water-miscible liquid continuous phase: the setting chemistry is essentially unaffected. (Incidentally, this gives the lie to the description of such products as 'pre-mixed' – quite clearly, they are not, as no reaction water is yet present. Such a presentation is a rather neat approach, so why is it trivialized by a nonsense label? This is advertising, not science.)

Whether or not a radio-opacifier is added to any of these does not affect the fundamental behaviour: the essential chemistry – hydraulic reaction – remains as the defining characteristic, whether or not that additive modifies the setting reaction rate or outcome in any way (whether deliberately or accidentally, and no matter how drastically) [20]. Indeed, whether any other additive is included or the formulation is tweaked for any reason (*e.g.* rate modification), the basic classification must remain if the key chemistry persists. Attempts to create 'generations' on a historical basis are as pointless as they are uninformative in the absence of logic, consistency, and relevance. There are no alternatives known at present for true HSCs, all of which are essentially based on CSs (as stressed elsewhere in this book).

The trouble is that what may reasonably be called 'fake HSCs' are also offered. Along the lines of compomer (*v.s.*), a PC material powder in a light-cured resin matrix has been produced: this is a filled (composite) resin (FR), no more, no less. It is simply irrational, and highly misleading (if not culpably misrepresented), to call this an HSC, or to imply that it is by association, irrespective of any beneficial effects, perceived or claimed, from a high pH at the surface, available calcium, and so on. If setting does not depend on water, it is not an HSC. In fact, water that does diffuse into the cured material (through the matrix, as is normal and expected for such resin systems, despite popular belief) must react with the PC material: such chemistry is unavoidable. Thus, one could reasonably expect this to expand (reaction product volume is necessarily greater than PC volume), with perhaps unfortunate results, albeit slowly – but this is not 'setting'.

Similarly, a PC- or CS-containing material to be mixed with a salicylate-containing second paste, setting by the usual acid–base (AB), salt-formation process of many other proper cementitious materials, and not in the first place by reaction with water, cannot rationally be described as an HSC; to do so would be chemically false representation. Such a material is not fundamentally different from the old silicate cements that were mixed with phosphoric acid for setting, although they may be nearer to setting calcium hydroxide liners in the primary reaction. But here, again, water that must and will diffuse in must and will react in the usual way with any remaining core (and again cause expansion), but the setting mechanism as such is not at all that of an HSC. They may not be called HSCs, or suggested to be such.

1.7 Conclusion

It is possible to go on and dissect many more aspects of endodontic materials and treatments from a materials science perspective, most especially for the chemistry that is abused, ignored, or imagined. Were one not inured to a working life exposed to such, despair would follow rather promptly. Given that the role of all dentists, and thus of nonclinical teachers as well, is ultimately to ensure patient well-being, the plea now is for the underlying science (and its practitioners, therefore) to be respected, given credit, and adopted as the means of supporting that motivation.

Critical reading and informed thinking can reveal much about the dogma, unwarranted assumptions, and wishful thinking (despite perhaps the best of intentions) that pervade endodontics at least as much as anywhere else in dentistry. Challenge it all – *nullius in verba* – and in so doing, with an open mind and sound advice, take the subject forward: true evidence-based dentistry awaits your contribution.

References

1 Smith, R.M. and Hansen, D.E. (1998). The pH-rate profile for the hydrolysis of a peptide bond. *J. Am. Chem. Soc.* 120: 8910–8913.

2 Kohli, M.R. and Karabucak, B. (2019). Bioceramic usage in endodontics. Available from http://www.aae.org/specialty/2019/07/08/bioceramic-usage-in-endodontics (accessed 10 August 2020).

3 Lee, S.-J., Monsef, M., and Torabinejad, M. (1993). Sealing ability of a mineral trioxide aggregate for repair of lateral root perforations. *J. Endod.* 19 (11): 541–544.

4 Torabinejad, M., Watson, T.F., and TRP, F. (1993). Sealing ability of a mineral trioxide aggregate when used as a root end filling material. *J. Endod.* 19 (12): 591–595.

5 Torabinejad, M., Hong, C., McDonald, F., and Pitt Ford, T.R. (1995). Physical and chemical properties of a new root-end filling material. *J. Endod.* 21 (7): 349–353.

6 Darvell, B.W. and Wu, R.C.T. (2011). 'MTA' – an hydraulic silicate cement: review update and setting reaction. *Dent. Mater.* 27 (6): 407–422.

7 Fleisher, R.M. and Heintz, C.E. (1977). A plastic tube technique for direct vision of endodontic procedures. *J. Dent. Educ.* 4 (10): 630–632.

8 Prado, M., Santos Júnior, H.M., Rezende, C.M. et al. (2013). Interactions between irrigants commonly used in endodontic practice: a chemical analysis. *J. Endod.* 39: 505–510.

9 Basrani, B.R., Manek, S., Sodhi, R.N. et al. (2007). Interaction between sodium hypochlorite and chlorhexidine gluconate. *J. Endod.* 33: 966–969.

10 Zollinger, A., Mohn, D., Zeltner, M., and Zehnder, M. (2018). Short-term storage stability of NaOCl solutions when combined with dual rinse HEDP. *Int. Endod. J.* 51 (6): 691–696.

11 Welsh, A.H., Townsend Peterson, A., and Altman, S.A. (1988). The fallacy of averages. *Am. Nat.* 132 (2): 277–288.

12 Musanje, L. and Darvell, B.W. (2003). Aspects of water sorption from the air, water and artificial saliva in resin composite restorative materials. *Dent. Mater.* 19 (5): 414–422.

13 Musanje, L., Shu, M., and Darvell, B.W. (2001). Water sorption and mechanical behaviour of cosmetic direct restorative materials in artificial salvia. *Dent. Mater.* 17: 394–401.

14 Şanlı, S., Dündar Çömlekoğlu, M., Çömlekoğlu, E. et al. (2015). Influence of surface treatment on the resin-bonding of zirconia. *Dent. Mater.* 31: 657–668.

15 Darvell, B.W. (2020) Misuse of ISO standards in dental materials research. *Dent. Mater.* 36 (12): 1493–1494.

16 http://www.chemspider.com/Chemical-Structure.5826.html?rid=4a01b359-c38c-4e4a-9bce-487b6c2b5176

17 Yelamanchili, A. and Darvell, B.W. (2008). Network competition in a resin-modified glass-ionomer cement. *Dent. Mater.* 24: 1065–1069.

18 Ruse, N.D. (1999). What is a 'compomer'? *J. Can. Dent. Assoc.* 65: 500–504.

19 Camilleri, J. (2020). Hydraulic calcium silicate-based endodontic cements. In: *Endodontic Advances and Evidence-Based Clinical Guidelines; Section 2: Advances in Materials and Technology* (eds. H.M.A. Ahmed and P.M.H. Dummer). London: Wiley.

20 Camilleri, J. (2007). Hydration mechanisms of mineral trioxide aggregate. *Int. Endod. J.* 40: 462–470.

2

Pulp Capping Materials for the Maintenance of Pulp Vitality

Phillip L. Tomson[1] and Henry F. Duncan[2]

[1] *School of Dentistry, Institute of Clinical Sciences, University of Birmingham, Birmingham, UK*
[2] *Division of Restorative Dentistry and Periodontology, Dublin Dental University Hospital, Trinity College Dublin, Dublin, Ireland*

TABLE OF CONTENTS

Endodontic Materials in Clinical Practice, First Edition. Edited by Josette Camilleri.
© 2021 John Wiley & Sons Ltd. Published 2021 by John Wiley & Sons Ltd.

2.1 Introduction

Preserving the health of the dental pulp, or at least part of it, is important when treating a vital tooth with a deep unexposed cavity or exposed pulp, particularly if the root formation is incomplete. There is a long tradition of treating deep cavities and exposed dental pulp by performing procedures such as pulp capping and partial and complete pulpotomy. An improved understanding of the regenerative capacity of the dentine–pulp complex and the introduction of new hydraulic calcium silicate cements (HCSCs) has stimulated a new wave of research and treatment strategies in this area. The aim of this chapter is to evaluate the pulpal healing response, the range of vital pulp treatment (VPT) procedures, and the nature of the materials employed in the management of deep caries and exposed pulp.

2.2 Maintaining Pulp Vitality

2.2.1 Why Maintain the Pulp?

Maintaining healthy pulp tissue is preferable to root canal treatment (RCT), which can be complex, destructive, time-consuming, and expensive for both patients and clinicians. Preserving all or at least part of the dental pulp is important after pulp exposure, especially when the tooth is immature and root formation is not yet complete [1]. The need for a more conservative approach to management of the inflamed pulp is a more biologically based and minimally invasive treatment strategy compared with pulpectomy and has recently been encouraged in editorials and position statements [1, 2]. Besides reducing intervention, this biological concept also maintains pulp developmental, defensive, and proprioceptive functions [3, 4]; VPT is generally considered technically easier to execute than RCT [5]. From a longitudinal perspective, advocating less aggressive dentistry reduces overtreatment and limits the 'restorative cycle'

concept [6], whilst also improving the cost-effectiveness of treatment [7]. Finally, with the surge in research and interest in regenerative endodontics [8], biomaterial developments [9], and the need to therapeutically utilize dental pulp stem cell (DPSC) populations [10], VPT has reemerged as an area of significant interest to both patients and dentists [11].

2.2.2 Pulpal Irritants

Although the pulp can be challenged by microbial, mechanical, and chemical stimuli, necrosis will not result without the presence of microorganisms [12]. Caries has traditionally been considered the principal cause of pulpal damage, and although falling in prevalence, it is now manifesting more commonly in disadvantaged and elderly populations [13–15]. Whilst inflammation of the pulp is evident even in shallow carious lesions [16, 17], it is not until the carious process is deep and comes within 0.5 mm of the pulp that the pulpitic response significantly intensifies [18]. As a result, before it reaches this stage, the damage is likely to be reversible. This forms the basis of predictable operative dentistry, in that the pulp should recover after removal of carious dentine and insertion of a suitable dental restorative material [19]. Microbial challenge, however, is not limited to caries, as bacterial microleakage is also a common cause of pulpitis and subsequent necrosis due to oral microorganisms colonizing the 'gap' between the restoration and the tooth [20]. Prevention of microleakage using lining material is no longer considered good practice [21], but dentine bonding agents and incremental placement of resin-based composites will reduce the risk of bacterial colonization [22], particularly if there is sufficient residual dentine thickness (RDT).

Views on the irritant effect of dental materials on the pulp have changed over the last 50 years. The idea that their toxicity to pulp tissue leads to pulpal necrosis has been questioned by several operators [20, 23, 24], who point to microbial contamination and leakage as the decisive factor in sustained pulpal inflammation. That said, there is also good evidence to suggest that some materials are more biocompatible and 'pulp-friendly' than others, with the adverse toxic effects of dental resins on pulp cells being repeatedly highlighted [25, 26]. Alternatively, the positive biological responses of HCSC [9] have led to recent suggestions that deep carious lesions should be lined with HCSC after deep caries removal [27]. Other nonmicrobial irritants such as bleaching procedures, particularly chairside 'power' techniques, can lead to rises in pulpal temperature and pulpitis [28]; however, whilst these are increasingly common as treatment strategies, the pulpal changes seen are generally reversible and are not catastrophic in nature [29, 30].

2.2.3 Pulpal Healing After Exposure

The odontoblast cell is responsible for forming primary dentine during tooth development, the more slowly deposited secondary dentine throughout the life of the tooth, and, when 'irritated', tertiary dentine in the pulp tissue adjacent to the source of challenge [31]. Dependent on the stimulant severity, tertiary dentine deposition can be either reactionary or reparative (Figure 2.1) [32]. Reactionary dentine is formed by an upregulation of existing odontoblast activity when the dentine–pulp complex is exposed to a relatively mild stimulus (e.g. shallow or slowly progressing carious disease process), whilst reparative dentine is formed generally after a stronger stimulus has led to odontoblast cell death (e.g. deep caries or traumatic exposure) [32, 33]. At a cellular level, reparative dentine is believed to be produced following cytodifferentiation of pulpal progenitor cells (DSPCs or other progenitor cells) and the formation of a new generation of odontoblast-like cells [1, 32, 33]. Although this description of reparative dentinogenesis represents the currently accepted theory, others have highlighted the influence of other cells such as fibroblasts or fibrocytes as secretory cells [34, 35]. The cellular differentiation is guided by the influence of growth factors and other bioactive molecules released from both the dentine matrix and the pulp cells

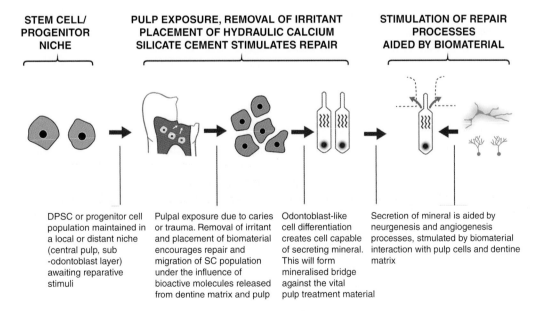

| STEM CELL/ PROGENITOR NICHE | PULP EXPOSURE, REMOVAL OF IRRITANT PLACEMENT OF HYDRAULIC CALCIUM SILICATE CEMENT STIMULATES REPAIR | STIMULATION OF REPAIR PROCESSES AIDED BY BIOMATERIAL |

| DPSC or progenitor cell population maintained in a local or distant niche (central pulp, sub-odontoblast layer) awaiting reparative stimuli | Pulpal exposure due to caries or trauma. Removal of irritant and placement of biomaterial encourages repair and migration of SC population under the influence of bioactive molecules released from dentine matrix and pulp | Odontoblast-like cell differentiation creates cell capable of secreting mineral. This will form mineralised bridge against the vital pulp treatment material | Secretion of mineral is aided by neurgenesis and angiogenesis processes, stmulated by biomaterial interaction with pulp cells and dentine matrix |

Figure 2.1 Schematic representation of the reparative process after pulp exposure, vital pulp treatment, and the potential influence of the material.

themselves [36, 37]. Whilst for didactic purposes the processes of reactionary and reparative dentinogenesis are considered separately in the event of pulp exposure, both are likely to occur simultaneously [38].

Inflammation is also an important stimulus that drives the reparative process [39], with odontoblasts involved in initial sensory stimulus transmission from the dentine and possessing an immunocompetent role in cellular defence [40]. Indeed, the low-level release of inflammatory mediators such as interleukins-2 and -6 in mineralizing cells in contact with an HCSC such as mineral trioxide aggregate (MTA) supports the need for a degree of inflammation in promoting regenerative processes [41].

A wide range of bioactive dentine matrix components are 'fossilized' in the mineralized tissue and released into the pulp during caries or trauma [38, 42]. Demineralization of dentine, and indeed contact with materials such as MTA [43], calcium hydroxide [44], and other agents [45], releases a plethora of bioactive molecules, including members of the transforming growth factor-β (TGF-β1) superfamily, which can stimulate a complex cascade of molecular events that promote pulp repair [36, 44]. These materials liberate dentine matrix components to varying degrees, highlighting the influence of the material in the biological response [46].

Using biologically based dental materials that promote the healing process is paramount in VPT [47]. Other strategies using irrigants to enhance the release of bioactive molecules from dentine in order to improve wound repair are also being developed [48]. Over the last 10 years, HCSCs have shown superior histological response compared with the gold-standard material, calcium hydroxide, in VPT [9, 49]. HCSCs work in a similar way to calcium hydroxide but are more efficient in their interaction with dental pulp cells and dentine extracellular matrix (dECM) [50]. In reality, both their mechanisms of action remain nonspecific and untargeted in nature (Figure 2.1) [49, 51].

2.2.4 Classifications of Pulpitis and Assessing the Inflammatory State of the Pulp

An accurate assessment of the inflammatory condition of the pulp has a large bearing on the success of VPT procedures, as teeth with carious exposures have a poorer outcome than those with traumatic ones [52, 53]. Pulpitis is generally classified as being either reversible or irreversible [54, 55]; however, in light of the development of predictable VPT solutions, such as pulpotomy in teeth with signs and symptoms indicative of irreversible pulpitis, alternative classifications have been proposed in order to more accurately reflect the true state of the pulp [2, 27]. New classification systems have tried to link diagnosis and management and to use more descriptive terms including 'mild', 'moderate', and 'severe' pulpitis [2], but their usefulness in effectively replacing the current classification system remains speculative. Pulpal status is routinely determined after pain history, a clinical/radiographic examination, and pulp tests. Unfortunately, clinical signs, symptoms, and tests are relatively nonspecific and generally do not accurately reflect the histopathological status of the pulp [56, 57] – although this assertion has recently been queried, as a strong correlation between pulp histology and the signs and symptoms of reversible and irreversible pulpitis has been demonstrated [34].

Reversible pulpitis can present either with no patient complaint or with symptoms that can extend to a sharp pain sensation with thermal stimuli. Notably, the pain resolves rapidly once the stimulus is removed. Spontaneous pain and sleep disturbance tend to indicate irreversible pulpitis [1, 57], with the symptoms lingering after stimulus removal. Unfortunately, patient symptoms are at best a guideline and can even mislead the clinician, with irreversible pulpitis being symptomless in the majority of cases [54, 58]. During the early stages, teeth presenting with signs and symptoms of irreversible pulpitis usually exhibit significant pulpal damage only in the area of the coronal pulp under the carious lesion, with a largely uninflamed radicular pulp [1, 34]. Invariably, without intervention, the partial irreversible pulpitis will progress until the entire pulp is irreversibly inflamed and necrosis ensues. Although treatment decisions are largely based on patient signs and symptoms, current tools are insufficient to accurately determine the threshold between reversible and irreversible forms [59]. As a result, it is critical to identify more discriminative tests based on molecular analysis of pulpal biomarkers [1].

2.2.5 Is Pulpal Exposure a Negative Prognostic Factor?

A traumatic pulpal exposure in a mature tooth, treated by pulp capping or pulpotomy, is a predictable procedure with a similar prognosis to RCT of >90% success [60, 61]. By contrast, if the pulp is cariously exposed, it has by its very nature been subjected to a sustained bacterial onslaught for a considerable period of time; this reduces the predictability of the VPT procedure, with quoted success rates ranging from as low as 20% [52, 62] to over 80% [11, 63]. The wide range of success highlights the difficulties in treating carious exposures and comparing individual pulp-capping studies, which show heterogeneous data, with some defining patient symptoms and pulpal diagnosis [11] and others including a mixed sample of both carious and traumatic exposures [64].

Although there is general agreement when managing deep lesions that the margins of the cavity should be clear of caries, there is less concurrence over whether all carious dentine overlying the pulp should be removed [63, 65]. In a tooth with a deep carious lesion which responds within normal limits to sensibility testing, selective (or partial) caries removal and avoidance of pulp exposure is recommended in preference to nonselective (or complete) removal and subsequent risk of exposure [1, 62, 66, 67]. This management strategy for deep caries can be carried out in one visit as indirect pulp therapy, or in two as a stepwise excavation technique [21]. There are a small number randomized controlled trials investigating caries management strategies in permanent teeth, but recent five-year results of a previously published trial [66] showed that selective (partial) caries removal and stepwise excavation increased the number of teeth that remained vital compared with a nonselective (complete) removal technique [62]. However, this assumes that pulp exposure is the principal problem, which is not convincingly shown in either study [62, 66]. Other conflicting prospective studies have demonstrated opposing results, with high success rates for conservative treatment of the cariously exposed pulp in an endodontic practice setting [63], general practice setting [68], and university setting investigating teeth with signs and symptoms of irreversible pulpitis [11]. All these studies used HCSCs such as MTA and Biodentine, but notably were not randomized in design.

At present, it appears that careful aseptic handling of the pulp tissue under magnification, judicious removal of pulpal tissue, and appropriate restoration of the tooth exposure may produce results comparable with or better than RCT [62, 63, 69].

2.2.6 Soft Tissue Factors Unique to the Tooth

Inflammation is a response to injury, and the presence of polymorphonuclear leucocytes and chronic inflammatory cells is indicative of failure of VPT. Swelling is also a feature of the inflammatory response, but the unique anatomy of the dentine–pulp complex and the rigidity of the surrounding dentine prevent expansion of the pulp. Additionally, after pulpal exposure, the buffering effect of the dentine is lost and the pulp tissue is rendered sensitive to potential adverse interactions from materials or microbes [70]. Notably, inflammation is also important in driving the soft tissue response during healing following

(a)

(b)

(c)

(d)

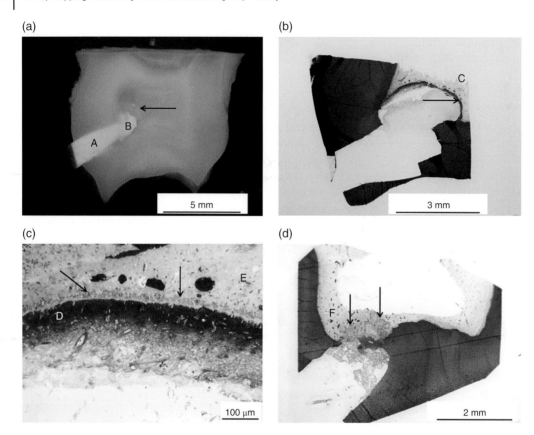

Figure 2.2 Histological response to pulp capping. (a) Macrophotographic view of the mesial half of a human maxillary third molar demonstrating the remnants of the restorative material (A) and ProRoot MTA capping material (B) at one month. Note the distinct hard tissue bridge (arrow). Original magnification ×8. (b) Photomicrograph of histological section of the specimen in (a) of an MTA pulp cap at one month. Note that the mineralized barrier (arrow) stretches across the entire width of the exposed pulp (C). Original magnification ×16. (c) Higher-magnification photomicrograph from (a) and (b). Cuboidal cells (arrows) line the hard tissue barrier (D). Note the absence of inflammatory cells in the pulp (E). Original magnification ×85. (d) Photomicrograph of a selected serial section of hard-setting calcium hydroxide cement (Dycal) at one month. Engorged blood vessels are prominent and inflammatory cells are present. Note the presence of Dycal particles (arrows) in the pulp (F). Original magnification ×16. *Source:* Images adapted from Nair, P.N., Duncan, H.F., Pitt Ford, T.R., Luder, H.U. Histological, ultrastructural and quantitative investigations on the response of healthy human pulps to experimental capping with mineral trioxide aggregate: a randomized controlled trial. Int. Endod. J. 2008; 41(2):128–50.

placement of a pulp-capping material [39]. Calcium hydroxide produces a mild irritation of the pulp and stimulates repair. If pulp capping is successful, then after a few days there will be a reduction in the number of inflammatory cells present under the necrotic zone, whilst under the capping material, the pulpal cells will proliferate, migrate, and form new collagen in contact with the necrotic zone [71].

Although the process is similar with HCSC, the pulpal irritation is less than that with calcium hydroxide (Figure 2.2) [9]. Tertiary reparative dentinogenesis is then initiated, odontoblast cells are formed, and mineralized matrix is secreted [72]. This matrix forms the so called 'hard tissue' bridge, which walls off the pulp and offers further protection to the soft tissue adjacent to the wound site.

2.3 Clinical Procedures for Maintaining Pulp Vitality

2.3.1 Managing the Unexposed Pulp

Regardless of the many years spent researching the ideal restorative material, there is no such thing as a permanent restoration: all have a limited lifetime [73]. As soon as the integrity of a tooth is broken, it must be replaced, setting it on a 'restorative cycle' [74]. And each time a restoration is placed, the pulp is made vulnerable and put under threat.

Clinicians carrying out an operative procedure on a vital tooth should be mindful of the heat generated by dental handpieces, the potential damage caused by overdehydrating dentine, and the use of caustic agents in tooth restoration, all of which can result in unnecessary iatrogenic pulp damage. Often, prevention is better than cure, so care and attention should be taken when removing tooth tissue and selecting materials to prevent injury to the pulp. The most influential variables in terms of causing injury to the unexposed pulp are considered the cavity's RDT and preparation of the cavity in the absence of coolant [75]. This confirms the observation that excessive heat is the most injurious event to pulp tissue [76]. Other potential sources of pulp injury during restoration of a cavity include etching of the dentin [77] and the choice of restorative material [78].

Any therapeutic process for the benefit of pulp survival that is adopted during the restoration of a tooth with a deep cavity, but unexposed pulp is an indirect pulp cap. Classically, this procedure is carried out when dentine is lost due to caries, trauma, or a previous iatrogenic intervention, and when a cavity exists close to the pulp but dentine remains over the pulp tissue. Indirect pulp capping can be defined as an application of a material on to a thin layer of dentine located close to the pulp with the aim of producing a positive biological response so that the pulp can protect itself.

2.3.2 Tooth Preparation to Avoid Exposure

The tooth should be isolated with a rubber dam and asepsis should be maintained throughout cavity preparation. The cavity should be disinfected using cotton pellets soaked with sodium hypochlorite (0.5–5%). Less invasive carious tissue-removal techniques are generally carried out using sterile round burs and excavators [79], but other self-limiting chemomechanical methods (e.g. Carisolv gel) have also been advocated for the management of deep carious lesions [80]. Regardless of the technique employed, carious tissue should be removed from the periphery of the cavity to hard dentine (i.e. nonselective removal), leaving soft or leathery dentine only on the pulpal aspect of the cavity. As RDT over the pulp cannot be accurately assessed clinically, the use of a biologically based biomaterial is recommended. Ideally, an HCSC or a glass ionomer cement (GIC) should be routinely applied to the dentine barrier prior to definitive restoration (Figure 2.3) [1, 27].

2.3.3 Managing the Exposed Pulp

If there is a suspicion that the pulp is exposed, the tooth should be immediately isolated with a rubber dam to ensure an aseptic environment and prevent any of the consequences that would result if the pulp were to become infected [12]. Magnification should ideally be used throughout the procedure to ensure removal of all softened dentine and to allow visual inspection of the pulp tissue in order to determine the degree of inflammation. The dentine should be carefully manipulated using sterile burs and sharp instruments. A high-speed bur and water coolant should be used for pulp tissue removal [81], followed by disinfection and control of pulpal bleeding. Haemostasis and disinfection should be achieved using cotton pellets soaked ideally with sodium hypochlorite (0.5–5%) or

(a)　　　　　(b)　　　　　(c)　　　　　(d)　　　　　(e)

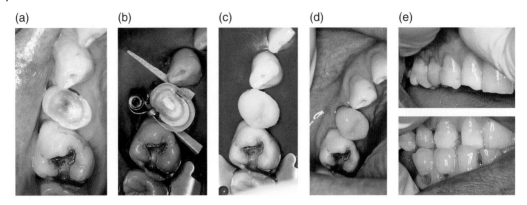

Figure 2.3 Intraoral photographs of an indirect pulp-capping procedure. (a) Preoperative image of a grossly broken-down upper right first premolar, showing a deep lesion with unexposed pulp. (b) Indirect pulp cap with a thin layer of Biodentine interfacing with dentine overlying the pulp, leaving the maximum amount of bonding tooth tissue available for a direct composite resin restoration. (c) Direct composite resin build-up. (d) Occlusal view of completed restoration. (e) Buccal view of composite resin restoration. *Source:* Phillip L. Tomson.

chlorhexidine (0.2–2%) [64, 82, 83]. If haemostasis cannot be controlled after five minutes, further pulp tissue should be removed (partial or full pulpotomy). In cases with signs and symptoms indicative of irreversible pulpitis (i.e. partial irreversible pulpitis confined to the coronal pulp tissue), a full coronal pulpotomy can be carried out to the level of the root canal orifices, with bleeding arrested as detailed previously [84]. This procedure may be easier for general dental practitioners without access to magnification than either partial pulpotomy or even direct pulp capping. Ideally, an HCSC should be placed directly on to the pulp tissue and the tooth immediately definitively restored to prevent further microleakage [61, 83, 85]. If bleeding cannot be controlled after full pulpotomy, a pulpectomy and RCT should be carried out, provided the tooth is restorable. Four different VPTs can be carried out: direct pulp capping, partial pulpotomy, full pulpotomy, and pulpectomy.

2.3.3.1 Direct Pulp Capping

This procedure is carried out if dentine is lost due to caries, trauma, or a previous iatrogenic intervention and a cavity exists where the soft tissue of the pulp is exposed (≤ 2.5 mm) and (in most cases) bleeding. Direct pulp capping is defined as application of a material directly on to the pulp with the aim of producing a positive biological response so that the pulp can protect itself. This treatment strategy may be applied out if a tooth is symptomless or has relatively mild symptoms (Figure 2.4).

2.3.3.2 Partial Pulpotomy

This procedure is carried out if dentine is lost due to caries, trauma, or a previous iatrogenic intervention and a cavity exists where the soft tissue of the pulp is exposed and bleeding, suggesting it is inflamed. The amount of bleeding is used as a surrogate marker of inflammation. Partial pulpotomy is defined as removal of a small portion of superficial coronal pulp tissue followed by application of a material directly on to the pulp with the aim of producing a positive biological response so that the pulp can protect itself. With this treatment strategy, pulp tissue is removed approximately 2 mm at a time and then an attempt is made to obtain haemostasis as previously described. If haemostasis is not achieved, the process is repeated (Figure 2.5).

2.3.3.3 Full Pulpotomy

This procedure is carried out when there is gross loss of dentine due to caries, trauma, or

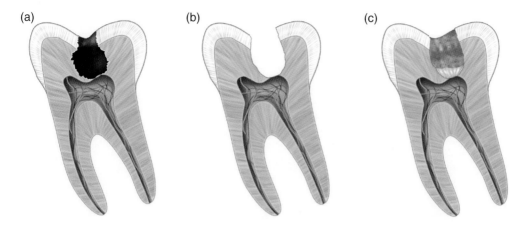

Figure 2.4 Direct pulp capping. (a) Deep carious lesion extending to the pulp. (b) Carious exposure of the pulp following cavity preparation. (c) Calcium silicate cement directly interfacing with the pulp following definitive restoration.

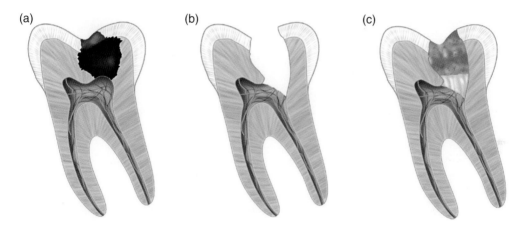

Figure 2.5 Partial pulpotomy. (a) Deep carious lesion extending to the pulp. (b) Removal of the superficial pulp tissue where it is inflamed. (c) Calcium silicate cement directly interfacing with the pulp following definitive restoration.

previous iatrogenic intervention and a cavity exists where a large portion of the soft tissue of the pulp is exposed and bleeding, suggesting inflammation or contamination, or where it is not possible to obtain haemostasis at a superficial level. Full pulpotomy is defined as complete removal of the coronal pulp to the root canal orifice level, followed by application of a material directly on to the remaining pulp with the aim of producing a positive biological response so that the pulp can protect itself (Figure 2.6).

2.3.3.4 Pulpectomy

For completeness, this procedure is considered here as it is a form of VPT. In treating cases where it is determined that the pulp is not viable as it appears to be severely inflamed or contaminated and haemostasis is unachievable or the pulp appears necrotic, a pulpectomy may be indicated. It has been shown that success rates are higher when the pulpectomy and RCT are completed in one visit, and the clinician should adopt a cautious approach with length control. Pulpectomy is defined as total

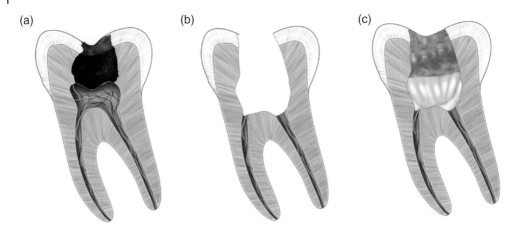

Figure 2.6 Full pulpotomy. (a) Deep carious lesion extending to the pulp. (b) Removal of the whole of the coronal portion of the pulp. (c) Calcium silicate cement directly interfacing with pulp stumps at the canal orifice following definitive restoration.

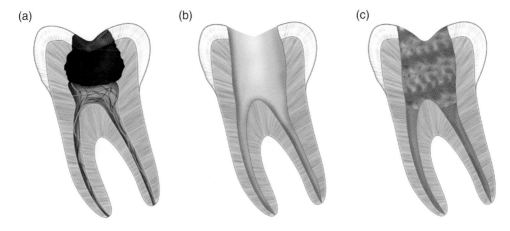

Figure 2.7 Pulpectomy. (a) Deep carious lesion extending to the pulp, resulting in irreversible change. (b) Complete removal of the pulp tissue and cleaning and preparation of the root canal system prior to root filling. (c) Obduration of the root canals with gutta-percha following definitive restoration.

removal of the pulp from the root canal system followed by RCT (Figure 2.7).

2.3.4 Immature Roots

VPT is of particular importance in immature permanent teeth where root formation is not complete and the root structure is weak. Successful maintenance of pulp vitality will allow root formation to continue in a process known as apexogenesis. In reality, the term 'apexogenesis' is seldom used in modern endodontics, first because it is often confused with apexification, and second because it simply refers to pulp capping: a partial or full pulpotomy procedure carried out in a tooth with an immature root structure. VPT on immature teeth is most commonly carried out following trauma on the anterior teeth, which for practical reasons may be better treated with a partial or 'Cvek' pulpotomy, where part of the exposed pulp tissue is removed and a capping material is placed [60]. Young patients presenting with an open apex will have a greater blood supply and increased cellularity of their pulps, which has been suggested to result in more predictable healing [86]. However, the influence of age has not generally been linked to improved healing in VPT [64, 87].

2.4 Materials Used in Vital Pulp Treatment

2.4.1 The Role of the Material

For predictable and successful VPT, careful material selection is required. The demands on the material itself are numerous, as it is situated in a unique environment in which it must interface with vital tissue that has a blood supply, hard dental tissues, and other restorative materials. Historically, numerous different materials have been used in VPT, including gold foil [88], aqueous calcium hydroxide [89], commercial preparations of calcium hydroxide [90], glycyrrhetinic acid/antibiotic mixture [91], resin bonding agents [92], corticosteroid/antibiotic mixture [93], isobutyl cyanoacrylate [94], resin-modified glass ionomer [95], and, more recently, HCSC [96].

The fundamental aim of any material used in VPT is to maintain a viable pulp so that it can continue normal homeostatic and protective functions of the tooth. As the pulp has the ability to lay down dental hard tissue in the form of reactionary or reparative dentine, the chosen material should promote this response in order to increase the thickness of dentine between the pulp and the deepest part of any cavity (Figure 2.2). The production of a thicker layer of mineralized tissue over the pulp renders it well protected from future noxious stimuli. Any pulp-capping material should also have antimicrobial properties, as it is well established that pulp necrosis will not result without the presence of microorganisms [12].

Materials used in VPT should have the following characteristics:

- Antimicrobial activity
- Creation of a bacterial tight seal and prevention of microleakage

- Promotion of tertiary dentinogenesis and control of hard tissue barrier formation
- Biocompatibility (prevention of 'over'-irritation and avoidance of induction of a severe inflammatory response
- Radiopacity
- Clinical ease of handling
- Resistant to forces of displacement following the subsequent application of a further material over the agent used in VPT
- Lack of induction of tooth discolouration

No one material demonstrates all of these properties, but in recent years significant advances have been made. Recently used pulp-capping agents will be considered in this section.

2.4.2 Calcium Hydroxide

Numerous different materials have been used as pulp-capping agents over the years, with varying degrees of success. However, generations of clinicians have gone back to using calcium hydroxide, which until recently was considered the gold standard [9], and is probably still one of the most common materials found in dental surgeries all over the world. This material has been in use for over 100 years [97], and it has been intensively researched during that time [71, 90, 98–103]. Indeed, direct pulp-capping studies using calcium hydroxide on nonexperimental pulp exposures that are carious or induced by trauma have demonstrated clinical success rates of 80–90% [87, 104].

There is still considerable debate about its mode of action; numerous animal studies have shown histological dentine bridge formation in 50–87% of treated teeth [89, 105–108], but this is less predictable in humans [9, 109, 110]. It has been suggested that the action of calcium hydroxide is related to its caustic nature; it has a high pH of 11–12, which initially induces tissue irritation and superficial necrosis (known as a zone of coagulation necrosis) [98].

For clinical application, calcium hydroxide is either mixed as a pure powder with an aqueous solution (water or saline) or, more commonly, used as a commercially available hard-setting wound dressing/lining material, such as Dycal (Denstply Caulk, Milford, DE, USA) or Life (Kerr, Boggio, Switzerland). Dycal and Life set through an acid–base reaction leading to the formation of Ca-salicylate chelate, although they use different setting activators (butyleneglycol disalicylate and methyl salicylate, respectively). Both show a marked calcium release.

Aqueous suspensions have been shown to induce wider zones of necrosis compared with commercial preparations [89]. In a histological study in rhesus monkeys [89], wound healing occurred at the material interface when commercial preparations were used, but for calcium hydroxide paste made with saline, the reparative tissue formation was some distance away from the material itself, leaving a persistent vacant zone. The hard-setting materials resulted in less evidence of caustic damage, and it appears that the necrotic zone was removed by phagocytosis and replaced with granulation tissue [90]. In a more recent study in humans [111], one week of pulp capping with calcium hydroxide resulted in a moderate inflammatory infiltrate, disorganized tissue with hyperaemia, and no evidence of a hard tissue barrier. At one month, the majority of samples showed a reduced inflammatory response with evidence of dECM components secretion and partial hard tissue repair. This is consistent with earlier reports suggesting that hard tissue healing next to calcium hydroxide was unpredictable and not complete across the wound, with numerous tunnel defects present [112].

The mechanisms by which calcium hydroxide induces hard tissue repair are not entirely understood [113]. It has been suggested that the superficial necrotic layer separates the vital tissue from the wound so that the pulp can repair itself [71]. Others have postulated that it is the creation of a supersaturated environment of calcium ions adjacent to the pulp that induces hard tissue healing, but this hypothesis was disproved when it was demonstrated that the calcium ions which were incorporated into the mineralized hard tissue bridge originated from the underlying tissues rather than from the pulp-capping material itself [114, 115]. It has also been proposed that the tissue may respond favourably to the high-pH environment created by the release of hydroxyl ions [116]. Without doubt, the bactericidal nature of calcium hydroxide, brought about by its high pH, provides an environment which is conducive to pulp survival [12, 117]. Dentine bridges were still formed in a high percentage of cases when exposed pulps were purposely infected with bacteria prior to pulp capping with calcium hydroxide [107, 108]. This suggests that the bactericidal nature of calcium hydroxide is an important property of the material. As with HCSCs, it has been shown that calcium hydroxide can solubilize growth factors sequestered in dentine; this is thought to initiate the sequence of reparative events which leads to tertiary dentine formation [44].

Although numerous studies have demonstrated successful pulp healing with calcium hydroxide, many clinicians view its use in pulp capping with scepticism. A 5- and 10-year retrospective analysis of 123 calcium hydroxide pulp-capping procedures performed on carious exposures showed that 45% had failed in the 5-year group and 80% in the 10-year one [52]. In another retrospective analysis of 248 teeth, with follow-up of 0.4–16.6 years (mean 6.1 ± 4.4 years), the overall survival rate was found to be 76.3% after 13.3 years [118]. Pulp capping in patients aged over 60 years showed a considerably less favourable outcome than in patients younger than 40 years.

All forms of calcium hydroxide, including the hard-setting variants, are easily solubilized. This poses a challenge for long-term restorative success, because even the best restorative materials available will inevitably undergo some form of microleakage. Under amalgam restorations, Dycal has been shown to be relatively soft in 70% of cases [119]; furthermore, it undergoes significant washout [120], so although it is bactericidal, it does not maintain a durable seal against bacterial microleakage [121].

2.4.3 Resin-Based Adhesives

Resin-based systems were first suggested for pulp capping in the mid-1990s [122] and remained fashionable for the next 10–15 years. The initial interest came from non-primate studies, which showed that mechanical exposures treated with adhesive systems led to pulp healing [123, 124]. Primate studies using uncontaminated mechanically-induced exposures also showed positive results, demonstrating that resin-based systems led to healing responses similar to those obtained with calcium hydroxide, the gold standard at the time [125, 126]. Further studies were conducted which reproduced more realistic conditions, such as capping of bacterial contaminated pulps. These represented the most common clinical situations, as most exposures result from a deep carious lesion or are treated when an operative field is not controlled with a rubber dam [127]. Between 2005 and 2008, seven human studies compared the histological response between resin-based systems and calcium hydroxide, with between 16 and 40 teeth in each. All showed a more favourable response in the calcium hydroxide group compared to the resin-based one irrespective of whether an etch-and-rinse or a self-etch system was used [128].

Resin-based adhesive systems are not suitable candidates for VPT due to their cytotoxic effects [129]; the challenge of obtaining a bacterial tight seal when there is likely to be moisture (open wound of the pulp), which will reduce polymerization [130]; the amount of unpolymerized material with a high prevalence of toxic components at the wound site; and certain components in the resin that reduce the pulp's immune response, leading to reduced microbial clearance [131]. It is thus well established that resin-based adhesives should not be used for VPT [1].

2.4.4 Hydraulic Calcium Silicate Cements

The first clinically available HCSC was MTA, which was developed in the 1990s by Mahmoud Torabinejad [132, 133] and is now widely thought of as the material of choice for managing endodontic problems that require a soft tissue interface with the pulp [9] or periradicular tissues [134]. It was ostensibly developed as an agent to seal the root canal from the periradicular tissues, but was also found to be biocompatible when interfacing with pulpal tissue and showed promise as a therapeutic pulp-capping material. The first commercially available MTA was ProRoot MTA (Dentsply Tulsa Dental, Tulsa, OK, USA). Its original grey version caused aesthetic problems when it was used for VPT in anterior teeth. A white variety was therefore developed, receiving FDA approval in 2001. It has since become apparent, however, that both versions of ProRoot MTA cause discolouration, and it is recommended that neither be used in the aesthetic zone [135, 136]. MTA is composed of Portland cement (tricalcium silicate, dicalcium silicate, tricalcium aluminate, calcium sulphate, and tetracalcium aluminoferrite in the grey version) and bismuth oxide [137–139].

This material has a number of drawbacks which limit its clinical use, particularly for VPT. These include its tendency to discolour tooth structure [135, 136], its 'sandy' consistency, and its long setting time. MTA Angelus (Angelus Soluções Odontológicas, Londrina, Brazil) was the first material to address the latter; it lacks calcium sulphate [137, 138], giving it a shorter setting time of 10–15 minutes [139, 140]. As ProRoot MTA and MTA Angelus are based on Portland cement and thus manufactured from naturally occurring raw materials, it is conceivable that they contain traces of heavy metals such as arsenic, lead, and chromium [138, 141, 142]. In an attempt to prevent this contamination, other manufacturers use pure laboratory-grade materials. The HCSCs Bioaggregate (Innovative Bioceramix Inc., Vancouver, Canada) and Biodentine (Septodont, Saint Maur des Fosses, France) have been manufactured using this approach. Bioaggregate is composed predominantly of tricalcium silicate, with additions of calcium phosphate, silicon dioxide, and tantalum oxide used as a radiopacifier. Biodentine powder predominantly consists of tricalcium silicate as the core material, along with dicalcium silicate, calcium carbonate (filler), iron oxide (shade), and zirconium oxide (radiopacifier) [143]. It differs from other HCSCs in that its liquid phase has active components, namely calcium chloride (accelerator) and a hydrosoluble polymer (water-reducing agent) [144]. The manufacturer approximates its setting time at between 9 and 12 minutes [145]. It has been suggested that it is longer in reality, however.

A workable mix of HCSC requires the addition of more water than is necessary for hydration. This results in a system of pores which reduces over time as the water is used up in hydration [146]. Generally, the total pore space is equivalent to the initial water-to-powder ratio; therefore, increasing the water-to-powder ratio increases the pore space [146, 147]. Ionic exchange between the cement surface and the fluid surrounding it leads to the liberation of a number of different leachable ions from the surface in an aqueous environment.

In order for a material to be regarded as clinically successful as a pulp-capping agent, it should demonstrate a number of important characteristics, as outlined earlier. Since their introduction, HCSCs have undergone extensive *in vitro* and *in vivo* analysis [148]. Their antimicrobial and antifungal effects show conflicting results, with an antibacterial effect found on some facultative bacteria, but no effect on any strict anaerobes; however, the same study showed that zinc oxide-eugenol-based materials tested in parallel led to inhibition of growth

amongst both types of bacteria [149]. An assessment using single-strain and polymicrobial broths of bacteria and fungi showed that MTA inhibited fungal and microbial growth in both [150]. Interestingly, grey MTA was shown to inhibit similar amounts of growth of *Streptococcus sanguis* to white MTA at lower concentrations, suggesting that it may have greater antibacterial activity [151]. Attempts have been made to enhance the antibacterial properties of HCSCs by combining them with chlorhexidine instead of water, at concentrations of 0.12% [152] and 2% [153] – both proved successful, but other authors have expressed doubts about their utility in terms of biocompatibility [154] and deterioration of physical characteristics [153]. Although *in vitro* microleakage studies are frequently viewed with scepticism [155–157], they are the main means of determining the ability of a material to create a barrier against bacterial penetration in a given clinical scenario. Numerous different *in vitro* techniques have been used to compare the sealing ability of HCSCs to other materials used in the same clinical situation, with HCSCs showing superior to amalgam, super EBA (ethoxy benzoic acid), and intermediate restorative material (IRM) with techniques including dye leakage [158, 159], fluid filtration [160, 161], and bacterial penetration studies [149, 162, 163].

MTA has been shown to exhibit excellent biocompatibility when it is in contact with pulp wounds in animals [164–168] and humans [9, 109, 169, 170]. Histological studies of iatrogenic exposures in human teeth, managed in aseptic conditions, compared teeth capped with MTA with those capped with calcium hydroxide. Notably, the ones capped with MTA demonstrated greater reparative dentine formation in terms of thickness and quality, less inflammation, and more predictable healing [9, 109, 170]. The precise mechanism by which HCSCs work is not well understood, however. They have been shown to induce key stages in pulp repair, namely pulp cell proliferation [171], migration [168], and differentiation [172]. Immunohistochemical analysis of

(a)   (b)   (c)

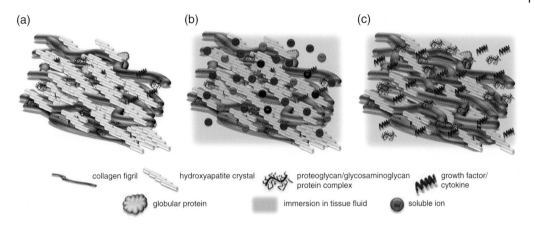

Figure 2.8 (a) Diagrammatic representation of dentine, including inorganic and organic components, at a nanometre scale. (b) Immersion of dentine in tissue fluid or extracellular exudate that has interacted locally with calcium silicate cement and has a unique ionic composition. (c) Ionic exchange between dentine and soluble components of calcium silicate cements, resulting in disruption of hydroxyapatite crystals, leading to solubilization and release of bioactive molecules from dECM, including noncollagenous proteins, glycosaminoglycans, and growth factors. (Components in diagrams not to scale.)

pulp wounds that had been capped with MTA for up to 11 weeks showed expression of DSPP and collagen type I in those odontoblasts in direct contact with the MTA. There was also evidence of dentine secretion by those same cells [173]. Biodentine has been shown to induce pulp cells to release TGF-β1, suggesting that this action induces reparative dentine formation [174]. The surface of MTA has been reported to form hydroxyapatite when it is in contact with synthetic body fluids [175, 176]. It is suggested that this biologically accepted surface layer allows for excellent cell/material adhesion and enables superior sealing characteristics when compared with other materials.

HCSCs show many of the properties expected of a VPT agent. It has been clearly demonstrated that they are biocompatible, and even bioinductive. Their interaction with local tissue fluids on the hydrated surface layer is a crucial aspect of this characteristic. Both grey and white MTA leach multiple different cations. From their setting and set phases *in vitro* and *in vitro*, this would modify adjacent local tissue fluids. Such fluids have the ability to interact with dentine and can solubilize dECM [43], which contains powerful signal molecules such as TGF-β1, hepatocyte growth

factor, and adrenomedullin (Figure 2.8) [177, 178]. The release of these soluble dECM components leads to cellular events such as proliferation, cell homing, and differentiation in pulp stem cells [177, 178], which are crucial for tissue repair and regeneration. Such a hypothesis is a plausible explanation for the positive reactionary and reparative dentinogenic responses which occur adjacent to HCSCs.

2.4.5 Resin-Based Hydraulic Calcium Silicate Cements

In an attempt to overcome the long setting time of HCSCs, command-set light-cured HCSCs have been developed. TheraCal LC (Bisco, Schaumburg, IL, USA) is one of the most researched. It consists of a mixture of Portland cement, strontium glass, fumed silica, barium-based radiopacifier, and a light-activated resin made up of Bis-GMA and polyethylene glycol dimethacrylate [179]. Although it is claimed to be an HCSC, the reaction of the Portland cement component requires the imbibition of fluids from its surroundings, which may be limited [180]. TheraCal cures through photopolymerization, and the water-based reaction is slow as the liquid required for the setting of the cement depends on the porosity of the resin. A number of organic components are not declared on the material safety data sheet [181]. Leaching of calcium hydroxide is negligible [182] or significantly less than that of other CSCs [183]. The alkaline pH of TheraCal is similar to that of Dycal [184] and significantly lower than that of ProRoot MTA at both short- and longer-term intervals [185].

Several *in vitro* studies have been carried out comparing TheraCal to other VPT agents. It has been demonstrated to be cytotoxic with pulp cells [186, 187], and it shows more significant inflammation and less bioactive potential than Biodentine [187]. The authors of the latter study even suggested it should not be considered a candidate for direct interfacing with the pulp.

TheraCal does not perform as well as conventional water-based HCSCs when interfacing with the pulp itself [188]. In a study of partial pulpotomies in dogs, it induced pulp inflammation in 90% of cases, compared with 18% of those treated with ProRoot MTA [188]. A histological study of partial pulpotomy of third molars in humans compared the use of Theracal, ProRoot MTA, and Biodentine. TheraCal treatment resulted in pulp disorganization beneath the material in 66.67% of cases and of the entire pulp in 22.2%. Discontinued dentinal bridge was noted in most cases treated, and the authors stated that Biodentine and ProRoot MTA were more reliable for long-term protection of dental pulp [189].

Based on the limited research to date, it does seem that TheraCal is a poor candidate for VPT when directly interfacing with the exposed dental pulp. It may be that it is more suitable for use as an indirect pulp-capping agent, but there is scant evidence for this indication.

2.4.6   Glass Ionomer Cements

GICs form as a result of an acid–base reaction between a weak polymeric acid and powdered glass, which is basic in nature. Curing occurs in concentrated solutions of water, and the final structure contains unreacted glass particles, which act as a filler, reinforcing the material. Resin-modified glass ionomer cements (RMGICs) were developed to provide command set in an attempt to decrease setting time/moisture sensitivity [190]. Ostensibly, they are a hybrid of glass ionomers and resin composite.

These materials are not traditionally thought of as an option for directly interfacing with the vital pulp tissue, due to their cytotoxicity. Conventional glass ionomers tend to be less toxic than the resin-modified formulations [191, 192]. Due to their ability to chemically bond to tooth structures, they provide an excellent bacterial seal [193] and show good biocompatibility when used in close approximation – but not direct contact – with the pulp [75].

When RMGICs were compared to calcium hydroxide in deep nonexposed cavities, a quantitative systematic review could not demonstrate superiority in terms of pulp response with either agent [194], and although histologically RMGICs showed more damage in the short term, this decreased over time, with both RMGICs and conventional GICs performing similarly [195].

Activa Bioactive base/liner (Pulpdent, Watertown, MA, USA) was launched in 2014. It has the mechanical strength, aesthetics, and physical properties of composites and the increased release and recharge of calcium, phosphate, and fluoride. Pulpdent suggests that it is a light-cured resin-modified calcium silicate, but this is misleading – it is much more indicative of an RMGIC [196]. The material has three setting mechanisms: glass ionomer (acid–base reaction), light composite resin, and self-cure composite resin; however, there is a suggestion that the self-cure reaction does not occur [197]. The bioactive properties of this material are based on a mechanism whereby changes in pH result in the release and recharge of significant amounts of calcium, phosphate, and fluoride [198]. Although this material is suggested for use in indirect and direct pulp therapies, there is insufficient evidence at this stage to support its placement directly against the pulp.

GICs are thus considered indirect pulp-capping agents rather than as suitable for direct placement on to the pulp itself. A high-quality randomized controlled clinical trial has shown them to be as effective as Biodentine in treating a deep carious lesion with reversible pulpitis when used in the former mode [27, 199]. Meanwhile, the European Society of Endodontology recommends either a glass ionomer or an HCSC be used as an indirect pulp-capping agent [1].

2.4.7 Experimental Agents Used in Vital Pulp Treatment

In order to improve the clinical outcomes of VPT, several experimental therapies that have shown promise in tissue regeneration elsewhere have been explored. Bioactive glasses composed of silica, sodium oxide, calcium oxide, and phosphorus pentoxide are well studied in biomaterials [200]. Originally, such glasses were used to repair bone fractures in order to stimulate the body's own regenerative capacity. Bioactive glass dissolves in the normal physiological environment and activates genes controlling osteogenesis and growth factor production [201], leading to bone growth of equivalent quality to that of natural bone [202]. Attempts have been made to assess bioactive glasses as pulp-capping materials [203], but they have never been significantly more successful than their controls [204].

Emdogain is an enamel matrix derivative originating from unerupted porcine tooth buds which contain amelogenins of various weights. It has proved successful in regenerating periodontal tissues when treating infrabony defects caused by periodontal disease [205]. However, the evidence is less convincing for pulpal tissues: the limited animal and human research conducted to this point shows that, at best, it is no better than calcium hydroxide or MTA [206].

There are several different growth factors and naturally occurring bioactive signalling molecules that are sequestered in dentine during tooth development [178] which have been considered for use as pulp-capping agents [207]. Bone morphogenetic protein-2 (BMP-2), a member of the TGF-β super family, has been approved by the US Food and Drug Administration (FDA) for clinical use in bone grafting [208] and is known to induce differentiation of DPSCs to an odontoblast phenotype [209]. However, very few other recombinant cytokines have made it past the animal research stage to become candidates for clinical trials. Fibroblast growth factor-2 (FGF-2)-incorporated gelatin hydrogels with collagen sponge have been used on the amputated pulp surface of a rat upper first molar [210, 211]; controlled release of FGF-2 from the hydrogel induced regeneration of pulp tissue and osteodentin-like hard tissue in the defect area. *In vitro* research shows that there is huge promise in the use of these naturally occurring bioactive signalling molecules [38].

The therapeutic use of pharmacological inhibitors to modulate epigenetic 'marks' on cellular chromatin has also been shown to alter mineralization response, with inhibitors targeted at DNA-methylation [212] and histone acetylation shown to promote odontoblast-like cell differentiation and mineralized tissue formation [51, 213]. Acetylation of histone tails on chromatin is controlled by histone deacetylase (HDAC) and histone acetyl-transferase enzymes, which if altered by HDAC-inhibitors (HDACis) result in the promotion of gene expression and a change in cell phenotype [214]. Application of HDACis to rat and human DPSC cultures enhanced mineralization processes, accompanied by an upregulation of genes associated with odontoblast differentiation and mineralization, such as TGF-β1, BMPs, and DSPP [213, 215, 216]. In addition to the direct regulation of cellular processes, HDACis also induced bioactive DMC release from dentine [45]. Finally, an *in vivo* study analysed the development of the dentine–pulp complex after systemic injection of trichostatin A (TSA) into prenatal mice and highlighted an increase in odontoblasts and dentine thickness compared with control samples [217].

2.4.8 Tooth Restoration After VPT

One of the main disadvantages of the use of MTA is its extended setting time, as this makes tooth restoration in one visit difficult. In order to circumvent this problem, the tooth can be definitively restored at a subsequent visit, or else GIC can be placed over the material to prevent washout during definitive restoration placement. A moist barrier should be used between the unset MTA and the temporary restorative material.

The shorter setting time of Biodentine compared to other HCSCs means that it is an excellent candidate for use in VPT. It also has the advantage of having a much higher compressive strength compared to other HCSCs, making it resilient enough to be exposed in the oral cavity, at least as a temporary material, or even as an intermediate restoration [145]. It can later be cut back in order to create space for a definitive restorative with a composite resin and treated like a traditional base.

2.5 Clinical Outcome and Practicalities

2.5.1 Vital Pulp Treatment Outcome

The outcome of VPT should be assessed clinically after six months and with additional radiographic assessment at one year. If symptoms dictate, the observation period should be extended annually for four years [1]. The tooth should be responsive to pulp sensibility testing, but this may be heightened or diminished during the review period. Notably, although teeth which have had a partial pulpotomy will respond positively to testing, those which have undergone full pulpotomy will be unresponsive [218]. There should be no history of pain or other symptoms, and there should be evidence of continued root formation in immature teeth radiographically, as well as absence apical periodontitis [219]. A successful outcome in mature permanent teeth with symptoms no worse than reversible pulpitis indicates that a pulp-capping procedure using an HCSC will be successful in approximately 80–90% of cases [63, 68, 82]. However, success is likely to be affected by the location (interproximal, occlusal) [79] and depth [66] of the carries, as well as operator skill [52, 63, 69] and material used [66, 68]. Other factors have not been consistently shown to be critical in determining outcome; these include patient age [83, 85, 196] and size of exposure [53, 118]. Interestingly, recent evidence highlights the potential of full pulpotomy to be as effective as pulpectomy in teeth with signs and symptoms suggestive of irreversible pulpitis [11, 84, 220–222]. That said, there is a lack of prospective controlled trials using standardized materials, irrigants, caries depth symptoms, and so on in this area; this will need to be addressed moving forward. Damaged immature teeth treated aseptically by VPT that remain vital will display continued root growth through the physiological processes of primary and ongoing secondary dentinogenesis.

2.5.2 Discolouration

Crown discolouration as a result of VPT does not constitute a biological failure of the procedure [219]; however, from the patient's perspective, it may be of genuine concern. Initially, commercial MTA was available as ProRoot in a grey formulation, which was later superseded by a white product, marketed as being superior in aesthetic areas. For many endodontic applications such as apexification and perforation repair, the discolouration risk of MTA is not critical; however, this is not the case for applications in which the cement in placed in contact with pulp cells in the coronal aspect of the tooth (Figure 2.9). Notably, white ProRoot

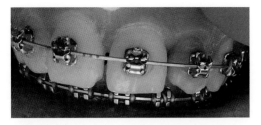

Figure 2.9 Discoloured maxillary left lateral incisor one year after a partial pulpotomy procedure using a hydraulic calcium silicate material containing bismuth oxide.
Source: Henry F. Duncan.

MTA has also been demonstrated to discolour teeth [135] – a process accentuated in the presence of irrigants such as sodium hypochlorite [223] and fluids like blood [224]. This discolouration has been attributed to the radiopacifier bismuth oxide, which forms a precipitate in the presence of collagen and sodium hypochlorite creating stains [225]. Other hydraulic calcium silicate materials contain other radiopacifiers, including zirconium oxide, which has been linked to a reduced colour change in Biodentine-treated teeth [226–228]. Tooth discolouration is possible with all HCSCs, particularly in the presence of blood products, but next-generation materials induce significantly less staining than ProRoot MTA [229], perhaps due to the removal of bismuth oxide. However, radiopacity is often reduced as a result. Interestingly, Biodentine's radiopacity is consistently reported as being below ISO standards [230, 231], and indeed operators cannot clearly visualize it as distinct to dentine.

2.5.3 Setting Time and Handling

ProRoot MTA is limited clinically by a prolonged setting time [232, 233], which lasts several hours. As a result, the manufacturer claims the material should be applied over two visits – a feature which is not ideal for vital pulp applications. Newer HCSCs, including MTA Angelus, Biodentine, and resin-modified calcium silicates such as TheraCal LC, advertise significantly shorter or instant setting times, facilitating completion of treatment in one visit. Notably, the setting time of Biodentine is not always predictable, with it often taking significantly longer than the advertised time even for initial setting to occur [145, 230]; however, it is still much quicker than ProRoot MTA. It has been reported that MTA Angelus and Biodentine have similar setting times [234]. Light-cured HCSCs, whilst offering an instantly setting material, have been shown to be cytotoxic and are not recommended for use as direct pulp-capping materials [187]. Traditionally, MTA has been reported to be difficult to handle because of its consistency and formulation [232, 235], whilst Biodentine is considered easier to mix and use [234]. A recent questionnaire-based study investigated Biodentine and MTA in VPT and highlighted that many dentists avoided using any calcium silicate materials, citing reasons of cost, lack of training, and difficulties in material handling [236].

2.6 Conclusion

Preserving the health of the dental pulp is an important aspect of modern endodontics. If successful, pulp preservation is a minimally invasive, biologically based, and technically undemanding alternative to pulpectomy. Therefore, selective caries removal, stepwise excavation, pulp capping, and pulpotomy are an essential part of the treatment armamentarium of every dentist. The advent of HCSCs has provided renewed impetus in VPT, and they are the current material of choice in this area. Although the exact mechanisms remain to be elucidated, pulp-capping materials like calcium hydroxide and MTA appear to stimulate the release of biologically active molecules from pulp cells and the dECM, stimulating dentinogenesis. Although the future of this area may involve molecular diagnostic biomarker assays and targeted third-generation biomaterials, prospective randomized trials using modern materials are required to support promising preliminary clinical data in the meantime.

References

1 Duncan, H.F., Galler, K.M., Tomson, P.L. et al. (2019). European Society of Endodontology position statement: management of deep caries and the exposed pulp. *Int. Endod. J.* 52 (7): 923–934.

2 Wolters, W.J., Duncan, H.F., Tomson, P.L. et al. (2017). Minimally invasive endodontics: a new diagnostic system for assessing pulpitis and subsequent treatment needs. *Int. Endod. J.* 50 (9): 825–829.

3 Randow, K. and Glantz, P.O. (1986). On cantilever loading of vital and non-vital teeth. An experimental clinical study. *Acta Odontol. Scand.* 44 (5): 271–277.

4 Paphangkorakit, J. and Osborn, J.W. (1998). Discrimination of hardness by human teeth apparently not involving periodontal receptors. *Arch. Oral Biol.* 43 (1): 1–7.

5 Stanley, H.R. (1989). Pulp capping: conserving the dental pulp – can it be done? Is it worth it? *Oral Surg. Oral Med. Oral Pathol.* 68 (5): 628–639.

6 Elderton, R.J. (1993). Overtreatment with restorative dentistry: when to intervene? *Int. Dent. J.* 43 (1): 17–24.

7 Schwendicke, F. and Stolpe, M. (2014). Direct pulp capping after a carious exposure versus root canal treatment: a cost-effectiveness analysis. *J. Endod.* 40 (11): 1764–1770.

8 Murray, P.E., Garcia-Godoy, F., and Hargreaves, K.M. (2007). Regenerative endodontics: a review of current status and a call for action. *J. Endod.* 33 (4): 377–390.

9 Nair, P.N., Duncan, H.F., Pitt Ford, T.R., and Luder, H.U. (2008). Histological, ultrastructural and quantitative investigations on the response of healthy human pulps to experimental capping with mineral trioxide aggregate: a randomized controlled trial. *Int. Endod. J.* 41 (2): 128–150.

10 Gronthos, S., Mankani, M., Brahim, J. et al. (2000). Postnatal human dental pulp stem cells (DPSCs) in vitro and in vivo. *Proc. Natl. Acad. Sci. U. S. A.* 97 (25): 13625–13630.

11 Taha, N.A. and Khazali, M.A. (2017). Partial pulpotomy in mature permanent teeth with clinical signs indicative of irreversible pulpitis: a randomized clinical trial. *J. Endod.* 43 (9): 1417–1421.

12 Kakehashi, S., Stanley, H.R., and Fitzgerald, R.J. (1965). The effects of surgical exposures of dental pulps in germ-free and conventional laboratory rats. *Oral Surg. Oral Med. Oral Pathol. Oral Radiol. Endod.* 20: 340–349.

13 Bernabe, E. and Sheiham, A. (2014). Age, period and cohort trends in caries of permanent teeth in four developed countries. *Am. J. Public Health* 104 (7): e115–e121.

14 Kassebaum, N.J., Bernabe, E., Dahiya, M. et al. (2015). Global burden of untreated caries: a systematic review and metaregression. *J. Dent. Res.* 94 (5): 650–658.

15 Sengupta, K., Christensen, L.B., Mortensen, L.H. et al. (2017). Trends in socioeconomic inequalities in oral health among 15-year-old Danish adolescents during 1995–2013: a nationwide, register-based, repeated cross-sectional study. *Community Dent. Oral Epidemiol.* 45 (5): 458–468.

16 Warfvinge, J. and Bergenholtz, G. (1986). Healing capacity of human and monkey dental pulps following experimentally-induced pulpitis. *Endod. Dent. Traumatol.* 2 (6): 256–262.

17 Brannstrom, M. and Lind, P.O. (1965). Pulpal response to early dental caries. *J. Dent. Res.* 44 (5): 1045–1050.

18 Reeves, R. and Stanley, H.R. (1966). The relationship of bacterial penetration and pulpal pathosis in carious teeth. *Oral Surg. Oral Med. Oral Pathol.* 22 (1): 59–65.

19 Mjor, I.A. and Tronstad, L. (1974). The healing of experimentally induced pulpitis. *Oral Surg. Oral Med. Oral Pathol.* 38 (1): 115–121.

20 Bergenholtz, G., Cox, C.F., Loesche, W.J., and Syed, S.A. (1982). Bacterial leakage around dental restorations: its effect on the dental pulp. *J. Oral Pathol.* 11 (6): 439–450.

21 Schwendicke, F., Frencken, J.E., Bjorndal, L. et al. (2016). Managing carious lesions: consensus recommendations on carious tissue removal. *Adv. Dent. Res.* 28 (2): 58–67.

22 El-Helali, R., Dowling, A.H., McGinley, E.L. et al. (2013). Influence of resin-based composite restoration technique and endodontic access on cuspal deflection and cervical microleakage scores. *J. Dent.* 41 (3): 216–222.

23 Browne, R.M., Tobias, R.S., Crombie, I.K., and Plant, C.G. (1983). Bacterial microleakage and pulpal inflammation in experimental cavities. *Int. Endod. J.* 16 (4): 147–155.

24 Cox, C.F., Keall, C.L., Keall, H.J. et al. (1987). Biocompatibility of surface-sealed dental materials against exposed pulps. *J. Prosthet. Dent.* 57 (1): 1–8.

25 Krifka, S., Seidenader, C., Hiller, K.A. et al. (2012). Oxidative stress and cytotoxicity generated by dental composites in human pulp cells. *Clin. Oral Investig.* 16 (1): 215–224.

26 Paranjpe, A., Cacalano, N.A., Hume, W.R., and Jewett, A. (2008). Mechanisms of N-acetyl cysteine-mediated protection from 2-hydroxyethyl methacrylate-induced apoptosis. *J. Endod.* 34 (10): 1191–1197.

27 Hashem, D., Mannocci, F., Patel, S. et al. (2015). Clinical and radiographic assessment of the efficacy of calcium silicate indirect pulp capping: a randomized controlled clinical trial. *J. Dent. Res.* 94 (4): 562–568.

28 Buchalla, W. and Attin, T. (2007). External bleaching therapy with activation by heat, light or laser – a systematic review. *Dent. Mater.* 23 (5): 586–596.

29 Leonard, R.H. Jr., Smith, L.R., Garland, G.E. et al. (2007). Evaluation of side effects and patients' perceptions during tooth bleaching. *J. Esthet. Restor. Dent.* 19 (6): 355–364; disc. 65–66.

30 Robertson, W.D. and Melfi, R.C. (1980). Pulpal response to vital bleaching procedures. *J. Endod.* 6 (7): 645–649.

31 Simon, S., Copper, P.R., Berdal, A. et al. (2009). Understanding pulp biology for routine clinical practice. *ENDO Endodontic Pract. Today* 3 (3): 171–184.

32 Lesot, H., Smith, A.J., Tziafas, D. et al. (1994). Biologically active molecules and dental tissue repair: a comparative review of reactionary and reparative dentinogenesis with the induction of odontoblast differentiation in vitro. *Cells Mater.* 4: 199–218.

33 Smith, A.J., Cassidy, N., Perry, H. et al. (1995). Reactionary dentinogenesis. *Int. J. Dev. Biol.* 39 (1): 273–280.

34 Ricucci, D., Loghin, S., and Siqueira, J.F. Jr. (2014). Correlation between clinical and histologic pulp diagnoses. *J. Endod.* 40 (12): 1932–1939.

35 Yoshiba, N., Edanami, N., Tohma, A. et al. (2018). Detection of bone marrow-derived fibrocytes in human dental pulp repair. *Int. Endod. J.* 51 (11): 1187–1195.

36 Cassidy, N., Fahey, M., Prime, S.S., and Smith, A.J. (1997). Comparative analysis of transforming growth factor-beta isoforms 1–3 in human and rabbit dentine matrices. *Arch. Oral Biol.* 42 (3): 219–223.

37 Smith, A.J. (2003). Vitality of the dentin–pulp complex in health and disease: growth factors as key mediators. *J. Dent. Educ.* 67 (6): 678–689.

38 Smith, A.J., Duncan, H.F., Diogenes, A. et al. (2016). Exploiting the bioactive properties of the dentin–pulp complex in regenerative endodontics. *J. Endod.* 42 (1): 47–56.

39 Cooper, P.R., Takahashi, Y., Graham, L.W. et al. (2010). Inflammation–regeneration interplay in the dentine–pulp complex. *J. Dent.* 38 (9): 687–697.

40 Couve, E., Osorio, R., and Schmachtenberg, O. (2013). The amazing odontoblast: activity, autophagy, and aging. *J. Dent. Res.* 92 (9): 765–772.

41 Huang, T.H., Yang, C.C., Ding, S.J. et al. (2005). Inflammatory cytokines reaction elicited by root-end filling materials. *J. Biomed. Mater. Res. B Appl. Biomater.* 73 (1): 123–128.

42 Rutherford, R.B., Wahle, J., Tucker, M. et al. (1993). Induction of reparative dentine

formation in monkeys by recombinant human osteogenic protein-1. *Arch. Oral Biol.* 38 (7): 571–576.

43 Tomson, P.L., Grover, L.M., Lumley, P.J. et al. (2007). Dissolution of bio-active dentine matrix components by mineral trioxide aggregate. *J. Dent.* 35 (8): 636–642.

44 Graham, L., Cooper, P.R., Cassidy, N. et al. (2006). The effect of calcium hydroxide on solubilisation of bio-active dentine matrix components. *Biomaterials* 27 (14): 2865–2873.

45 Duncan, H.F., Smith, A.J., Fleming, G.J. et al. (2017). Release of bio-active dentine extracellular matrix components by histone deacetylase inhibitors (HDACi). *Int. Endod. J.* 50 (1): 24–38.

46 Giraud, T., Jeanneau, C., Rombouts, C. et al. (2019). Pulp capping materials modulate the balance between inflammation and regeneration. *Dent. Mater.* 35 (1): 24–35.

47 Ferracane, J.L., Cooper, P.R., and Smith, A.J. (2010). Can interaction of materials with the dentin-pulp complex contribute to dentin regeneration? *Odontology* 98 (1): 2–14.

48 Galler, K.M. and Widbiller, M. (2017). Perspectives for cell-homing approaches to engineer dental pulp. *J. Endod.* 43 (9S): S40–S45.

49 Tran, X.V., Gorin, C., Willig, C. et al. (2012). Effect of a calcium-silicate-based restorative cement on pulp repair. *J. Dent. Res.* 91 (12): 1166–1171.

50 Sangwan, P., Sangwan, A., Duhan, J., and Rohilla, A. (2013). Tertiary dentinogenesis with calcium hydroxide: a review of proposed mechanisms. *Int. Endod. J.* 46 (1): 3–19.

51 Duncan, H.F., Smith, A.J., Fleming, G.J., and Cooper, P.R. (2013). Histone deacetylase inhibitors epigenetically promote reparative events in primary dental pulp cells. *Exp. Cell Res.* 319 (10): 1534–1543.

52 Barthel, C.R., Rosenkranz, B., Leuenberg, A., and Roulet, J.F. (2000). Pulp capping of carious exposures: treatment outcome after 5 and 10 years: a retrospective study. *J. Endod.* 26 (9): 525–528.

53 Mejare, I. and Cvek, M. (1993). Partial pulpotomy in young permanent teeth with deep carious lesions. *Endod. Dent. Traumatol.* 9 (6): 238–242.

54 Seltzer, S., Bender, I.B., and Ziontz, M. (1963). The interrelationship of pulp and periodontal disease. *Oral Surg. Oral Med. Oral Pathol.* 16: 1474–1490.

55 AAE (2012). *Glossary of Endodontic Terms*, 8e. Chicago, IL: American Association of Endodontists.

56 Garfunkel, A., Sela, J., and Ulmansky, M. (1973). Dental pulp pathosis. Clinicopathologic correlations based on 109 cases. *Oral Surg. Oral Med. Oral Pathol.* 35 (1): 110–117.

57 Dummer, P.M., Hicks, R., and Huws, D. (1980). Clinical signs and symptoms in pulp disease. *Int. Endod. J.* 13 (1): 27–35.

58 Michaelson, P.L. and Holland, G.R. (2002). Is pulpitis painful? *Int. Endod. J.* 35 (10): 829–832.

59 Bjorndal, L., Simon, S., Tomson, P.L., and Duncan, H.F. (2019). Management of deep caries and the exposed pulp. *Int. Endod. J.* 52 (7): 949–973.

60 Cvek, M. (1978). A clinical report on partial pulpotomy and capping with calcium hydroxide in permanent incisors with complicated crown fracture. *J. Endod.* 4 (8): 232–237.

61 Al-Hiyasat, A.S., Barrieshi-Nusair, K.M., and Al-Omari, M.A. (2006). The radiographic outcomes of direct pulp-capping procedures performed by dental students: a retrospective study. *J. Am. Dent. Assoc.* 137 (12): 1699–1705.

62 Bjorndal, L., Fransson, H., Bruun, G. et al. (2017). Randomized clinical trials on deep carious lesions: 5-year follow-up. *J. Dent. Res.* 96 (7): 747–753.

63 Marques, M.S., Wesselink, P.R., and Shemesh, H. (2015). Outcome of direct pulp capping with mineral trioxide aggregate: a prospective study. *J. Endod.* 41 (7): 1026–1031.

64 Mente, J., Hufnagel, S., Leo, M. et al. (2014). Treatment outcome of mineral trioxide aggregate or calcium hydroxide direct pulp capping: long-term results. *J. Endod.* 40 (11): 1746–1751.

65 Ricketts, D.N., Kidd, E.A., Innes, N., and Clarkson, J. (2006). Complete or ultraconservative removal of decayed tissue in unfilled teeth. *Cochrane Database Syst. Rev.* (3): CD003808.

66 Bjorndal, L., Reit, C., Bruun, G. et al. (2010). Treatment of deep caries lesions in adults: randomized clinical trials comparing stepwise vs. direct complete excavation, and direct pulp capping vs. partial pulpotomy. *Eur. J. Oral Sci.* 118 (3): 290–297.

67 Innes, N.P., Frencken, J.E., Bjorndal, L. et al. (2016). Managing carious lesions: consensus recommendations on terminology. *Adv. Dent. Res.* 28 (2): 49–57.

68 Hilton, T.J., Ferracane, J.L., and Mancl, L. (2013). Comparison of CaOH with MTA for direct pulp capping: a PBRN randomized clinical trial. *J. Dent. Res.* 92 (7 Suppl): 16s–22s.

69 Bogen, G., Kim, J.S., and Bakland, L.K. (2008). Direct pulp capping with mineral trioxide aggregate: an observational study. *J. Am. Dent. Assoc.* 139 (3): 305–315; quiz 315.

70 Bergenholtz, G. (2000). Evidence for bacterial causation of adverse pulpal responses in resin-based dental restorations. *Crit. Rev. Oral Biol. Med.* 11 (4): 467–480.

71 Schroder, U. (1985). Effects of calcium hydroxide-containing pulp-capping agents on pulp cell migration, proliferation, and differentiation. *J. Dent. Res.* 64: 541–548.

72 Cvek, M., Granath, L., Cleaton-Jones, P., and Austin, J. (1987). Hard tissue barrier formation in pulpotomized monkey teeth capped with cyanoacrylate or calcium hydroxide for 10 and 60 minutes. *J. Dent. Res.* 66 (6): 1166–1174.

73 Burke, F.J.T. and Lucarotti, P.S.K. (2018). The ultimate guide to restoration longevity in England and Wales. Part 10: Key findings from a ten million restoration dataset. *Br. Dent. J.* 225 (11): 1011–1018.

74 Elderton, R.J. and Nuttall, N.M. (1983). Variation among dentists in planning treatment. *Br. Dent. J.* 154 (7): 201–206.

75 Murray, P.E., Hafez, A.A., Smith, A.J., and Cox, C.F. (2002). Hierarchy of pulp capping and repair activities responsible for dentin bridge formation. *Am. J. Dent.* 15 (4): 236–243.

76 Zach, L. (1972). Pulp lability and repair; effect of restorative procedures. *Oral Surg. Oral Med. Oral Pathol.* 33 (1): 111–121.

77 Murray, P.E., Smyth, T.W., About, I. et al. (2002). The effect of etching on bacterial microleakage of an adhesive composite restoration. *J. Dent.* 30 (1): 29–36.

78 Hilton, T.J. (1996). Cavity sealers, liners, and bases: current philosophies and indications for use. *Oper. Dent.* 21 (4): 134–146.

79 Maltz, M., Jardim, J.J., Mestrinho, H.D. et al. (2013). Partial removal of carious dentine: a multicenter randomized controlled trial and 18-month follow-up results. *Caries Res.* 47 (2): 103–109.

80 Ali, A.H., Koller, G., Foschi, F. et al. (2018). Self-limiting versus conventional caries removal: a randomized clinical trial. *J. Dent. Res.* 97 (11): 1207–1213.

81 Granath, L.E. and Hagman, G. (1971). Experimental pulpotomy in human bicuspids with reference to cutting technique. *Acta Odontol. Scand.* 29 (2): 155–163.

82 Kundzina, R., Stangvaltaite, L., Eriksen, H.M., and Kerosuo, E. (2017). Capping carious exposures in adults: a randomized controlled trial investigating mineral trioxide aggregate versus calcium hydroxide. *Int. Endod. J.* 50 (10): 924–932.

83 Harms, C.S., Schafer, E., and Dammaschke, T. (2019). Clinical evaluation of direct pulp capping using a calcium silicate cement-treatment outcomes over an average period of 2.3 years. *Clin. Oral Investig.* 23 (9): 3491–3499.

84 Cushley, S., Duncan, H.F., Lappin, M.J. et al. (2019). Pulpotomy for mature carious teeth with symptoms of irreversible pulpitis: a systematic review. *J. Dent.* 88: 103158.

85 Mente, J., Geletneky, B., Ohle, M. et al. (2010). Mineral trioxide aggregate or calcium hydroxide direct pulp capping: an analysis of the clinical treatment outcome. *J. Endod.* 36 (5): 806–813.

86 Massler, M. (1972). Therapy conductive to healing of the human pulp. *Oral Surg. Oral Med. Oral Pathol.* 34 (1): 122–130.

87 Matsuo, T., Nakanishi, T., Shimizu, H., and Ebisu, S. (1996). A clinical study of direct pulp capping applied to carious-exposed pulps. *J. Endod.* 22 (10): 551–556.

88 Pfaf, P. (1756). *Abhandlung von den Zähnen des menschlichen Körpers und deren Krankheiten*. Berlin: Haude und Spener.

89 Heys, D.R., Cox, C.F., Heys, R.J., and Avery, J.K. (1981). Histological considerations of direct pulp capping agents. *J. Dent. Res.* 60 (7): 1371–1379.

90 Stanley, H.R. and Lundy, T. (1972). Dycal therapy for pulp exposures. *Oral Surg. Oral Med. Oral Pathol.* 34 (5): 818–827.

91 Shovelton, D.S., Friend, L.A., Kirk, E.E., and Rowe, A.H. (1971). The efficacy of pulp capping materials. A comparative trial. *Br. Dent. J.* 130 (9): 385–391.

92 Horsted-Bindslev, P., Vilkinis, V., and Sidlauskas, A. (2003). Direct capping of human pulps with a dentin bonding system or with calcium hydroxide cement. *Oral Surg. Oral Med. Oral Pathol. Oral Radiol. Endod.* 96 (5): 591–600.

93 Cowan, A. (1966). Treatment of exposed vital pulps with a corticosteroid antibiotic agent. *Br. Dent. J.* 120 (11): 521–532.

94 Bhaskar, S.N., Beasley, J.D., Ward, J.P., and Cutright, D.E. (1972). Human pulp capping with isobutyl cyanoacrylate. *J. Dent. Res.* 51 (1): 58–61.

95 do Nascimento, A.B., Fontana, U.F., Teixeira, H.M., and Costa, C.A. (2000). Biocompatibility of a resin-modified glass-ionomer cement applied as pulp capping in human teeth. *Am. J. Dent.* 13 (1): 28–34.

96 Torabinejad, M. and Chivian, N. (1999). Clinical applications of mineral trioxide aggregate. *J. Endod.* 25 (3): 197–205.

97 Hermann, B. (1920). Calcium hydroxyd als mitten zum behandeln und fullen von Wurzelkanallen. Dissertation. Wursburg. (Printed in: Malo, P.R.T., Kessler Nieto, F., and Vadillo, M.V.M. (1987). Hidroxido de calcio y apicoformacion. *Revista Espanola de Endodoncia* 5: 41–61).

98 Glass, R.L. and Zander, H.A. (1949). Pulp healing. *J. Dent. Res.* 28 (2): 97–107.

99 Schroder, U. (1972). Evaluation of healing following experimental pulpotomy of intact human teeth and capping with calcium hydroxide. *Odontol. Revy* 23 (3): 329–340.

100 Schroder, U. (1973). Effect of an extra-pulpal blood clot on healing following experimental pulpotomy and capping with calcium hydroxide. *Odontol. Revy* 24 (3): 257–268.

101 Tronstad, L. (1974). Reaction of the exposed pulp to Dycal treatment. *Oral Surg. Oral Med. Oral Pathol.* 38 (6): 945–953.

102 Pitt Ford, T.R. (1979). Pulpal response to Procal for capping exposures in dog's teeth. *J. Br. Endod. Soc.* 12 (2): 67–72.

103 Pitt Ford, T.R. and Roberts, G.J. (1991). Immediate and delayed direct pulp capping with the use of a new visible light-cured calcium hydroxide preparation. *Oral Surg. Oral Med. Oral Pathol.* 71 (3): 338–342.

104 Baume, L.J. and Holz, J. (1981). Long term clinical assessment of direct pulp capping. *Int. Dent. J.* 31 (4): 251–260.

105 Brannstrom, M., Nyborg, H., and Stromberg, T. (1979). Experiments with pulp capping. *Oral Surg. Oral Med. Oral Pathol.* 48 (4): 347–352.

106 Cox, C.F., Bergenholtz, G., Fitzgerald, M. et al. (1982). Capping of the dental pulp mechanically exposed to the oral microflora – a 5 week observation of wound healing in the monkey. *J. Oral Pathol.* 11 (4): 327–339.

107 Cox, C.F., Bergenholtz, G., Heys, D.R. et al. (1985). Pulp capping of dental pulp mechanically exposed to oral microflora: a 1–2 year observation of wound healing in the monkey. *J. Oral Pathol.* 14 (2): 156–168.

108 Pitt Ford, T.R. (1985). Pulpal response to a calcium hydroxide material for capping exposures. *Oral Surg. Oral Med. Oral Pathol.* 59 (2): 194–197.

109 Aeinehchi, M., Eslami, B., Ghanbariha, M., and Saffar, A.S. (2003). Mineral trioxide aggregate (MTA) and calcium hydroxide as pulp-capping agents in human teeth: a preliminary report. *Int. Endod. J.* 36 (3): 225–231.

110 Chacko, V. and Kurikose, S. (2006). Human pulpal response to mineral trioxide aggregate (MTA): a histologic study. *J. Clin. Pediatr. Dent.* 30 (3): 203–209.

111 Lu, Y., Liu, T., Li, H., and Pi, G. (2008). Histological evaluation of direct pulp capping with a self-etching adhesive and calcium hydroxide on human pulp tissue. *Int. Endod. J.* 41 (8): 643–650.

112 Cox, C.F., Subay, R.K., Ostro, E. et al. (1996). Tunnel defects in dentin bridges: their formation following direct pulp capping. *Oper. Dent.* 21 (1): 4–11.

113 Smith, A.J. (2002). Pulpal responses to caries and dental repair. *Caries Res.* 36 (4): 223–232.

114 Pisanti, S. and Sciaky, I. (1964). Origin of calcium in the repair wall after pulp exposure in the dog. *J. Dent. Res.* 43: 641–644.

115 Sciaky, I. and Pisanti, S. (1960). Localization of calcium placed over amputated pulps in dogs' teeth. *J. Dent. Res.* 39: 1128–1132.

116 Kardos, T.B., Hunter, A.R., Hanlin, S.M., and Kirk, E.E. (1998). Odontoblast differentiation: a response to environmental calcium? *Endod. Dent. Traumatol.* 14 (3): 105–111.

117 Kakehashi, S., Stanley, H.R., and Fitzgerald, R. (1969). The exposed germ-free pulp: effects of topical corticosteroid medication and restoration. *Oral Surg. Oral Med. Oral Pathol.* 27 (1): 60–67.

118 Dammaschke, T., Leidinger, J., and Schafer, E. (2010). Long-term evaluation of direct pulp capping – treatment outcomes over an average period of 6.1 years. *Clin. Oral Investig.* 14 (5): 559–567.

119 Pereira, J.C., Manfio, A.P., Franco, E.B., and Lopes, E.S. (1990). Clinical evaluation of Dycal under amalgam restorations. *Am. J. Dent.* 3 (2): 67–70.

120 Novickas, D., Fiocca, V.L., and Grajower, R. (1989). Linings and caries in retrieved permanent teeth with amalgam restorations. *Oper. Dent.* 14 (1): 33–39.

121 Cox, C.F. and Suzuki, S. (1994). Re-evaluating pulp protection: calcium hydroxide liners vs. cohesive hybridization. *J. Am. Dent. Assoc.* 125 (7): 823–831.

122 Kanca, J. 3rd. (1996). Replacement of a fractured incisor fragment over pulpal exposure: a long-term case report. *Quintessence Int.* 27 (12): 829–832.

123 Olmez, A., Oztas, N., Basak, F., and Sabuncuoglu, B. (1998). A histopathologic study of direct pulp-capping with adhesive resins. *Oral Surg. Oral Med. Oral Pathol. Oral Radiol. Endod.* 86 (1): 98–103.

124 Tsuneda, Y., Hayakawa, T., Yamamoto, H. et al. (1995). A histopathological study of direct pulp capping with adhesive resins. *Oper. Dent.* 20 (6): 223–229.

125 Cox, C.F., Hafez, A.A., Akimoto, N. et al. (1998). Biocompatibility of primer, adhesive and resin composite systems on non-exposed and exposed pulps of non-human primate teeth. *Am. J. Dent.* 11: S55–S63.

126 Fujitani, M., Shibata, S., Van Meerbeek, B. et al. (2002). Direct adhesive pulp capping: pulpal healing and ultra-morphology of the resin-pulp interface. *Am. J. Dent.* 15 (6): 395–402.

127 Pameijer, C.H. and Stanley, H.R. (1998). The disastrous effects of the 'total etch' technique in vital pulp capping in primates. *Am. J. Dent.* 11: S45–S54.

128 Hilton, T.J. (2009). Keys to clinical success with pulp capping: a review of the literature. *Oper. Dent.* 34 (5): 615–625.

129 de Souza Costa, C.A., do Nascimento, A.B., and Teixeira, H.M. (2002). Response of human pulps following acid conditioning and application of a bonding agent in deep cavities. *Dent. Mater.* 18 (7): 543–551.

130 Abebe, W., Pashley, D.H., and Rueggeberg, F.A. (2005). Vasorelaxant effect of resin-based, single-bottle dentin bonding systems. *J. Endod.* 31 (3): 194–197.

131 Jontell, M., Hanks, C.T., Bratel, J., and Bergenholtz, G. (1995). Effects of unpolymerized resin components on the function of accessory cells derived from the rat incisor pulp. *J. Dent. Res.* 74 (5): 1162–1167.

132 Lee, S.J., Monsef, M., and Torabinejad, M. (1993). Sealing ability of a mineral trioxide aggregate for repair of lateral root perforations. *J. Endod.* 19 (11): 541–544.

133 Torabinejad, M., White, D.J., inventors; Loma Linda University, assignee. (1995). Tooth filling material and method of use. US patent 5415547.

134 Parirokh, M. and Torabinejad, M. (2010). Mineral trioxide aggregate: a comprehensive literature review – Part III: Clinical applications, drawbacks, and mechanism of action. *J. Endod.* 36 (3): 400–413.

135 Lenherr, P., Allgayer, N., Weiger, R. et al. (2012). Tooth discoloration induced by endodontic materials: a laboratory study. *Int. Endod. J.* 45 (10): 942–949.

136 Ioannidis, K., Mistakidis, I., Beltes, P., and Karagiannis, V. (2013). Spectrophotometric analysis of coronal discolouration induced by grey and white MTA. *Int. Endod. J.* 46 (2): 137–144.

137 Oliveira, M.G., Xavier, C.B., Demarco, F.F. et al. (2007). Comparative chemical study of MTA and Portland cements. *Braz. Dent. J.* 18 (1): 3–7.

138 Camilleri, J., Kralj, P., Veber, M., and Sinagra, E. (2012). Characterization and analyses of acid-extractable and leached trace elements in dental cements. *Int. Endod. J.* 45 (8): 737–743.

139 Song, J.S., Mante, F.K., Romanow, W.J., and Kim, S. (2006). Chemical analysis of powder and set forms of Portland cement, gray ProRoot MTA, white ProRoot MTA, and gray MTA-Angelus. *Oral Surg. Oral Med. Oral Pathol. Oral Radiol. Endod.* 102 (6): 809–815.

140 Santos, A.D., Araujo, E.B., Yukimitu, K. et al. (2008). Setting time and thermal expansion of two endodontic cements. *Oral Surg. Oral Med. Oral Pathol. Oral Radiol. Endod.* 106 (3): e77–e79.

141 Duarte, M.A., De Oliveira Demarchi, A.C., Yamashita, J.C. et al. (2005). Arsenic release provided by MTA and Portland cement. *Oral Surg. Oral Med. Oral Pathol. Oral Radiol. Endod.* 99 (5): 648–650.

142 De-Deus, G., de Souza, M.C., Sergio Fidel, R.A. et al. (2009). Negligible expression of arsenic in some commercially available brands of Portland cement and mineral trioxide aggregate. *J. Endod.* 35 (6): 887–890.

143 Camilleri, J., Sorrentino, F., and Damidot, D. (2015). Characterization of un-hydrated and hydrated BioAggregate™ and MTA Angelus™. *Clin. Oral Investig.* 19 (3): 689–698.

144 Camilleri, J., Sorrentino, F., and Damidot, D. (2013). Investigation of the hydration and bioactivity of radiopacified tricalcium silicate cement, Biodentine and MTA Angelus. *Dent. Mater.* 29 (5): 580–593.

145 Grech, L., Mallia, B., and Camilleri, J. (2013). Investigation of the physical properties of tricalcium silicate cement-based root-end filling materials. *Dent. Mater.* 29 (2): e20–e28.

146 Odler, I. (1993). Hydration, setting and hardening of Portland cement. In: *Lea's Chemistry of Cement on Concrete* (ed. P.C. Hewlett), 241–297. Oxford: Elsevier Butterworth-Heinemann.

147 Fridland, M. and Rosado, R. (2003). Mineral trioxide aggregate (MTA) solubility and porosity with different water-to-powder ratios. *J. Endod.* 29 (12): 814–817.

148 Torabinejad, M. and Parirokh, M. (2010). Mineral trioxide aggregate: a comprehensive literature review – Part II: Leakage and biocompatibility investigations. *J. Endod.* 36 (2): 190–202.

149 Torabinejad, M., Hong, C.U., Pitt Ford, T.R., and Kettering, J.D. (1995). Antibacterial effects of some root end filling materials. *J. Endod.* 21 (8): 403–406.

150 Estrela, C., Bammann, L.L., Estrela, C.R. et al. (2000). Antimicrobial and chemical study of MTA, Portland cement, calcium hydroxide paste, Sealapex and Dycal. *Braz. Dent. J.* 11 (1): 3–9.

151 Al-Hezaimi, K., Al-Shalan, T.A., Naghshbandi, J. et al. (2006). Antibacterial effect of two mineral trioxide aggregate (MTA) preparations against *Enterococcus faecalis* and *Streptococcus sanguis* in vitro. *J. Endod.* 32 (11): 1053–1056.

152 Stowe, T.J., Sedgley, C.M., Stowe, B., and Fenno, J.C. (2004). The effects of chlorhexidine gluconate (0.12%) on the antimicrobial properties of tooth-colored ProRoot mineral trioxide aggregate. *J. Endod.* 30 (6): 429–431.

153 Holt, D.M., Watts, J.D., Beeson, T.J. et al. (2007). The anti-microbial effect against enterococcus faecalis and the compressive strength of two types of mineral trioxide aggregate mixed with sterile water or 2% chlorhexidine liquid. *J. Endod.* 33 (7): 844–847.

154 Hernandez, E.P., Botero, T.M., Mantellini, M.G. et al. (2005). Effect of ProRoot MTA mixed with chlorhexidine on apoptosis and cell cycle of fibroblasts and macrophages in vitro. *Int. Endod. J.* 38 (2): 137–143.

155 Rechenberg, D.K., De-Deus, G., and Zehnder, M. (2011). Potential systematic error in laboratory experiments on microbial leakage through filled root canals: review of published articles. *Int. Endod. J.* 44 (3): 183–194.

156 Wu, M.K. and Wesselink, P.R. (1993). Endodontic leakage studies reconsidered. Part I. Methodology, application and relevance. *Int. Endod. J.* 26 (1): 37–43.

157 De-Deus, G. (2008). New directions in old leakage methods. *Int. Endod. J.* 41 (8): 720–721; disc. 1–3.

158 Torabinejad, M., Higa, R.K., McKendry, D.J., and Pitt Ford, T.R. (1994). Dye leakage of four root end filling materials: effects of blood contamination. *J. Endod.* 20 (4): 159–163.

159 Martell, B. and Chandler, N.P. (2002). Electrical and dye leakage comparison of three root-end restorative materials. *Quintessence Int.* 33 (1): 30–34.

160 Wu, M.K., Kontakiotis, E.G., and Wesselink, P.R. (1998). Long-term seal provided by some root-end filling materials. *J. Endod.* 24 (8): 557–560.

161 Karlovic, Z., Pezelj-Ribaric, S., Miletic, I. et al. (2005). Erbium:YAG laser versus ultrasonic in preparation of root-end cavities. *J. Endod.* 31 (11): 821–823.

162 Fischer, E.J., Arens, D.E., and Miller, C.H. (1998). Bacterial leakage of mineral trioxide aggregate as compared with zinc-free amalgam, intermediate restorative material, and Super-EBA as a root-end filling material. *J. Endod.* 24 (3): 176–179.

163 Tang, H.M., Torabinejad, M., and Kettering, J.D. (2002). Leakage evaluation of root end filling materials using endotoxin. *J. Endod.* 28 (1): 5–7.

164 Ford, T.R., Torabinejad, M., Abedi, H.R. et al. (1996). Using mineral trioxide aggregate as a pulp-capping material. *J. Am. Dent. Assoc.* 127 (10): 1491–1494.

165 Keiser, K., Johnson, C.C., and Tipton, D.A. (2000). Cytotoxicity of mineral trioxide aggregate using human periodontal ligament fibroblasts. *J. Endod.* 26 (5): 288–291.

166 Faraco, I.M. Jr. and Holland, R. (2001). Response of the pulp of dogs to capping with mineral trioxide aggregate or a calcium hydroxide cement. *Dent. Traumatol.* 17 (4): 163–166.

167 Asgary, S., Eghbal, M.J., Parirokh, M. et al. (2008). A comparative study of histologic response to different pulp capping materials and a novel endodontic cement. *Oral Surg. Oral Med. Oral Pathol. Oral Radiol. Endod.* 106 (4): 609–614.

168 Kuratate, M., Yoshiba, K., Shigetani, Y. et al. (2008). Immunohistochemical analysis of nestin, osteopontin, and proliferating cells in the reparative process of exposed dental pulp capped with mineral trioxide aggregate. *J. Endod.* 34 (8): 970–974.

169 Accorinte Mde, L., Holland, R., Reis, A. et al. (2008). Evaluation of mineral trioxide aggregate and calcium hydroxide cement as pulp-capping agents in human teeth. *J. Endod.* 34 (1): 1–6.

170 Min, K.S., Park, H.J., Lee, S.K. et al. (2008). Effect of mineral trioxide aggregate on dentin bridge formation and expression of dentin sialoprotein and heme oxygenase-1 in human dental pulp. *J. Endod.* 34 (6): 666–670.

171 Moghaddame-Jafari, S., Mantellini, M.G., Botero, T.M. et al. (2005). Effect of ProRoot MTA on pulp cell apoptosis and proliferation in vitro. *J. Endod.* 31 (5): 387–391.

172 Masuda-Murakami, Y., Kobayashi, M., Wang, X. et al. (2010). Effects of mineral trioxide aggregate on the differentiation of rat dental pulp cells. *Acta Histochem.* 112 (5): 452–458.

173 Simon, S., Cooper, P., Smith, A. et al. (2008). Evaluation of a new laboratory model for pulp healing: preliminary study. *Int. Endod. J.* 41 (9): 781–790.

174 Laurent, P., Camps, J., and About, I. (2012). Biodentine(TM) induces TGF-beta1 release from human pulp cells and early dental pulp mineralization. *Int. Endod. J.* 45 (5): 439–448.

175 Sarkar, N.K., Caicedo, R., Ritwik, P. et al. (2005). Physicochemical basis of the biologic properties of mineral trioxide aggregate. *J. Endod.* 31 (2): 97–100.

176 Reyes-Carmona, J.F., Felippe, M.S., and Felippe, W.T. (2009). Biomineralization ability and interaction of mineral trioxide aggregate and white Portland cement with dentin in a phosphate-containing fluid. *J. Endod.* 35 (5): 731–736.

177 Tomson, P.L., Lumley, P.J., Alexander, M.Y. et al. (2013). Hepatocyte growth factor is sequestered in dentine matrix and promotes regeneration-associated events in dental pulp cells. *Cytokine* 61 (2): 622–629.

178 Tomson, P.L., Lumley, P.J., Smith, A.J., and Cooper, P.R. (2016). Growth factor release from dentine matrix by pulp capping agents promote pulp tissue repair-associated events. *Int. Endod. J.* 50 (3): 281–292.

179 Gandolfi, M.G., Siboni, F., and Prati, C. (2012). Chemical-physical properties of TheraCal, a novel light-curable MTA-like material for pulp capping. *Int. Endod. J.* 45 (6): 571–579.

180 Camilleri, J., Laurent, P., and About, I. (2014). Hydration of Biodentine, Theracal LC, and a prototype tricalcium silicate-based dentin replacement material after pulp capping in entire tooth cultures. *J. Endod.* 40 (11): 1846–1854.

181 Nilsen, B.W., Jensen, E., Ortengren, U., and Michelsen, V.B. (2017). Analysis of organic components in resin-modified pulp capping materials: critical considerations. *Eur. J. Oral Sci.* 125 (3): 183–194.

182 Gomes-Filho, J.E., de Faria, M.D., Bernabe, P.F. et al. (2008). Mineral trioxide aggregate but not light-cure mineral trioxide aggregate stimulated mineralization. *J. Endod.* 34 (1): 62–65.

183 Koutroulis, A., Kuehne, S.A., Cooper, P.R., and Camilleri, J. (2019). The role of calcium ion release on biocompatibility and antimicrobial properties of hydraulic cements. *Sci. Rep.* 9 (1): 19019.

184 Gandolfi, M.G., Siboni, F., Botero, T. et al. (2015). Calcium silicate and calcium hydroxide materials for pulp capping: biointeractivity, porosity, solubility and bioactivity of current formulations. *J. Appl. Biomater. Funct. Mater.* 13 (1): 43–60.

185 Yamamoto, S., Han, L., Noiri, Y., and Okiji, T. (2017). Evaluation of the Ca ion release, pH and surface apatite formation of a prototype tricalcium silicate cement. *Int. Endod. J.* 50 (Suppl. 2): e73–e82.

186 Hebling, J., Lessa, F.C., Nogueira, I. et al. (2009). Cytotoxicity of resin-based light-cured liners. *Am. J. Dent.* 22 (3): 137–142.

187 Jeanneau, C., Laurent, P., Rombouts, C. et al. (2017). Light-cured tricalcium silicate toxicity to the dental pulp. *J. Endod.* 43 (12): 2074–2080.

188 Lee, H., Shin, Y., Kim, S.O. et al. (2015). Comparative study of pulpal responses to pulpotomy with ProRoot MTA, RetroMTA, and TheraCal in dogs' teeth. *J. Endod.* 41 (8): 1317–1324.

189 Bakhtiar, H., Nekoofar, M.H., Aminishakib, P. et al. (2017). Human pulp responses to partial pulpotomy treatment with TheraCal as compared with biodentine and ProRoot MTA: a clinical trial. *J. Endod.* 43 (11): 1786–1791.

190 Berzins, D.W., Abey, S., Costache, M.C. et al. (2010). Resin-modified glass-ionomer setting reaction competition. *J. Dent. Res.* 89 (1): 82–86.

191 Schmalz, G., Schweikl, H., Esch, J., and Hiller, K.A. (1996). Evaluation of a dentin barrier test by cyctotoxicity testing of various dental cements. *J. Endod.* 22 (3): 112–115.

192 de Souza Costa, C.A., Hebling, J., Garcia-Godoy, F., and Hanks, C.T. (2003). In vitro cytotoxicity of five glass-ionomer cements. *Biomaterials* 24 (21): 3853–3858.

193 Heys, R.J. and Fitzgerald, M. (1991). Microleakage of three cement bases. *J. Dent. Res.* 70 (1): 55–58.

194 Mickenautsch, S., Yengopal, V., and Banerjee, A. (2010). Pulp response to resin-modified glass ionomer and calcium hydroxide cements in deep cavities: a quantitative systematic review. *Dent. Mater.* 26 (8): 761–770.

195 Ribeiro, A.P.D., Sacono, N.T., Soares, D.G. et al. (2019). Human pulp response to conventional and resin-modified glass ionomer cements applied in very deep cavities. *Clin. Oral Invest.* 24: 1739–1748.

196 Kunert, M. and Lukomska-Szymanska, M. (2020). Bio-inductive materials in direct and indirect pulp capping – a review article. *Materials (Basel)* 13 (5): 1204.

197 Benetti, A.R., Michou, S., Larsen, L. et al. (2019). Adhesion and marginal adaptation of a claimed bioactive, restorative material. *Biomater. Investig. Dent.* 6 (1): 90–98.

198 May, E. and Donly, K.J. (2017). Fluoride release and re-release from a bioactive restorative material. *Am. J. Dent.* 30 (6): 305–308.

199 Hashem, D., Mannocci, F., Patel, S. et al. (2019). Evaluation of the efficacy of calcium silicate vs. glass ionomer cement indirect pulp capping and restoration assessment criteria: a randomised controlled clinical trial – 2-year results. *Clin. Oral Investig.* 23 (4): 1931–1939.

200 Hench, L.L. (2006). The story of Bioglass. *J. Mater. Sci. Mater. Med.* 17 (11): 967–978.

201 Hench, L.L., Xynos, I.D., Buttery, L.D., and Polak, J.M. (2000). Bioactive materials to control cell cycle. *Mater. Res. Innovat.* 3 (6): 313–323.

202 Xynos, I.D., Hukkanen, M.V., Batten, J.J. et al. (2000). Bioglass 45S5 stimulates osteoblast turnover and enhances bone formation in vitro: implications and applications for bone tissue engineering. *Calcif. Tissue Int.* 67 (4): 321–329.

203 Stanley, H.R., Clark, A.E., Pameijer, C.H., and Louw, N.P. (2001). Pulp capping with a modified bioglass formula (#A68-modified). *Am. J. Dent.* 14 (4): 227–232.

204 Hanada, K., Morotomi, T., Washio, A. et al. (2019). In vitro and in vivo effects of a novel bioactive glass-based cement used as a direct pulp capping agent. *J. Biomed. Mater. Res. B Appl. Biomater.* 107 (1): 161–168.

205 Esposito, M., Grusovin, M.G., Papanikolaou, N. et al. (2009). Enamel matrix derivative (Emdogain(R)) for periodontal tissue regeneration in intrabony defects. *Cochrane Database Syst. Rev.* (4): CD003875.

206 Torabinejad, M., Parirokh, M., and Dummer, P.M.H. (2018). Mineral trioxide aggregate and other bioactive endodontic cements: an updated overview – Part II: Other clinical applications and complications. *Int. Endod. J.* 51 (3): 284–317.

207 Rutherford, B. and Fitzgerald, M. (1995). A new biological approach to vital pulp therapy. *Crit. Rev. Oral Biol. Med.* 6 (3): 218–229.

208 McKay, W.F., Peckham, S.M., and Badura, J.M. (2007). A comprehensive clinical review of recombinant human bone morphogenetic protein-2 (INFUSE Bone Graft). *Int. Orthop.* 31 (6): 729–734.

209 Iohara, K., Nakashima, M., Ito, M. et al. (2004). Dentin regeneration by dental pulp stem cell therapy with recombinant human bone morphogenetic protein 2. *J. Dent. Res.* 83 (8): 590–595.

210 Kikuchi, N., Kitamura, C., Morotomi, T. et al. (2007). Formation of dentin-like particles in dentin defects above exposed pulp by controlled release of fibroblast growth factor 2 from gelatin hydrogels. *J. Endod.* 33 (10): 1198–1202.

211 Ishimatsu, H., Kitamura, C., Morotomi, T. et al. (2009). Formation of dentinal bridge on surface of regenerated dental pulp in dentin defects by controlled release of fibroblast growth factor-2 from gelatin hydrogels. *J. Endod.* 35 (6): 858–865.

212 Zhang, D., Li, Q., Rao, L. et al. (2015). Effect of 5-Aza-2′-deoxycytidine on odontogenic differentiation of human dental pulp cells. *J. Endod.* 41 (5): 640–645.

213 Paino, F., La Noce, M., Tirino, V. et al. (2014). Histone deacetylase inhibition with valproic acid downregulates osteocalcin gene expression in human dental pulp stem cells and osteoblasts: evidence for HDAC2 involvement. *Stem Cells* 32 (1): 279–289.

214 Yamauchi, Y., Cooper, P.R., Shimizu, E. et al. (2020). Histone acetylation as a

regenerative target in the dentine–pulp complex. *Front. Genet.* 11: 1.

215 Duncan, H.F., Smith, A.J., Fleming, G.J., and Cooper, P.R. (2012). Histone deacetylase inhibitors induced differentiation and accelerated mineralization of pulp-derived cells. *J. Endod.* 38 (3): 339–345.

216 Duncan, H.F., Smith, A.J., Fleming, G.J. et al. (2016). The histone-deacetylase-inhibitor suberoylanilide hydroxamic acid promotes dental pulp repair mechanisms through modulation of matrix metalloproteinase-13 activity. *J. Cell. Physiol.* 231 (4): 798–816.

217 Jin, H., Park, J.Y., Choi, H., and Choung, P.H. (2013). HDAC inhibitor trichostatin A promotes proliferation and odontoblast differentiation of human dental pulp stem cells. *Tissue Eng. Part A* 19 (5–6): 613–624.

218 Careddu, R. and Duncan, H.F. (2018). How does the pulpal response to Biodentine and ProRoot mineral trioxide aggregate compare in the laboratory and clinic? *Br. Dent. J.* 225: 743–749.

219 ESE (2006). Quality guidelines for endodontic treatment: consensus report of the European Society of Endodontology. *Int. Endod. J.* 39 (12): 921–930.

220 Galani, M., Tewari, S., Sangwan, P. et al. (2017). Comparative evaluation of postoperative pain and success rate after pulpotomy and root canal treatment in cariously exposed mature permanent molars: a randomized controlled trial. *J. Endod.* 43 (12): 1953–1962.

221 Linsuwanont, P., Wimonsutthikul, K., Pothimoke, U., and Santiwong, B. (2017). Treatment outcomes of mineral trioxide aggregate pulpotomy in vital permanent teeth with carious pulp exposure: the retrospective study. *J. Endod.* 43 (2): 225–230.

222 Qudeimat, M.A., Alyahya, A., and Hasan, A.A. (2017). Mineral trioxide aggregate pulpotomy for permanent molars with clinical signs indicative of irreversible pulpitis: a preliminary study. *Int. Endod. J.* 50 (2): 126–134.

223 Camilleri, J. (2014). Color stability of white mineral trioxide aggregate in contact with hypochlorite solution. *J. Endod.* 40 (3): 436–440.

224 Felman, D. and Parashos, P. (2013). Coronal tooth discoloration and white mineral trioxide aggregate. *J. Endod.* 39 (4): 484–487.

225 Marciano, M.A., Costa, R.M., Camilleri, J. et al. (2014). Assessment of color stability of white mineral trioxide aggregate angelus and bismuth oxide in contact with tooth structure. *J. Endod.* 40 (8): 1235–1240.

226 Camilleri, J. (2015). Staining potential of Neo MTA Plus, MTA Plus, and Biodentine used for pulpotomy procedures. *J. Endod.* 41 (7): 1139–1145.

227 Kohli, M.R., Yamaguchi, M., Setzer, F.C., and Karabucak, B. (2015). Spectrophotometric analysis of coronal tooth discoloration induced by various bioceramic cements and other endodontic materials. *J. Endod.* 41 (11): 1862–1866.

228 Valles, M., Roig, M., Duran-Sindreu, F. et al. (2015). Color stability of teeth restored with biodentine: a 6-month in vitro study. *J. Endod.* 41 (7): 1157–1160.

229 Keskin, C., Demiryurek, E.O., and Ozyurek, T. (2015). Color stabilities of calcium silicate-based materials in contact with different irrigation solutions. *J. Endod.* 41 (3): 409–411.

230 Kaup, M., Schafer, E., and Dammaschke, T. (2015). An in vitro study of different material properties of Biodentine compared to ProRoot MTA. *Head Face Med.* 11: 16.

231 Lucas, C.P., Viapiana, R., Bosso-Martelo, R. et al. (2017). Physicochemical properties and dentin bond strength of a tricalcium silicate-based retrograde material. *Braz. Dent. J.* 28 (1): 51–56.

232 Kogan, P., He, J., Glickman, G.N., and Watanabe, I. (2006). The effects of various additives on setting properties of MTA. *J. Endod.* 32 (6): 569–572.

233 Lee, J.B., Park, S.J., Kim, H.H. et al. (2014). Physical properties and biological/ odontogenic effects of an experimentally developed fast-setting alpha-tricalcium phosphate-based pulp capping material. *BMC Oral Health* 14: 87.

234 Butt, N., Talwar, S., Chaudhry, S. et al. (2014). Comparison of physical and mechanical properties of mineral trioxide aggregate and Biodentine. *Indian J. Dent. Res.* 25 (6): 692–697.

235 Ma, J., Shen, Y., Stojicic, S., and Haapasalo, M. (2011). Biocompatibility of two novel root repair materials. *J. Endod.* 37 (6): 793–798.

236 Chin, J.S., Thomas, M.B., Locke, M., and Dummer, P.M. (2016). A survey of dental practitioners in Wales to evaluate the management of deep carious lesions with vital pulp therapy in permanent teeth. *Br. Dent. J.* 221 (6): 331–338.

3

Treatment of Immature Teeth with Pulp Necrosis

Paul R. Cooper[1], Henry F. Duncan[2], Matthias Widbiller[3], and Kerstin M. Galler[3]

[1] Sir John Walsh Research Institute, Department of Oral Sciences, Faculty of Dentistry, University of Otago, Dunedin, New Zealand
[2] Division of Restorative Dentistry and Periodontology, Trinity College Dublin, Dublin Dental University Hospital, Dublin, Ireland
[3] Department of Conservative Dentistry and Periodontology, University Hospital Regensburg, Regensburg, Germany

TABLE OF CONTENTS

Endodontic Materials in Clinical Practice, First Edition. Edited by Josette Camilleri.
© 2021 John Wiley & Sons Ltd. Published 2021 by John Wiley & Sons Ltd.

3.1 Introduction

In immature teeth, if left untreated, carious lesions, traumatic injuries, and developmental anomalies (dens invaginatus, dens evaginatus) may lead to pulpitis, pulp necrosis, and eventually apical periodontitis. Once the crown of an erupting tooth appears in the oral cavity, it will still take approximately three years before root formation is complete. Depending on the stage of root development, conventional root canal treatment (RCT) may not be possible due to several anatomical characteristics: a wide-open apical foramen with blunderbuss shape, thin root canal walls, and an unfavourable crown-root ratio, all of which increase the risk of fracture. Whereas a vital pulp should be preserved and receive vital pulp treatment (VPT) [1], therapies for immature teeth with pulp necrosis aim at resolving signs and symptoms of infection, and at the long-term preservation of affected teeth.

Two treatment modalities are currently considered suitable for immature teeth with pulp necrosis: an apical plug with mineral trioxide aggregate (MTA) and revitalization. Placement of MTA or another hydraulic calcium silicate cement (HCSC) in contact with the periapical tissue enables osseous healing and induces mineralized tissue formation adjacent to the material [2–5]. The core procedural detail for revitalization is the induction of bleeding into the root canal, where the blood clot serves as a starting point for healing. Thus, revitalization offers the potential to enable root lengthening and thickening, and may thus be advantageous in stabilizing the thin dentinal walls of immature teeth, reducing the risk of fracture.

This idea of provocation of bleeding into the root canal dates back to the 1960s, when Nygaard-Østby conducted studies in animals and patients to show that new tissue formation was possible after allowing the root canal to fill with blood [6]. In dental traumatology, it was observed early on that, following avulsion, immature teeth could present with a newly formed vascular network throughout the canal only 30 days after replantation [7]. The term 'revascularization' was thus used for the first cases published on the provocation of bleeding into immature teeth with pulp necrosis. As expectations grew to include the idea of inducing regeneration with this protocol, the term 'regenerative endodontic procedure' was coined [8]. 'Revitalization' reflects the formation of new tissue inside the root canal without specifying the type [9], whilst the term 'guided endodontic repair' takes into account that the procedure is controlled and aimed at tissue repair and healing [10].

The radiographically observed response to revitalization shows a wide range, including unaltered apical anatomy, apical closure, narrowing of the root canal, increased root length and thickness, root canal obliteration, and completion of root formation [11–15]. A multitude of parameters influence the outcome after revitalization. Non-operator-dependent factors include the patient's individual anatomy, the stage of root development, the pathosis, the type of injury and tissue damage, the extent of infection and inflammation, and the patient's healing capacity. Operator-dependent factors, meanwhile, include the determination of indication, the procedural details (particularly the use of certain agents and materials, concentrations, and durations of action), and, importantly, the disinfection protocol. Whilst the clinician must take the non-operator-dependent factors into account and make a reasonable decision regarding the choice of treatment in each individual case, these factors cannot be altered. However, the use of biomaterials during the procedure is the operator's choice and requires an in-depth knowledge of the agents and materials in question, their composition, and their effects on cells and tissues. In order to better understand the interactions of materials and tissue reactions, it is indispensable to have a deep knowledge of the healing process, inflammation, growth factor signalling, and potential epigenetic influences – all of which will be discussed in this chapter.

Whereas current clinical protocols induce tissue repair, true regeneration of the dentine–pulp complex is subject to continuous research efforts. Tissue engineering approaches for dental pulp regeneration have been applied in cell-based and cell-free systems, and proof of principle exists that dental pulp regeneration is possible. The development of increasingly sophisticated scaffold materials and the use of dentine-derived growth factors may enable us to implement such concepts in the clinic in the near future. Again, an in-depth understanding of the procedures, materials, and tissue responses will be required to conduct successful regenerative treatment in endodontics.

3.2 Apexification and Root-End Closure

If dental caries is allowed to proceed without remedial treatment, the microbial biofilm will advance and bacteria will invade the pulp tissue. This challenge leads to irreversible pulpits, pulp necrosis, and subsequent apical periodontitis [16]. Management of pulp necrosis in mature teeth requires RCT, but if the root formation is not complete, the combination of thin dentine walls and open apices will make completion of conventional RCT impossible [17]. Furthermore, immature teeth which have lost vitality are also more vulnerable to injury (losing the ability to sense environmental change) and more prone to root fracture compared to mature teeth [18, 19].

From a biological perspective, the treatment of nonvital immature teeth requires the same level of disinfection and removal of necrotic tissue as conventional RCT, albeit with a reduction or absence of root canal instrumentation. Traditional treatment of immature teeth is by apexification, a technique that induces an apical mineralized barrier using nonsetting calcium hydroxide (CH) over a period of a few months. During the apexification procedure, the necrotic tissue is removed via chemomechanical disinfection, whilst the canal is dried

and dressed with a nonsetting CH paste placed carefully on to the tooth apex with an endodontic plugger or spiral filler in order to ensure good contact with the apical tissues. The CH is generally changed after one month, and thereafter every three months, until an apical barrier forms. This barrier is usually a poor-quality cementum-like tissue that can be viewed radiographically, and its presence is confirmed by gentle palpation with a paper point. The entire process takes anywhere from 6 to 18 months to complete. Once confirmed, the teeth can be filled with thermoplastic gutta-percha. From a practical perspective, apexification is clearly time-consuming [20] and costly for both patients and dentists, whilst the predictable creation of a mineralized barrier is hard to achieve [21]. Notably, root fracture is significantly increased with long-term CH dressing in immature teeth [18].

As a result, root-end closure techniques, which involve placing an HCSC matrix at the apex [22, 23], have recently been preferred over long-term CH therapy. The use of an apical plug reduces treatment time to one or two visits, limiting the risk of loss of patient compliance and of root fracture (Figure 3.1). Although not essential, the use of magnifying loupes or an operating microscope facilitates this treatment, which (at least initially) is carried out in an identical manner to apexification using CH. An HCSC, ideally possessing a radioaopacity greater than dentine, is placed gently with an endodontic plugger or specialized MTA carrier until a thickness of 5 mm from the radiographic apex in achieved [23]. Thereafter, the tooth can be dressed with a moist cotton pellet or paper point prior to the placement of thermoplastic gutta-percha at a subsequent visit; alternatively, it may be filled in a single visit if the HCSC sets.

Notably, treatment outcome comparisons have highlighted a similar or improved response with root-end closure using MTA over traditional apexification techniques using CH [24, 25]. However, both these techniques are not designed to induce extension of root

(a)   (b)   (c)

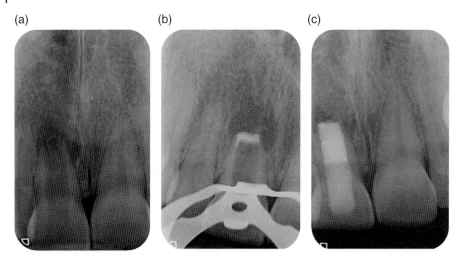

Figure 3.1 MTA root-end closure in a necrotic immature central incisor. (a) Immature incisor with apical radiolucency and wide root canal apically. (b) MTA plug placed following noninstrumentation protocol. (c) Remainder of canal filled with thermoplastic gutta-percha and resin-based composite extending below the CEJ. Note the relatively thin dentinal walls, particularly in the cervical area, which predisposes the tooth to subsequent fracture. *Source:* Paul Cooper, Henry F. Duncan, Matthias Widbiller, Kerstin M. Galler.

length or width [26, 27], and they generally have poor long-term prognosis [28]. Therefore, strategies to either maintain the healthy pulp or stimulate the development of new biological tissue are paramount, not only to promote minimally invasive solutions, but also to retain or reinstate the capacity of the pulp to generate tertiary dentine and respond to injurious stimuli [29].

3.3 Revitalization

Within the last few years, revitalization has been established as an alternative treatment to the apical plug, and sufficient evidence is available to show that the outcomes in terms of tooth survival and success rates are similar across both treatment modalities [2].

The first case reports from the early 2000s suggested provoking bleeding into the root canal and covering the blood clot with MTA instead of inducing an apical barrier or placing an apical plug with MTA. Follow-up in immature teeth after this procedure showed a completion of root formation where radiographically both root lengthening and root thickening were observed [15, 30]. These results sparked interest and raised the question whether pulp regeneration was possible using such an approach. More case reports, and then case series, were published. The verification of the presence of mesenchymal stem cells in the root canal led to the hypothesis that provocation of bleeding would induce an influx of stem cells from the apical papilla, which could differentiate and form new pulp and tubular dentine [31]. A more realistic evaluation of revitalization indicates that repair rather than regeneration takes place after this procedure. This is based on results from animal studies and histological analysis of human teeth following revitalization [32–34].

3.3.1 Indications

Revitalization is indicated in immature teeth with pulp necrosis, with or without a periapical lesion. Thus, this treatment is an alternative to the apical plug. Recently, it has been suggested that revitalization is beneficial in teeth at stages 1–3 of root development according to Cvek (less than half to over two-thirds of root development with open apex), whilst at stage 4 (nearly completed root formation with open apex) either revitalization or an MTA plug can be performed [35]. Immature permanent teeth with a necrotic pulp requiring a post to ensure an adequate coronal restoration are not suitable for revitalization and should be treated with an apical plug and root canal filling.

Whereas revitalization is easier to perform from a technical perspective when compared to the placement of an apical plug, it requires high compliance of the patient, as the induction of bleeding may cause discomfort or even pain despite the anaesthesia.

3.3.2 Procedure

The European Society of Endodontology (ESE) and American Association of Endodontists (AAE) have put forward recommendations on the procedural details of revitalization therapy. Whereas minor differences can be found between the protocols, single details may not be critical for success; rather, it is the clinician's understanding of the procedure and the response of the involved tissues and cells to manipulation that are important.

The procedure is undertaken in two visits. The first includes proper diagnostics, field isolation, preparation of an access cavity, and disinfection by 1.5–3.0% sodium hypochlorite (NaOCl) and then saline, followed by 17% ethylenediaminetetraacetic acid (EDTA). The root canal walls should be minimally or not at all instrumented. CH can be used as an intracanal medicament and a restoration, providing a tight seal is placed. Saline and EDTA may reduce the cytotoxic effects of NaOCl on the periapical tissues. Antibiotics have been used as an intracanal medicament in early case reports, case series, and clinical studies, but the routine use of antibiotic pastes (ciprofloxacin, metronidazole, and minocycline or cefuroxim) is no longer recommended due to sensitization, bacterial resistance, and limited removability. Signs and symptoms of inflammation should have receded before the next steps are executed.

During the second visit, the tooth is reopened and the canal is rinsed with 17% EDTA and dried. Note that NaOCl is no longer indicated at this point, as it may interfere with the desired effects of EDTA, namely exposure of collagen and dentine-derived growth factors on the surface [36]. Bleeding is induced by mechanical irritation of the periapical tissues and should reach up below the cementoenamel junction (CEJ). Placement of a collagenous material is optional. The blood clot is then covered with HCSC, followed by a permanent restoration. Regular follow-up is recommended. For further details on the procedure, see the ESE and AAE guidelines [37, 38].

3.3.3 Outcome

To date, the level of evidence for revitalization procedures is quite high. Besides case reports, case series, and laboratory and animal studies, retrospective and prospective cohort studies [14, 39] have been published, together with randomized controlled clinical studies [13, 40–42], systematic reviews, and meta-analyses [2, 43, 44]. Survival rates and healing are similar for the apical plug and revitalization. Apical closure can be observed after both procedures, but increased root length and thickness is seen only after revitalization. However, this finding is infrequent and unpredictable (Figure 3.2). Comparative clinical studies show higher success rates for the apical plug and revitalization compared to CH apexification [26], with similar results across the former two modalities [14, 27].

Failure with recurrent signs and symptoms of inflammation is a possible outcome after revitalization [34, 45]. Insufficient disinfection may be considered the main cause. Illustrative animal studies show that the presence of bacteria in the root canal after revitalization, which may not manifest in periapical lesions, will cause an absence of root lengthening and thickening [46].

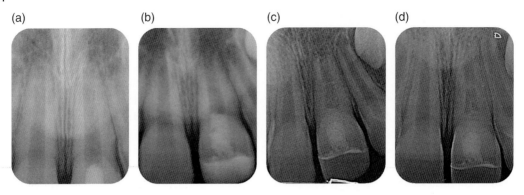

(a) (b) (c) (d)

Figure 3.2 Revitalization in a necrotic immature central incisor. (a) Preoperative radiograph. (b) Postoperative radiograph after provocation of bleeding and application of hydraulic tricalcium silicate (Biodentine, Septodont, Saint-Maur-des-Fossés, France). (c) 12-month and (d) 24-month follow-up. Completion of root formation cannot be observed. The tooth responds to cold testing. *Source:* Paul Cooper, Henry F. Duncan, Matthias Widbiller, Kerstin M. Galler.

3.3.4 Limitations

Initial expectations for revitalization procedures were high, and true regeneration of the dentine–pulp complex with differentiation of odontoblasts from stem cells of the apical papilla and formation of tubular dentine was assumed. When the first animal studies, along with human teeth extracted after revitalization procedures, showed ectopic tissue formation in the root canal [32–34] – including fibrous tissue and apposition of cementum or ingrowth of bone – disillusion began to spread. Diogenes et al. [10] separated patient-based, clinician-based, and scientist-based expected outcomes, and gave rise to a different perspective. Nowadays, the absence of signs and symptoms of inflammation, together with the healing of periapical lesions, is considered the primary goal of revitalization [38], and this can be achieved reliably in 91–94% of cases [2, 43].

Further limitations arise from the risk of discolouration, which may be induced by the different irrigants and materials used during the procedure. Stringent material selection (e.g. nondiscolouring intracanal medicaments and HCSC without bismuth oxide as radioopacifier) can help, and colour changes may be prevented by sealing the dentine in the access cavity with a dentine-bonding agent [47, 48].

As revitalization is a fairly new treatment modality, long-term results are not available, and the clinical protocol is still in a state of flux. Additional information will lead to slight changes to the recommended procedure. This is made explicit in the ESE position statement: 'As . . . new evidence is still emerging, this position statement will be updated at appropriate intervals. This might lead to changes to the protocol provided here' [37].

3.4 Material Requirements

3.4.1 Materials and Applications

The treatment of nonvital immature teeth presents a range of challenges. The disadvantageous crown-to-root ratio, thin root canal walls, and wide-open apices make it technically difficult to place a root canal filling, as an apical stop against which filling materials can be condensed is absent. Therefore, the traditional apexification method (described in Section 3.2) aims to induce a mineralized tissue barrier at the root canal end through long-term application of CH. The mechanical barrier facilitates root canal obturation and compaction of root filling materials without extrusion of materials into the periapical tissues.

CH used as an intracanal dressing is a mixture of a powder and a vehicle. The white odourless powder exhibits basic properties (~pH 12.5) and dissociates into calcium and hydroxyl ions when in contact with aqueous fluids. Besides water-soluble substances (water, saline, etc.), viscous (glycerin, polyethylene glycol, etc.) and oil-based (silicone oil, olive oil, eugenol, etc.) solvents have been used as vehicles [49, 50]. The vehicle with which the CH powder is mixed determines the physical and chemical properties of the resulting paste. In general, the low viscosity of water-soluble substances provides high and rapid ion liberation, whereas more viscous vehicles prolong this action. Viscous CH preparations can remain in the root canal for several months with a stable pH and a slow-ion release, but their action may be compromised by negative side effects and limited antibacterial activity [49, 50]. Notably, the application of CH over a prolonged time span comes with mechanical weakening of the dentine and an increased risk of cervical root fractures in immature teeth [18, 51]. Furthermore, the required time for apical closure is unpredictable (6–24 months), and the risk of microleakage or bacterial contamination during the interappointment phase is high [49, 52]. CH formulations containing bismuth-based radiopacifers may thus lead to tooth discolouration and should therefore be avoided [53, 54].

For these reasons, the apical plug technique using MTA has proven the method of choice in recent years. Here, MTA is placed apically at open foramina of immature teeth to create an artificial barrier that allows for prompt root canal obturation. Treatment time appears to be shorter compared with CH apexification, improving patient compliance, and the mentioned disadvantages recede [25, 55]. An immediate adhesive seal of the root canal and access cavity may prevent potential fracture of immature teeth [56]. MTA is a type 1 HCSC and is composed of Portland cement with bismuth oxide as radiopacifier, which characteristically sets in a moist environment. Its main components, tricalcium silicate and dicalcium silicate, react with water and form calcium silicate hydrate and CH during the setting reaction [57]. However, original commercial formulations of MTA exhibit considerable drawbacks, including a long setting time (up to three hours), difficult handling, high cost, and risk of tooth discolouration [58].

To overcome these drawbacks, improved formulations of HCSCs have been introduced over the last few years. Natural raw materials such as Portland cement are avoided in order to prevent contamination with trace elements or unwanted substances [58, 59]. Instead, manufacturers rely on pure, laboratory-grade tricalcium silicate, which shows a similar hydration pattern to MTA and similarly forms CH [60]. Furthermore, the radiopaque bismuth oxide is substituted, because of the risk of tooth discolouration [58, 61]. Bismuth oxide interacts with collagen in the tooth structure [62] and blood [63], and also with sodium hypochlorite [64, 65] used as an irrigant, leading to the development of a dark brown/black precipitate that penetrates the tooth structure [62]. Zirconium oxide and tantalum oxide have been used as alternatives, but they exert a lower radiopacity. These radiopacifiers are inert during the setting reaction and do not leach out from the cements as described for bismuth oxide [58], and thus pose a lower risk of discolouration. Mixing liquids are supplemented with calcium chloride or calcium nitrite in order to accelerate setting, and addition of water-soluble polymers improve their handling [58].

HCSC formulations are clinically available in powder–liquid-set, preencapsulated, and other delivery systems. Recently, light-curable cement preparations have been developed to simplify application through a quicker and defined setting. However, light-curable products are generally resin-based, meaning cement hydration and therefore CH release are limited by polymerization [66, 67]. Furthermore, resin-based materials are disadvantageous in contact with vital tissue because of their resinous constituents, which may compromise cellular viability and biological activity [68, 69]. Other additives, such as calcium phosphates and microsilicia, have been used, but these can affect formation of CH and compromise biocompatibility [70]. The treatment outcome after the use of CH and MTA in immature teeth with pulp necrosis has been well documented. Although apical plug therapy provides several practical advantages over CH apexification, such as a lower risk of root fractures and a shorter treatment time, systematic reviews did not find any significant differences in terms of clinical success [55, 71].

A novel biology-based alternative for immature teeth with pulp necrosis is revitalization. Here, bleeding into the root canal is induced and a blood clot forms, which serves as a biological scaffold to guide the ingrowth of reparative tissue. This regenerative endodontic approach can facilitate healing of periapical lesions and enable further development of the fragile tooth roots, providing biological and mechanical advantages [51, 72]. In this specific application, HCSCs are suitable for covering the intracanal blood clot before the access cavity is sealed with an adhesive composite restoration. In contrast to apical plug therapy, bioactive cements do not come in contact with vascularized and structured connective tissue, but instead with a loose fibrin-based coagulum and blood cells. This may require different qualities of bioactive materials, both biologically and mechanically.

3.4.2 Biological Requirements

3.4.2.1 Bioactivity

Bioactivity describes the controlled interaction of materials with a tissue in order to initiate desired biological reactions, such as biomineralization, hydroxyapatite formation, antibacterial effects, or an immune response [73]. Thus, the goal of CH apexification is a stimulation of the vital periapical tissue in order to form a mineralized barrier. When CH contacts connective tissue, its high pH causes a superficial coagulation necrosis. Starting from a localized and mild inflammatory reaction, periapical cells begin to form osteocementum or bone-like tissue [49]. Interestingly, MTA and other HCSCs form CH by hydrolysis of tri- and dicalcium silicate [58, 74]. Thus, the bioactivity of HCSCs can partly be tracked back to similar mechanisms to that of CH and lasts as long as their setting reaction is in progress. However, the abrupt ending of a setting reaction by light-curable formulation is likely to compromise the bioactivity of the material [66, 68].

3.4.2.2 Reaction with Tissue Fluids

Another aspect of bioactivity is founded in the precipitation of carbonated apatite on the material surface when it comes in contact with body fluids or tissues. *In vitro*, similar observations have been made upon immersing materials in a serum-like solution, the so-called simulated body fluid (SBF). Within the setting reaction of the cements, hydrolysis and ion exchange lead to the formation of CH, which creates an alkaline environment [58, 75]. At this basic pH, an amorphous calcium silicate hydrate gel layer develops on the surfaces of calcium silicate particles and binds calcium ions from surrounding fluids [76]. However, the bound Ca^{2+} from the set cements can be released again at a later stage and reacts with HPO_4^{2-} from phosphate-containing liquids. The resulting amorphous calcium phosphates, which are in solution at first, densify near the cement surface and finally deposit on the calcium silicate hydrate layer. Over time, the nucleated calcium phosphate undergoes maturation into carbonated apatite [76]. Since carbonated apatite represents the biological elements found in bone, cementum, and dentine, it plays a triggering role in cytocompatibility and the bioactive potential of HCSCs [75, 77]. *In vitro*, SBF corresponds to human blood or plasma, which is generally saturated with calcium and phosphate ions [76]. Following the implantation of a foreign material into the body, the material's surface is immediately coated with proteins derived from blood and interstitial fluids. In contrast to a bioinert material, which is encapsulated by fibrous tissue, bioactive materials create an interface that interacts with the host tissue biologically and mechanically [76–78]. Although the *in vitro* bioactivity of HCSCs has been demonstrated, data on the bioactive potential of HCSCs *in vivo* are sparse; however, recent studies indicate that the clinical situation is different between the two scenarios [76, 79, 80].

3.4.2.3 Release of Dentine Matrix Proteins

Another mechanism by which biological responses can be elicited is the release of bioactive molecules from the dentine matrix. HCSCs create an intimate interface with dentine and can solubilize signalling molecules from it by local demineralization [81, 82]. Dentine is a rich source of cytokines, bioactive proteins, and growth factors that have been fossilized during dentinogenesis [83, 84]. Once released, these can exert their biological effects on various cell types and promote, for example, differentiation of pulp cells into an odontoblast-like phenotype [85–87]. Like MTA, soluble components of setting and set HCSCs have a basic pH and are able to release calcium ions, which lead in turn to the release of dentine matrix components (DMCs) [88, 89]. These are likely to have an impact on reparative and regenerative processes during the treatment of immature teeth.

3.4.2.4 Blood Clot

HCSCs can be applied in various treatment strategies and environments. Not only can they be placed as an apical plug at the root tip, in direct contact with bone or connective tissue, but they can also be used to cover a blood clot at the CEJ during revitalization therapy. Thus, local conditions, as well as neighbouring tissues, may alter the material setting and formation of carbonated apatite. There is a paucity of literature, however, on the behaviour of HCSCs

in contact with blood or autoresorbable collagen plugs, which are usually placed on a clot to create an abutment for cement application. In this context, the status of Portland cement in teeth that had been extracted for orthodontic purposes after revitalization therapy was assessed chemically and micromechanically, showing a porous cement surface that was primarily enriched in calcium carbonate instead of CH or apatite [80]. Interestingly, very little attention has been paid to calcium carbonate products, and their role in bioactivity is yet to be determined [90]. Moreover, blood contamination can affect the antimicrobial properties of HCSCs, which may be clinically relevant [91].

Further studies are required to elucidate the behaviour of these materials in the context of revitalization, but it appears both desirable and necessary to develop materials with optimal properties for this specific purpose.

3.4.3 Mechanical Requirements

3.4.3.1 Impact on Microhardness

Although the setting reaction of calcium silicate cements is hydraulic and requires a wet environment, unwanted liquid contamination at the place of application can affect the mechanical characteristics of the restorative material. Indeed, failure of the setting reaction and reduction of microhardness have been described in the presence of serum or tissue fluids – the very environment that the material used as an apical plug is in contact with [92, 93]. Likewise, blood components that are unavoidable in revitalization therapy can compromise mechanical properties of HCSCs [58]. Contamination of MTA with blood has been shown to deteriorate compressive strength and microhardness [94, 95].

Besides mechanical properties, adhesion of HCSCs to dentine is also important. For both the apical plug and revitalization, a sufficient bond to the dentinal surface is crucial in order to stabilize immature teeth and prevent leakage and contamination [72, 96]. HCSCs interact with dentine through mineral exchange at the tooth–material interface and the formation of mineral tags along the dental tubules [97]. The interfacial gap is filled by calcium phosphate deposition [98]. Furthermore, alkaline hydration products denature collagenous proteins at the dentine interface, as well as in tubular dentine. The exact mechanism by which the mineral interaction occurs requires further investigation, since certain laboratory-related conditions may affect the conditions at the interface [98, 99].

In this context, newer HCSCs have demonstrated stronger bonds to dentine than conventional MTA [100, 101]. A better uniformity and a smaller size of the particles enable deeper material penetration, which generally results in cohesive failures – whereas adhesive modes prevail with MTA [100]. Interestingly, the irrigation solution applied before application of HCSCs can compromise the bond to dentine. Notably, when using MTA, chlorhexidine and EDTA were reported to affect the micromechanical adhesion; however, saline and sodium hypochlorite (NaOCl) allowed for a sufficient bond strength [100, 102, 103]. Similarly, intracanal dressing with CH increased bond strength, whilst antibiotic medicaments reduced it significantly [101]. Ultrasonic agitation during placement of HCSCs achieved better marginal adaption, which led to stronger adhesion [104].

Long-term contact of CH pastes with dentine alters the facture resistance of the tooth. Similarly, prolonged contact of HCSCs with mineralized dentine has adverse effects by affecting the collagenous matrix [105], resulting in reduced flexural strength [106].

Handling requirements (including fluidity and setting time) and environmental issues (such as wetness, existing fluids, and dentinal anatomy) are important factors affecting the specific clinical application of HCSCs. Therefore, the development of new and customized cements will be helpful in overcoming the current drawbacks and improving clinical outcomes. In addition to a demand-driven material design, treatment parameters such as irrigation, intracanal dressing, and application modality need to be considered and adapted. Thus, the use of CH as a medicament and a final irrigation with saline or NaOCl seem to be beneficial for an optimal dentine adhesion.

3.4.3.2 Discolouration

From a clinical perspective, discolouration of the tooth crown constitutes a major drawback that highly compromises the aesthetic result – and thus the outcome – of a procedure from the patient's perspective. Therefore, a decisive requirement of materials used for apical plug therapy and revitalization treatment is that they avoid staining the dentine and instead preserve the natural tooth shade. The discolouration potential of HCSCs varies widely. In this context, a multitude of factors have an impact, including material constituents, contamination with blood, and mixture with irrigants, as well as local environmental factors. As already stated, bismuth oxide serves as a radiopaque additive in the original MTA formulation. It can cause tooth discolouration on reaction with collagenous dentine components, irrespective of its concentration [62, 81]. Despite other factors, newer formulations of HCSC avoid bismuth oxide and thus successfully obviate dentine staining [58, 81]. Furthermore, contamination of MTA with blood leads to inclusion of blood components in the porous structure and darkening of the tooth. However, newly developed materials reportedly have fewer pores and thus a reduced risk of discolouration when they come in contact with blood [107]. Likewise, residues of NaOCl in dentine tubules can effect colour changes, although the exact chemical nature of these changes is still unclear [61, 64, 81]. Generally, light and oxygen affect bismuth compounds and lead to the formation of a dark-brown precipitate that can discolour the tooth [108, 109]. Interestingly, formulations without bismuth oxide have also been reported to discolour dentine when irrigated with NaOCl or CHX, but to a much lesser extent [61, 81].

These bioactive cements are placed primarily as plug materials within the root canal, but they can reach the aesthetic zone – especially in revitalization procedures, where the plug may reside at the level of the CEJ. In order to counteract discolouration, bismuth oxide should be avoided in material formulations, irrigant residues should be carefully removed before cement application, and blood contamination should be obviated. Further, the coronal dentine surface may be sealed with bonding agents [47, 48], and cements covered with opaque resin-based composite materials.

3.5 Healing Process and Cellular Responses

3.5.1 Biological Aspects

'Primary dentinogenesis' is the term used to describe the process of developmental dentine formation. The odontoblasts at the periphery of the pulp reportedly deposit the dentine at a relatively rapid rate of ~4 μm/day until tooth root formation is complete. The odontoblasts remain intimately associated with the dentine via their processes, which reside in tubules for the lifetime of the tooth. The pulp remains vital following tooth eruption and functions to support the tooth throughout its life. At the pulp core are fibroblasts, which are the most abundant cell type; these secrete the relatively soft spongy tissue matrix. Also within the pulp are complex and intricate structures of nerves and blood vessels that enter the tooth via the roots. These are more finely branched in the peripheral areas, where they intimately interact with the tissues and cells to provide the tooth with sensitivity and the nutrient supply to ensure its vitality. There are also several stem cell populations, which reportedly reside within the pulp and not only contribute to any repair and regenerative processes within it but also are capable of differentiating into other tissue cell types [110, 111].

The odontoblasts at the periphery of the tissue continue to lay down secondary dentine throughout the life of the tooth. This process reportedly occurs at a much slower rate of ~0.4 μm/day. Importantly, cells within the viable pulpal tissue have been shown to be able to detect and respond to infecting bacteria, pain stimuli, and temperature changes. Indeed, many of these irritations can lead to the stimulation of the formation of tertiary dentinogenesis, which represents the tooth's natural wound-healing response [112, 113]. Two forms are described (see Figure 3.3). Following relatively mild dental injury, such as in the early stages of dental caries, the original odontoblasts reactivate and secrete a reactionary dentine at an increased rate of deposition. This newly formed dentine exhibits tubular continuity with the original primary and secondary dentines. If the dental injury is of a greater extent and intensity – such as due to a rapidly progressing and deep carious lesion – then the original odontoblasts will die beneath the site of injury. However, if the disease and tissue damage can be arrested, potentially following clinical intervention, then stem/progenitor cells from within the pulp may be recruited to the site of the tissue damage, where they are signalled to differentiate into new odontoblast-like cells. These cells also deposit a tertiary reparative dentine matrix at a relatively rapid rate, seen clinically as a dentine or mineralized bridge which partially repairs the tooth's hard tissue and aims to 'wall off' any further invading bacteria. Quite clearly, these two tertiary dentinogenic processes exhibit different degrees of complexity (Figure 3.3). Reactionary dentinogenesis more simply requires only the upregulation of the activity of the surviving odontoblasts, whilst the reparative dentinogenic response comprises complex interactions between several cellular processes, including recruitment, differentiation, and activation of dentine synthetic and secretory activity [114, 115]. Notably, the reported upregulated rate of tertiary dentine deposition is ~4 μm/day – similar to that

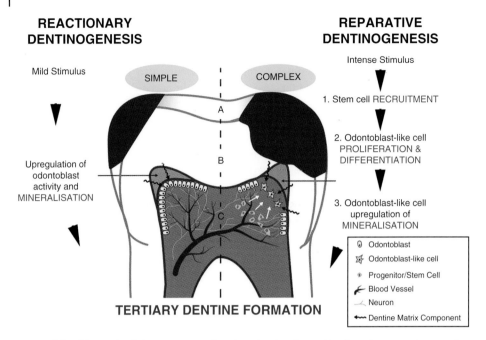

Figure 3.3 Schematic of the processes of tertiary dentine formation. Reactionary and reparative dentinogenesis processes differ in the source of the secreting cell. Reactionary dentinogenesis is a comparatively simple process undertaken by the existing primary odontoblasts when a relatively mild stimulation causes their upregulation of synthetic and secretory activity. Reparative dentine formation involves a more complex sequence of events in which a severe stimulus results in the death of the primary odontoblasts, which are subsequently replaced following differentiation of progenitor or stem cells into odontoblast-like cells under the influence of bioactive molecules (including dentine matrix components). (A) Enamel. (B) Dentine. (C) Pulp.

described for the primary dentinogenesis process [116].

Decades of study have demonstrated many aspects of similarity between primary and tertiary dentinogenesis. Both processes are signalled and driven by a similar array of bioactive molecules, many of which become sequestrated and bound within the dentine during its formation [84, 116, 117]. Notably, these bioactive molecules can be released from their inactive form by a variety of treatments to the dentine, including by carious bacterial acids and certain restorative materials such as CH and HCSCs [88, 89, 118]. When released, they stimulate the formation of a dentine or mineralized bridge beneath the lesion or restored area via a reparative dentinogenic mechanism.

Studies show not only that stem cells from the pulpal niche can be stimulated by these bioactive molecules but also that gradients of

many of these molecules result in their 'trafficking' to repair sites, as well as stimulating increases in their numbers to enable repopulation of the wounded area. Furthermore, it is clear that many of these bioactive molecules can stimulate the differentiation of the 'homed' stem cells into odontoblast-like cells and promote the upregulation of their dentine synthetic and secretory activity [1]. Notably, recent studies have also indicated that when degraded due to the relatively aggressive environment generated in the wound area, these bioactive molecules – including members of several growth factor families – are more potent in terms of signalling compared to their intact counterparts [119].

Neuropeptides and neurotrophic factors are expressed by odontoblasts, potentially due to their close association with the tooth's neuronal network (plexus of Raschkow) and to odontoblasts originating from cranial neural crest cells [120–122]. Indeed, several neuropeptides have been shown to play a role in pulpal disease pathogenesis. Studies have examined the presence and functionality of a range of these molecules within the dentine–pulp complex, including calcitonin (CT), calcitonin gene-related peptide (CGRP), neuropeptide Y (NPY), substance P (SP), and vasoactive intestinal polypeptide (VIP) [123]. Interestingly, some have been shown to be capable of stimulating regenerative dentinogenic processes. SP, CGRP, VIP, and NPY may represent novel regulators of pulpal angiogenesis, whilst CGRP and CT have been shown to stimulate osteodentine deposition [124, 125]. Furthermore, targeted studies on the neurotrophins of nerve growth factor (NGF) and brain-derived neurotrophic factor (BDNF) have demonstrated their expression in dental pulp cells and odontoblasts during tooth development [122]. NGF has been implicated in dentinogenesis and dental repair, and studies suggest that it may directly promote odontoblast differentiation [126–128]. Glial cell line-derived growth factor (GDNF) is a member of the transforming growth factor-β (TGF-β) superfamily and has been shown to be expressed in pulp cells and pre-odontoblasts [122, 129]. It is also implicated in dental tissue cytodifferentiation and can promote survival and proliferation of cultured dental pulp cells [130].

The molecular response within the pulp during infectious disease progression is complex. However, the processes involved are similar to those occurring at other sites within the body, and host cells and tissues recognize the infecting agents with a response aimed at elimination. Indeed, odontoblasts and core pulpal cells (fibroblasts, neurological, endothelial, and stem cells, and resident immune cells) express a range of receptors capable of detecting microbiological components, including molecules derived from bacterial cell walls such as lipopolysaccharides (LPSs) and lipoteichoic acid (LTA), as well as internal molecules such as bacterial DNA. The best

characterized family of pattern-recognition receptors is the Toll-like receptor family, of which there are nine human members (TLRs 1–9). Once the microbial ligand binds to the receptor, downstream signalling results in activation of key transcriptional regulatory pathways, such as those involving NF-κβ and MAP kinases [131]. These pathways lead to the release of a range of antimicrobial peptides (AMPs) and inflammation-regulating cytokines. Several groups have shown that diseased pulps express increased levels of cytokines, which regulate immune cell recruitment, extravasation, cell activation, differentiation, and antibody production. Within the pulp, there are now well characterized roles for many cytokines, including interleukins IL-1α, IL1-β, IL-4, IL-6, IL-8, and IL-10 and tissue necrosis factor alpha (TNF-α), which are known to orchestrate many aspects of the immune response according to their respective levels and profiles. It is only after the infection is removed (e.g. via clinical procedures) that levels of these cytokines return to those present during homeostasis. If levels remain high due to the presence of infection or a dysregulated host response then chronic inflammation will persist within the tooth, limiting the ability and activation of innate tissue-repair mechanisms [132, 133].

Pulpal inflammation is a double-edged sword, as whilst the inflammatory response is aimed at eliminating the invading bacteria via activation of immune cell function and associated antimicrobial activity, collateral host tissue damage also occurs. Notably, the inflammatory cells must degrade the tissue in order to traverse it, and many antimicrobial processes likewise subject host cells and tissue to significant stress. In particular, neutrophils, which provide a first line of defence against infection, are well known for releasing tissue-degradative enzymes such as matrix metalloproteinases (MMPs), as well as for generating molecular-damaging reactive oxygen species (ROS), which aim at extracellular antimicrobial killing. Notably, whilst ROS release can cause significant collateral tissue damage, it is also capable of stimulating further cellular cytokine release via activation of proinflammatory signalling mechanisms, such as those involving the aforementioned p38-MAPK and NF-κβ pathways [134, 135]. Recently, we have shown that the bacterial killing and containment mechanism known as neutrophil extracellular traps, which involves ROS-triggered release of cellular DNA adorned with AMPs, may also inadvertently cause cellular insult. This process may exacerbate the pulp's inflammatory response and instigate pulpal cell death, dependent upon local tissue levels of these toxic molecules [136, 137].

In recent decades, it has become more apparent that chronic inflammation impedes reparative and regenerative events within host tissues. Indeed, the accepted paradigm is that pulp healing can only occur after removal of the infecting bacteria and significant modulation of the inflammatory process [138–140]. Both animal studies and *in vitro* studies replicating pulpal inflammation demonstrate this association, as well as highlighting the biphasic effects of many proinflammatory mediators [141]. It is notable that at relatively low levels, cytokines such as TNF-α and TGF-β, as well as ROS and bacterial components such as LPS, can stimulate dental cell-mediated repair events. However, when these same molecules are present at relatively high levels, such as in chronic and infectious inflammation, they exert deleterious effects in the pulp, including induction of cell and tissue death. In addition, stem-cell differentiation events are directly regulated by several proinflammatory mediators [131].

Without the appropriate clinical intervention, the tooth may be lost due to rampant infection and chronic inflammation. Unchecked continuation of these processes will likely result in pulp necrosis, requiring urgent remedial dental treatment possibly involving RCT to preserve the tooth's functionality. Notably, such treatments are destructive and expensive and weaken the remaining tooth structure, likely limiting the life of the tooth [142]. Whilst RCT is a relatively common procedure, it is not always effective in the long term; 10–50% of cases will fail, with the likelihood of failure being higher in general dental practice [143]. This is reportedly due to compromise of the efficacy of chemomechanical debridement and to certain patients exhibiting an undesirable innate response to the treatment [144].

3.5.2 Mineralization

Treatment strategies for the regeneration of the dentine–pulp complex in necrotic immature teeth require the combination of a scaffold, morphogens, and a stem or progenitor cell population. This stem cell population may either be 'homed' into the necrotic root canal system directly from the periapical tissues and circulating blood supply or placed in the empty root canal space as part of a cell-based tissue engineering strategy to replace the cells of the dentine and pulp. The clinical translation of these biological strategies to replace vital tissue in the root canal system has recently attracted attention in the form of 'regenerative endodontic' procedures [8]. Despite this name, human studies have demonstrated a range of mineralized tissue deposits present in the root canal space after pulp revitalization procedures, including 'cementum-like' and 'bone-like' ones, as well as 'dentine-like' [34, 145, 146]. Notably, regeneration of biological tissue is possible if the periapical tissues, which contain Hertwig's epithelial root sheath and the apical papilla, remain in a healthy state prior to a tissue engineering approach being used [34, 145, 146]. However, if the root canal contains necrotic material and there is no pulp tissue remaining apically, a bone-like fibrous tissue rather than new pulp tissue tends to fill the space [34].

Although other cells such as fibroblasts are capable of producing mineral [147], stem cells are the most likely to be responsible for its secretion after cytodifferentiation into odontoblast-like cells in reparative dentinogenesis, or into other cell types capable of producing bone

Figure 3.4 Schematic representation showing the localization of stem cells relevant to revitalization and dental tissue regeneration.

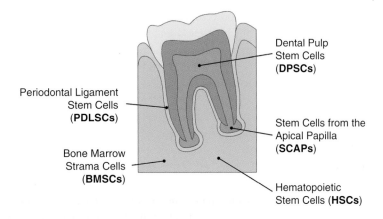

Dental Pulp Stem Cells (**DPSCs**)

Periodontal Ligament Stem Cells (**PDLSCs**)

Stem Cells from the Apical Papilla (**SCAPs**)

Bone Marrow Strama Cells (**BMSCs**)

Hematopoietic Stem Cells (**HSCs**)

or cementum within the root canal space. Stem cells are an essential component of regenerative mineralization procedures as they are self-renewable and possess the ability to differentiate into multiple tissue lineages [148, 149]. Various stem cell populations in dental and central niches (see Figure 3.4) are potentially important in contributing to revitalization procedures and dental tissue engineering, including dental pulp stem cells (DPSCs), stem cells for the apical papilla (SCAPs), human periodontal ligament stem cells (PDLSCs), and centrally-residing stem cell populations such as human bone marrow stromal stem cells (BMSSCs) and haematopoietic stem cells (HSCs) [150]. These migrating stem cells can be modulated and differentiated into a range of tissues, including blood vessels, nerves, and mineral-secreting cells under the influence of growth factors released from dentine [151] and other cells [152], or else in 'doped' scaffold materials [153].

DPSCs are located in the central region of the pulp space [154] and have the ability to migrate, proliferate, and differentiate into odontoblast-like cells following primary odontoblast death in reparative tertiary dentinogenesis [155]. Although they do not represent a significant stem cell population after pulp necrosis, they can survive inflammatory challenge and differentiate down osteogenic/dentinogenic lineages in irreversible pulpitis and early necrosis when at least some vital tissue persists apically [156].

Furthermore, growth factors such as stromal cell-derived factor-1 and basic fibroblast growth factor enhance DPSC migration *in vitro*, whilst another growth factor, bone morphogenetic protein 7 (BMP-7), induces osteogenic differentiation. This highlights the varying and complimentary roles of individual growth factors in dental regenerative processes.

SCAPs are another likely cell source for primary root formation [157], alongside DPSCs. After pulp necrosis, the recruitment of SCAPs or DPSCs migrating from the blood system becomes more important – but potentially more complex – than recruitment of DPSCs due to a loss of pulpal blood supply [158]. During apical periodontitis, SCAPs retain vitality and stemness, and can undergo osteogenic and angiogenic differentiation under the influence of growth factors [159]. Chemotactic growth factors, including stromal cell-derived factor-1, TGF-β1, platelet-derived growth factor (PDGF), and basic fibroblast growth factor, stimulate migration of SCAPs, whilst TGF-β1 significantly enhances mineralization responses [151]. From a translational perspective, SCAPs transplanted into the root canal form a vascularized pulp-like tissue and new dentine-like tissue at the dentinal wall, at least in a biological model [160]. PDLSCs are less likely to contribute to dentine–pulp regeneration as they are located between the bone and cementum, participating in the formation of the cementum as well as in bone formation [160].

During revascularisation procedures, it is necessary to increase the thickness and length of the root dentine wall and to stimulate an apical closure with cementum, and recruiting PDLSCs may contribute to this.

Finally, as BMSCs are capable of differentiation down the mesoderm lineage to osteoblasts, adipocytes, and chondrocytes, they are potentially a good cell source for pulp revitalization. Indeed, stem cell factor (SCF) enhances cell migration, proliferation, and osteogenic differentiation of BMSCs *in vivo* in a dental cell-homing model [161]. Angiogenesis and neovascularization are critical to HSC survival and migration with vascular endothelial growth factor (VEGF), stimulating bone marrow-derived endothelial cells and the recruitment of perivascular cells including CXCR4-positive cells via upregulation of CXCL12 [162, 163]. Both *in vitro* and *in vivo* studies have demonstrated that human recombinant VEGF treatment strongly induces mobilization of endothelial precursor cells [164], highlighting the importance of dentally derived growth factors in attracting BMSCs to injury sites in the root canal.

Several studies have shown that a host of signalling molecules are contained within dentine and predentine and are important in the regulation of dental tissue regenerative processes. The extracellular matrix (ECM) component of dentine comprises collagenous and noncollagenous proteins (NCPs) and is known to contain a significant number of well-characterized bioactive regulatory molecules. Several of these molecules are phosphorylated proteins, such as dentine sialoprotein (DSP), dentine phosphoprotein (DPP), bone sialoprotein, dentine matrix acidic phosphoprotein 1, osteopontin, and matrix extracellular phosphoglycoprotein. Members of this family are termed small integrin-binding ligand N-linked glycoproteins (SIBLINGs), and their triplet Arg-Gly-Asp domains function in signalling and act as nucleating factors for subsequent mineralization processes [165–168]. Several of these molecules, such as DSP and DPP, are regarded as being particularly characteristic of dentine [169, 170].

3.6 Future Directions: Tissue Engineering Approaches

3.6.1 Principles of Tissue Engineering

Tissue engineering concepts involve the combination of competent (stem) cells with a scaffold material as a structural matrix to support three-dimensional tissue formation, along with bioactive molecules to promote cell proliferation and differentiation. The goal is to improve or even restore the architecture and function of diseased tissues or organs. Whereas current clinical procedures induce repair, tissue engineering concepts may provide more control over cellular behaviour and allow for true regeneration of the dentine–pulp complex. The presence of stem cells in the dental pulp of permanent [111] and deciduous teeth [171], the periodontal ligament [172], the dental follicle [173], and the apical papilla [157], but also in the periapical tissues [159, 174], has been demonstrated. Thus, several sources of stem cells are available for potential regenerative therapies in the oral cavity. For the regeneration of the dentine–pulp complex, mesenchymal stem cells from pulp, apical papilla. and periapical tissues appear particularly interesting.

For tissue engineering approaches, the choice of an appropriate scaffold is a crucial step. Highly sophisticated techniques have been developed to generate biomimetic and tailor-made materials for specific applications. Scaffolds have transitioned from inert, passive cell carriers and mere delivery vehicles to inductive and instructive matrices that can be controlled in different aspects of material behaviour and elicit a desired cellular behaviour by means of stiffness, degradation rate and pattern, bioactive motifs, or controlled release of growth and differentiation signals. Materials such as collagen [175, 176], PLGA [177], chitosan [176, 178], polyethylene glycol [179], and self-assembling peptides [180] have been utilized for tissue engineering of dental pulp. More recently, composite materials have been explored in an attempt to benefit from the advantages of different types of materials, including combinations of polycaprolactone with bioactive glass [181], bioprinting of alginate/gelatin hydrogels [182], and chitosan-enriched fibrin hydrogels [183]. Furthermore, dental pulp or dentine matrix has come to be of interest as a scaffold material itself [184–186].

Eventually, bioactive molecules and motifs will be especially important in cellular signalling for chemotaxis, adhesion, proliferation, differentiation, and mineralization. Particularly relevant growth factor families for dental pulp development and regeneration include the TGF-βs [187–189] and the BMPs [190–192]. Molecules such as dentine matrix protein-1 [193], dexamethasone [194], and β-glycerophosphate [195] may stimulate the differentiation and mineralization of dental pulp cells. In the light of bacterial infection and inflammation of the dental pulp, antibacterial molecules and factors that modulate the inflammatory response may be particularly interesting for dentine–pulp tissue engineering. Whilst the addition of exogenous signalling molecules is one way of driving cell proliferation, differentiation, and tissue formation, questions and problems regarding the optimum concentrations and the possibility of undesirable side effects (including tumourigenesis) remain. An alternative is the recruitment of endogenous growth factors, which are present in the dentine matrix itself.

3.6.2 Dentine Matrix Proteins and Epigenetic Influences

3.6.2.1 Dentine Matrix Components
Dentine is a reservoir for a broad range of bioactive 'fossilized' DMCs, which are stored in the matrix during development. Several bioactive groups are present, including growth factors, chemokines, cytokines, and tissue proteases [196–199], and their release following carious processes or dental trauma is key to promoting regenerative processes [197, 200, 201]. Irrigant solutions, medicaments, biomaterials, and pharmacological inhibitors, including EDTA [202, 203], MTA [88], CH [118], histone deacetylase inhibitors [204], and dental adhesives [205], have been shown to facilitate the release of DMCs. Furthermore, the functionality of sequestered bioactive molecules in inducing both reactionary [202] and reparative dentinogenesis [206], including hard tissue bridge formation [190], has been highlighted.

Irrigant solutions, used as part of a chemo-mechanical disinfection protocol, have the potential to release a range of DMCs, including growth factors beneficial to cell migration, proliferation, and differentiation [203]. Indeed, irrigating with a 17% EDTA solution can release TGF-β family members from the dentine extracellular matrix (dECM) [118]. Sodium hypochlorite, on the other hand, may have a deleterious effect on stem cell survival and differentiation, leading to suggestions that the final rinse in cell-homing procedures should always be with 17% EDTA [207]. In VPT, the capping materials MTA [88] and CH [118] interact directly with dental pulp cells as well as the dentine matrix, highlighting a synergistic response to the promotion of pulpal repair processes after exposure [206].

3.6.2.2 Growth Factors and Molecular Modulators
The dECM contains a wealth of bioactive molecules which, when made bioavailable, have the ability to drive many aspects required for dental tissue regeneration. Studies over several decades have demonstrated their therapeutic potential, as well as possible routes for harnessing their regenerative abilities. The growth factor with arguably the best characterized action that is found in relative abundance in the dECM is TGF-β1. Studies in animal

models, as well as *ex vivo* tooth organ cultures using alginate hydrogel carrier systems, have demonstrated its ability to induce tertiary dentinogenic events on its own [116, 208]. Due to the complexity of the associated signalling that occurs within the pulp tissue as it attempts to defend itself from the infection and repair itself, more recent studies have aimed at obtaining a better understanding of the molecular response involved, including high-throughput gene-expression studies in diseased and healthy pulp tissue. Data indicate that during disease, tissue processes relating to inflammation are mainly invoked, with repair-associated molecular events only appearing to be instigated at a relatively low level [209]. Differential expression of several molecules previously not reported as being associated with dental disease has also been identified. In particular, the pleiotropic growth factor adrenomedullin (ADM) is identified, providing a candidate modulator of both inflammation and tooth tissue repair. Previously, this molecule was reported as having antibacterial and immunomodulatory activities, and as promoting angiogenesis and mineralized tissue repair processes [210, 211]. Interestingly, downstream characterization studies have indicated a role for ADM in dental tissue development. It is archived within the dECM, where it can be released later in the life of the tooth to play a role in both tissue defence and repair events [212]. The mining of high-throughput transcriptional data using well-characterized clinical samples can facilitate our understanding of the link between inflammation and regeneration and identify novel molecular targets for future clinical exploitation.

3.6.2.3 Epigenetic Influences

The number of studies in epigenetics relating to the dental pulp is rapidly expanding, providing an understanding of both the role of environmental factors such as inflammation and ageing on gene expression and the therapeutic benefit of epigenetic modulation during disease progression and tissue regeneration.

This knowledge provides opportunities for the identification of novel pulpal inflammatory diagnostic markers and the application of epigenetic-based therapies in regenerative endodontics [213]. In general, epigenetics encompasses the fields of noncoding RNAs (e.g. microRNAs (miRNAs) and long noncoding RNAs (lncRNAs)), as well as modifications of DNA-associated proteins by methylation and acetylation processes. These types of regulation have been demonstrated to control not only stem cell self-renewal but also regulation of mineralized tissue repair and inflammatory processes in the dental pulp and throughout the body [214].

lncRNAs and shorter miRNAs regulate gene expression and subsequent translational events through their ability to bind to complementary nucleic acid sequences, including both DNA and RNA. Recent studies comparing their expression profiles in diseased and healthy teeth have highlighted their potential importance in pulp biology. Data indicate that 752 lncRNAs are significantly differentially expressed in inflamed pulp compared with healthy pulp tissue [215]. miRNA expression has also been demonstrated to be altered in pulipitis, with 36 miRNAs being significantly differentially expressed in diseased compared with healthy tissue [216]. Notably, many of the previously characterized noncoding RNAs that are differentially expressed in the pulp have been associated with immune and stress responses.

The process of DNA methylation involves the transfer of a methyl group to a cytosine base in DNA, resulting in a 5-methylcytosine. In humans, this process is regulated by four DNA methyltransferase (DNMT) enzymes [217]. DNA acetylation, however, is balanced by histone acetyltransferases, which add a negatively charged acetyl group and weaken the interaction between DNA and histone residues. Histone deacetylases (HDACs) remove this acetyl group. Both processes regulate DNA accessibility and subsequently modulate gene-expression profiles in cells and tissues. Potential therapeutic applications of epigenetic-modifying agents are targeted at DNA methylation, DNA methyltransferase inhibitors (DNMTis), and histone acetylation. Indeed, histone deacetylase inhibitors (HDACis), at specific concentrations, have been shown to promote mineralization and repair processes in dental pulp cell cultures and to be able to release bioactive dentine matrix-derived components [204]. Both HDACis and DNMTis have the potential to enhance tertiary dentinogenesis by influencing the cellular and tissue processes at relatively low doses with minimal side effects. This approach potentially provides an opportunity to develop topical, inexpensive, bio-inductive restorative materials [204, 213].

So far, there has been only one study reporting the reparative mineralization inductive effects of the DNMTi 5-aza-2′-deoxycytidine in dental pulp cells [218]. The data show that this compound promoted induction of an odontoblast-like mineralizing cell phenotype. Notably, clinical studies have gone on to link changes in DNA methylation patterns with dental pulp inflammation, and *in vitro* work using pulp cell cultures has shown a potential role of DNA methylation enzymes in bacterial-induced inflammation. These data further highlight the increasing importance of epigenetic processes in dental pulp inflammation [219, 220].

There are significantly more studies on the role and application of HDACis in the field of dental pulp regeneration. Indeed, in *in vitro* studies, several HDACis have been applied to dental pulp cell cultures, and the data show that these compounds can promote migration of progenitor cells and stimulate their differentiation into an odontoblast-like mineralizing cell phenotype [221–223]. Whilst this suggests the promise of this epigenetic approach for application in regenerative endodontics, there is currently only one *in vivo* study examining the effect of HDACis on dental pulp. Results from this work indicate that HDACis

stimulated an increase in dentine deposition and increased the number of associated odontoblasts compared with controls [222].

3.6.3 Cell-Based and Cell-Free Dental Pulp Tissue Engineering

It is now broadly accepted that dental pulp tissue engineering is possible following transplantation of stem cells into the root canal [36, 177, 224–226]. Further, the feasibility of transplanting stem cells into empty root canals after pulpectomy or in the case of pulp necrosis has recently been demonstrated in clinical studies [227, 228]. It appears that the choice of scaffold material is of secondary importance in the development of a clinical procedure for stem cell transplantation for pulp regeneration, as the stem cells' inherent competence to form pulp tissue can be utilized. However, cell-based tissue engineering of dental pulp is afflicted with several problems, including its high cost and the requirement for facilities for cell storage and expansion following good manufacturing practice (GMP) guidelines. Regarding the clinical situation, the benefit currently does not outweigh the cost and effort, and therefore an alternative cell-free approach using cell homing for pulp regeneration has been proposed. In this scenario, a scaffold material in combination with growth factors is used to recruit local tissue-resident stem cells and attract them to populate the scaffold, proliferate, differentiate, and generate a three-dimensional tissue [229]. Notably, stem cells may be recruited either from remnant vital pulp tissue after pulpotomy or, if the pulp tissue is lost, from the periapical region [159, 174]. After migration into the scaffold via chemotaxis, the cells will degrade the material and replace it with cognate ECM. The scaffold plays a key role in this procedure and should be tailored towards this specific application. Indeed, promising scaffold materials with excellent cytocompatibility that can be inserted or injected into the root canal have already been generated [183, 184, 186, 230–232].

3.6.4 Clinical Approaches and Future Perspectives

In addition to the provocation of a blood clot by mechanical disruption of the apical tissues during revitalization procedures, blood-derived preparations have also been used. Following centrifugation of whole blood, usually extracted from veins in the arm, platelet-rich plasma (PRP) or, more recently, platelet-rich fibrin (PRF) has been isolated and subsequently inserted into the root canal. Whilst both PRP and PRF are fibrin-based preparations and contain PDGFs, it is reported that PRP releases these factors more rapidly. Indeed, PRF, which does not require anticoagulation, incorporates greater amounts of growth factors and demonstrates slower release kinetics [233]. Currently, the clinical outcomes following the use of PRP or PRF in comparison to the relatively simple blood clot-induction approach are somewhat controversial. A clinical case series reported an increase of root thickness with PRP [39], whilst animal experiments showed ectopic tissue formation in the root canal and no further root thickening [234, 235]. A systematic review of platelet concentrates for revitalization procedures stated that data are scarce but concluded that these preparations show promising results [236].

Tissue engineering approaches have also been tested in clinical studies. Transplantation of autologous stem cells from deciduous teeth [228] into immature incisors with pulp necrosis following dental trauma showed a completion of root formation in radiographs and cone-beam computed tomography (CBCT) [228]. Similarly, autologous pulp stem cells were transplanted into mature teeth of adult patients with irreversible pulpitis, where the development of functional tissue was demonstrated by mineral apposition detected by CBCT [227].

Recently, the concept of revitalization has been applied to teeth with complete root formation. Case reports [237], case series [238], and randomized clinical studies demonstrate favourable clinical and radiographical outcomes, including in comparison with RCT [40]. Histologically, the newly formed tissue in mature roots presents as a combination of fibrous connective tissue and bone-like tissue [239]. It is clear that research on and clinical approaches to dental pulp repair and regeneration are converging. A broadening of the indication for regenerative endodontic procedures can be expected in the near future, which ultimately will benefit patients.

3.7 Conclusion

Whilst the management of pulp necrosis in immature teeth remains a challenge, MTA apexification and revitalization are well-established treatment modalities with concise recommendations regarding the procedural details. With the use of bioactive materials, biology-based and regenerative approaches are becoming more pronounced in endodontics. This development is supported by recent scientific findings, where an in-depth understanding of the underlying cellular and molecular mechanisms, along with the generation of novel scaffolds and the utilization of bioactive molecules, is laying the foundation for future tissue engineering strategies and thus optimized therapies for our patients.

References

1 Duncan, H.F., Kobayashi, Y., and Shimizu, E. (2018). Growth factors and cell homing in dental tissue regeneration. *Curr. Oral Health Rep.* 5 (4): 276–285.

2 Torabinejad, M., Nosrat, A., Verma, P., and Udochukwu, O. (2017). Regenerative endodontic treatment or mineral trioxide aggregate apical plug in teeth with necrotic pulps and open apices: a systematic review and meta-analysis. *J. Endod.* 43 (11): 1806–1820.

3 Moore, A., Howley, M.F., and O'Connell, A.C. (2011). Treatment of open apex teeth using two types of white mineral trioxide aggregate after initial dressing with calcium hydroxide in children. *Dent. Traumatol.* 27 (3): 166–173.

4 Felippe, W.T., Felippe, M.C.S., and Rocha, M.J.C. (2006). The effect of mineral trioxide aggregate on the apexification and periapical healing of teeth with incomplete root formation. *Int. Endod. J.* 39 (1): 2–9.

5 Baek, S.-H., Plenk, H., and Kim, S. (2005). Periapical tissue responses and cementum regeneration with amalgam, SuperEBA, and MTA as root-end filling materials. *J. Endod.* 31 (6): 444–449.

6 Nygaard-Østby, B. (1961). The role of the blood clot in endodontic therapy. An experimental histologic study. *Acta Odontol. Scand.* 19: 324–353.

7 Skoglund, A., Tronstad, L., and Wallenius, K. (1978). A microangiographic study of vascular changes in replanted and autotransplanted teeth of young dogs. *Oral Surg. Oral Med. Oral Pathol.* 45 (1): 17–28.

8 Murray, P.E., Garcia-Godoy, F., and Hargreaves, K.M. (2007). Regenerative endodontics: a review of current status and a call for action. *J. Endod.* 33 (4): 377–390.

9 Galler, K.M. (2016). Clinical procedures for revitalization: current knowledge and considerations. *Int. Endod. J.* 49 (10): 926–936.

10 Diogenes, A.R., Ruparel, N.B., Shiloah, Y., and Hargreaves, K.M. (2016). Regenerative endodontics: a way forward. *J. Am. Dent. Assoc.* 147 (5): 372–380.

11 Nazzal, H., Kenny, K., Altimimi, A. et al. (2018). A prospective clinical study of regenerative endodontic treatment of traumatized immature teeth with necrotic pulps using bi-antibiotic paste. *Int. Endod. J.* 51 (Suppl. 3): e204–e215.

12 Kahler, B., Rossi-Fedele, G., Chugal, N., and Lin, L.M. (2017). An evidence-based review of the efficacy of treatment approaches for immature permanent teeth with pulp necrosis. *J. Endod.* 43 (7): 1052–1057.

13 Lin, J., Zeng, Q., Wei, X. et al. (2017). Regenerative endodontics versus apexification in immature permanent teeth with apical periodontitis: a prospective randomized controlled study. *J. Endod.* 43 (11): 1821–1827.

14 Nagy, M.M., Tawfik, H.E., Hashem, A.A.R., and Abu-Seida, A.M. (2014). Regenerative potential of immature permanent teeth with necrotic pulps after different regenerative protocols. *J. Endod.* 40 (2): 192–198.

15 Banchs, F. and Trope, M. (2004). Revascularization of immature permanent teeth with apical periodontitis: new treatment protocol? *J. Endod.* 30 (4): 196–200.

16 Reeves, R. and Stanley, H.R. (1966). The relationship of bacterial penetration and pulpal pathosis in carious teeth. *Oral Surg. Oral Med. Oral Pathol.* 22 (1): 59–65.

17 Luder, H.U. (2015). Malformations of the tooth root in humans. *Front. Physiol.* 6: 307.

18 Andreasen, J.O., Farik, B., and Munksgaard, E.C. (2002). Long-term calcium hydroxide as a root canal dressing may increase risk of root fracture. *Dent. Traumatol.* 18 (3): 134–137.

19 Caplan, D.J., Cai, J., Yin, G., and White, B.A. (2005). Root canal filled versus non-root canal filled teeth: a retrospective comparison of survival times. *J. Public Health Dent.* 65 (2): 90–96.

20 Dominguez Reyes, A., Muñoz Muñoz, L., and Aznar Martín, T. (2005). Study of calcium hydroxide apexification in 26 young permanent incisors. *Dent. Traumatol.* 21 (3): 141–145.

21 Finucane, D. and Kinirons, M.J. (1999). Non-vital immature permanent incisors: factors that may influence treatment outcome. *Endod. Dent. Traumatol.* 15 (6): 273–277.

22 Witherspoon, D.E. and Ham, K. (2001). One-visit apexification: technique for

inducing root-end barrier formation in apical closures. *Pract. Proced. Aesthet. Dent.* 13 (6): 455–460.

23 Simon, S., Rilliard, F., Berdal, A., and Machtou, P. (2007). The use of mineral trioxide aggregate in one-visit apexification treatment: a prospective study. *Int. Endod. J.* 40 (3): 186–197.

24 El-Meligy, O.A.S. and Avery, D.R. (2006). Comparison of apexification with mineral trioxide aggregate and calcium hydroxide. *Pediatr. Dent.* 28 (3): 248–253.

25 Damle, S.G., Bhattal, H., and Loomba, A. (2012). Apexification of anterior teeth: a comparative evaluation of mineral trioxide aggregate and calcium hydroxide paste. *J. Clin. Pediatr. Dent.* 36 (3): 263–268.

26 Jeeruphan, T., Jantarat, J., Yanpiset, K. et al. (2012). Mahidol study 1: comparison of radiographic and survival outcomes of immature teeth treated with either regenerative endodontic or apexification methods: a retrospective study. *J. Endod.* 38 (10): 1330–1336.

27 Alobaid, A.S., Cortes, L.M., Lo, J. et al. (2014). Radiographic and clinical outcomes of the treatment of immature permanent teeth by revascularization or apexification: a pilot retrospective cohort study. *J. Endod.* 40 (8): 1063–1070.

28 Katebzadeh, N., Dalton, B.C., and Trope, M. (1998). Strengthening immature teeth during and after apexification. *J. Endod.* 24 (4): 256–259.

29 Wolters, W.J., Duncan, H.F., Tomson, P.L. et al. (2017). Minimally invasive endodontics: a new diagnostic system for assessing pulpitis and subsequent treatment needs. *Int. Endod. J.* 50 (9): 825–829.

30 Iwaya, S.I., Ikawa, M., and Kubota, M. (2001). Revascularization of an immature permanent tooth with apical periodontitis and sinus tract. *Dent. Traumatol.* 17 (4): 185–187.

31 Lovelace, T.W., Henry, M.A., Hargreaves, K.M., and Diogenes, A.R. (2011). Evaluation of the delivery of mesenchymal stem cells into the root canal space of necrotic immature teeth after clinical regenerative endodontic procedure. *J. Endod.* 37 (2): 133–138.

32 Wang, X., Thibodeau, B., Trope, M. et al. (2010). Histologic characterization of regenerated tissues in canal space after the revitalization/revascularization procedure of immature dog teeth with apical periodontitis. *J. Endod.* 36 (1): 56–63.

33 da Silva, L.A.B., Nelson-Filho, P., da Silva, R.A.B. et al. (2010). Revascularization and periapical repair after endodontic treatment using apical negative pressure irrigation versus conventional irrigation plus triantibiotic intracanal dressing in dogs' teeth with apical periodontitis. *Oral Surg. Oral Med. Oral Pathol. Oral Radiol. Endod.* 109 (5): 779–787.

34 Shimizu, E., Ricucci, D., Albert, J. et al. (2013). Clinical, radiographic, and histological observation of a human immature permanent tooth with chronic apical abscess after revitalization treatment. *J. Endod.* 39 (8): 1078–1083.

35 Kim, S.G., Malek, M., Sigurdsson, A. et al. (2018). Regenerative endodontics: a comprehensive review. *Int. Endod. J.* 51 (12): 1367–1388.

36 Galler, K.M., D'Souza, R.N., Federlin, M. et al. (2011). Dentin conditioning codetermines cell fate in regenerative endodontics. *J. Endod.* 37 (11): 1536–1541.

37 Galler, K.M., Krastl, G., Simon, S. et al. (2016). European Society of Endodontology position statement: revitalization procedures. *Int. Endod. J.* 49 (8): 717–723.

38 American Association of Endodontists (AAE) (2018). Clinical considerations for a regenerative procedure. Available from https://f3f142zs0k2w1kg84k5p9i1o-wpengine.netdna-ssl.com/specialty/wp-content/uploads/sites/2/2018/06/ConsiderationsForRegEndo_AsOfApril2018.pdf (accessed 10 August 2020).

39 Jadhav, G., Shah, N., and Logani, A. (2012). Revascularization with and without

platelet-rich plasma in nonvital, immature, anterior teeth: a pilot clinical study. *J. Endod.* 38 (12): 1581–1587.

40 Arslan, H., Ahmed, H.M.A., Şahin, Y. et al. (2019). Regenerative endodontic procedures in necrotic mature teeth with periapical radiolucencies: a preliminary randomized clinical study. *J. Endod.* 45 (7): 863–872.

41 Botero, T.M., Tang, X., Gardner, R. et al. (2017). Clinical evidence for regenerative endodontic procedures: immediate versus delayed induction? *J. Endod.* 43 (9S): S75–S81.

42 Jiang, X., Liu, H., and Peng, C. (2017). Clinical and radiographic assessment of the efficacy of a collagen membrane in regenerative endodontics: a randomized, controlled clinical trial. *J. Endod.* 43 (9): 1465–1471.

43 Tong, H.J., Rajan, S., Bhujel, N. et al. (2017). Regenerative endodontic therapy in the management of nonvital immature permanent teeth: a systematic review-outcome evaluation and meta-analysis. *J. Endod.* 43 (9): 1453–1464.

44 Duggal, M., Tong, H.J., Al-Ansary, M. et al. (2017). Interventions for the endodontic management of non-vital traumatised immature permanent anterior teeth in children and adolescents: a systematic review of the evidence and guidelines of the European Academy of Paediatric Dentistry. *Eur. Arch. Paediatr. Dent.* 18 (3): 139–151.

45 Chaniotis, A. (2017). Treatment options for failing regenerative endodontic procedures: report of 3 cases. *J. Endod.* 43 (9): 1472–1478.

46 Verma, P., Nosrat, A., Kim, J.R. et al. (2017). Effect of residual bacteria on the outcome of pulp regeneration in vivo. *J. Dent. Res.* 96 (1): 100–106.

47 Akbari, M., Rouhani, A., Samiee, S., and Jafarzadeh, H. (2012). Effect of dentin bonding agent on the prevention of tooth discoloration produced by mineral trioxide aggregate. *Int. J. Dent.* 2012: 563203.

48 Shokouhinejad, N., Razmi, H., Farbod, M. et al. (2019). Coronal tooth discoloration induced by regenerative endodontic treatment using different scaffolds and intracanal coronal barriers: a 6-month ex vivo study. *Restor. Dent. Endod.* 44 (3): e25.

49 Mohammadi, Z. and Dummer, P.M.H. (2011). Properties and applications of calcium hydroxide in endodontics and dental traumatology. *Int. Endod. J.* 44 (8): 697–730.

50 Fava, L.R. and Saunders, W.P. (1999). Calcium hydroxide pastes: classification and clinical indications. *Int. Endod. J.* 32 (4): 257–282.

51 Cvek, M. (1992). Prognosis of luxated non-vital maxillary incisors treated with calcium hydroxide and filled with gutta-percha. A retrospective clinical study. *Dent. Traumatol.* 8 (2): 45–55.

52 Figini, L., Lodi, G., Gorni, F., and Gagliani, M. (2008). Single versus multiple visits for endodontic treatment of permanent teeth: a cochrane systematic review. *J. Endod.* 34 (9): 1041–1047.

53 Ordinola-Zapata, R., Bramante, C.M., Garcia-Godoy, F. et al. (2015). The effect of radiopacifiers agents on pH, calcium release, radiopacity, and antimicrobial properties of different calcium hydroxide dressings. *Microsc. Res. Tech.* 78 (7): 620–625.

54 Metzger, Z., Solomonov, M., and Mass, E. (2001). Calcium hydroxide retention in wide root canals with flaring apices. *Dent. Traumatol.* 17 (2): 86–92.

55 Chala, S., Abouqal, R., and Rida, S. (2011). Apexification of immature teeth with calcium hydroxide or mineral trioxide aggregate: systematic review and meta-analysis. *Oral Surg. Oral Med. Oral Pathol. Oral Radiol. Endod.* 112 (4): e36–e42.

56 Steinig, T.H., Regan, J.D., and Gutmann, J.L. (2003). The use and predictable placement of mineral trioxide aggregate in one-visit apexification cases. *Aust. Endod. J.* 29 (1): 34–42.

57 Camilleri, J. (2008). Characterization of hydration products of mineral trioxide aggregate. *Int. Endod. J.* 41 (5): 408–417.

58 Camilleri, J. (2015). Mineral trioxide aggregate: present and future developments. *Endod. Topics* 32 (1): 31–46.

59 Duarte, M.A.H., De Oliveira Demarchi, A.C.C., Yamashita, J.C. et al. (2005). Arsenic release provided by MTA and Portland cement. *Oral Surg. Oral Med. Oral Pathol. Oral Radiol. Endod.* 99 (5): 648–650.

60 Camilleri, J. (2011). Characterization and hydration kinetics of tricalcium silicate cement for use as a dental biomaterial. *Dent. Mater.* 27 (8): 836–844.

61 Keskin, C., Demiryurek, E.O., and Ozyurek, T. (2015). Color stabilities of calcium silicate-based materials in contact with different irrigation solutions. *J. Endod.* 41 (3): 409–411.

62 Marciano, M.A., Costa, R.M., Camilleri, J. et al. (2014). Assessment of color stability of white mineral trioxide aggregate angelus and bismuth oxide in contact with tooth structure. *J. Endod.* 40 (8): 1235–1240.

63 Schembri Wismayer, P., Lung, C.Y.K., Rappa, F. et al. (2016). Assessment of the interaction of Portland cement-based materials with blood and tissue fluids using an animal model. *Sci. Rep.* 6 (1): 34547–34549.

64 Camilleri, J. (2014). Color stability of white mineral trioxide aggregate in contact with hypochlorite solution. *J. Endod.* 40 (3): 436–440.

65 Marciano, M.A., Duarte, M.A.H., and Camilleri, J. (2015). Dental discoloration caused by bismuth oxide in MTA in the presence of sodium hypochlorite. *Clin. Oral Investig.* 19 (9): 2201–2209.

66 Camilleri, J. (2014). Hydration characteristics of Biodentine and Theracal used as pulp capping materials. *Dent. Mater.* 30 (7): 709–715.

67 Camilleri, J., Laurent, P., and About, I. (2014). Hydration of Biodentine, Theracal LC, and a prototype tricalcium silicate-based dentin replacement material after pulp capping in entire tooth cultures. *J. Endod.* 40 (11): 1846–1854.

68 Bortoluzzi, E.A., Niu, L.-N., Palani, C.D. et al. (2015). Cytotoxicity and osteogenic potential of silicate calcium cements as potential protective materials for pulpal revascularization. *Dent. Mater.* 31 (12): 1510–1522.

69 Collado-González, M., García-Bernal, D., Oñate-Sánchez, R.E. et al. (2017). Cytotoxicity and bioactivity of various pulpotomy materials on stem cells from human exfoliated primary teeth. *Int. Endod. J.* 50 (Suppl. 2): e19–e30.

70 Zhou, H.-M., Shen, Y., Zheng, W. et al. (2013). Physical properties of 5 root canal sealers. *J. Endod.* 39 (10): 1281–1286.

71 Lin, J.-C., Lu, J.-X., Zeng, Q. et al. (2016). Comparison of mineral trioxide aggregate and calcium hydroxide for apexification of immature permanent teeth: a systematic review and meta-analysis. *J. Formos. Med. Assoc.* 115 (7): 523–530.

72 Bucchi, C., Marcé-Nogué, J., Galler, K.M., and Widbiller, M. (2019). Biomechanical performance of an immature maxillary central incisor after revitalization: a finite element analysis. *Int. Endod. J.* 52 (10): 1508–1518.

73 Schmalz, G., Widbiller, M., and Galler, K.M. (2016). Material tissue interaction-from toxicity to tissue regeneration. *Oper. Dent.* 41 (2): 117–131.

74 Darvell, B.W. and Wu, R.C.T. (2011). 'MTA' – an hydraulic silicate cement: review update and setting reaction. *Dent. Mater.* 27 (5): 407–422.

75 Widbiller, M., Lindner, S.R., Buchalla, W. et al. (2016). Three-dimensional culture of dental pulp stem cells in direct contact to tricalcium silicate cements. *Clin. Oral Investig.* 20 (2): 237–246.

76 Niu, L.-N., Jiao, K., Wang, T.-D. et al. (2014). A review of the bioactivity of hydraulic calcium silicate cements. *J. Dent.* 42 (5): 517–533.

77 Okiji, T. and Yoshiba, K. (2009). Reparative dentinogenesis induced by mineral trioxide aggrcgate: a review from the biological and physicochemical points of view. *Int. J. Dent.* 2009 (3): 464280–464212.

78 Han, L. and Okiji, T. (2011). Uptake of calcium and silicon released from calcium silicate-based endodontic materials into root canal dentine. *Int. Endod. J.* 44 (12): 1081–1087.

79 Bohner, M. and Lemaitre, J. (2009). Can bioactivity be tested in vitro with SBF solution? *Biomaterials* 30 (12): 2175–2179.

80 Meschi, N., Li, X., Van Gorp, G. et al. (2019). Bioactivity potential of Portland cement in regenerative endodontic procedures: from clinic to lab. *Dent. Mater.* 35 (9): 1342–1350.

81 Torabinejad, M., Parirokh, M., and Dummer, P.M.H. (2018). Mineral trioxide aggregate and other bioactive endodontic cements: an updated overview – Part II: Other clinical applications and complications. *Int. Endod. J.* 51 (3): 284–317.

82 Ferracane, J.L., Cooper, P.R., and Smith, A.J. (2010). Can interaction of materials with the dentin–pulp complex contribute to dentin regeneration? *Odontology* 98 (1): 2–14.

83 Widbiller, M., Schweikl, H., Bruckmann, A. et al. (2019). Shotgun proteomics of human dentin with different prefractionation methods. *Sci. Rep.* 9 (1): 4457.

84 Smith, A.J., Scheven, B.A., Takahashi, Y. et al. (2012). Dentine as a bioactive extracellular matrix. *Arch. Oral Biol.* 57 (2): 109–121.

85 Widbiller, M., Eidt, A., Lindner, S.R. et al. (2018). Dentine matrix proteins: isolation and effects on human pulp cells. *Int. Endod. J.* 51 (Suppl. 4): e278–e290.

86 Sadaghiani, L., Gleeson, H.B., Youde, S. et al. (2016). Growth factor liberation and DPSC response following dentine conditioning. *J. Dent. Res.* 95 (11): 1298–1307.

87 Tziafas, D., Alvanou, A., Panagiotakopoulos, N. et al. (1995). Induction of odontoblast-like cell differentiation in dog dental pulps after in vivo implantation of dentine matrix components. *Arch. Oral Biol.* 40 (10): 883–893.

88 Tomson, P.L., Grover, L.M., Lumley, P.J. et al. (2007). Dissolution of bio-active dentine matrix components by mineral trioxide aggregate. *J. Dent.* 35 (8): 636–642.

89 Wattanapakkavong, K. and Srisuwan, T. (2019). Release of transforming growth factor beta 1 from human tooth dentin after application of either ProRoot MTA or Biodentine as a coronal barrier. *J. Endod.* 45 (6): 701–705.

90 Mozafari, M., Banijamali, S., Baino, F. et al. (2019). Calcium carbonate: adored and ignored in bioactivity assessment. *Acta Biomater.* 91: 35–47.

91 Farrugia, C., Baca, P., Camilleri, J., and Arias Moliz, M.T. (2017). Antimicrobial activity of ProRoot MTA in contact with blood. *Sci. Rep.* 7 (1): 41359–41310.

92 Kim, Y., Kim, S., Shin, Y.S. et al. (2012). Failure of setting of mineral trioxide aggregate in the presence of fetal bovine serum and its prevention. *J. Endod.* 38 (4): 536–540.

93 Kang, J.S., Rhim, E.M., Huh, S.Y. et al. (2012). The effects of humidity and serum on the surface microhardness and morphology of five retrograde filling materials. *Scanning* 34 (4): 207–214.

94 Nekoofar, M.H., Oloomi, K., Sheykhrezae, M.S. et al. (2010). An evaluation of the effect of blood and human serum on the surface microhardness and surface microstructure of mineral trioxide aggregate. *Int. Endod. J.* 43 (10): 849–858.

95 Nekoofar, M.H., Stone, D.F., and Dummer, P.M.H. (2010). The effect of blood contamination on the compressive strength and surface microstructure of mineral trioxide aggregate. *Int. Endod. J.* 43 (9): 782–791.

96 Belli, S., Eraslan, O., and Eskitaşcıoğlu, G. (2018). Effect of different treatment options on biomechanics of immature teeth: a finite element stress analysis study. *J. Endod.* 44 (3): 475–479.

97 Atmeh, A.R., Chong, E.Z., Richard, G. et al. (2012). Dentin-cement interfacial interaction: calcium silicates and polyalkenoates. *J. Dent. Res.* 91 (5): 454–459.

98 Li, X., Pongprueksa, P., Van Landuyt, K. et al. (2016). Correlative micro-Raman/EPMA analysis of the hydraulic calcium silicate cement interface with dentin. *Clin. Oral Investig.* 20 (7): 1663–1673.

99 Hadis, M., Wang, J., Zhang, Z.J. et al. (2020). Interaction of hydraulic calcium silicate and glass ionomer cements with dentine. *Materialia* 9: 100515.

100 Guneser, M.B., Akbulut, M.B., and Eldeniz, A.U. (2013). Effect of various endodontic irrigants on the push-out bond strength of biodentine and conventional root perforation repair materials. *J. Endod.* 39 (3): 380–384.

101 Nagas, E., Cehreli, Z.C., Uyanik, M.O. et al. (2016). Effect of several intracanal medicaments on the push-out bond strength of ProRoot MTA and Biodentine. *Int. Endod. J.* 49 (2): 184–188.

102 Hong, S.-T., Bae, K.-S., Baek, S.-H. et al. (2010). Effects of root canal irrigants on the push-out strength and hydration behavior of accelerated mineral trioxide aggregate in its early setting phase. *J. Endod.* 36 (12): 1995–1999.

103 Uyanik, M.O., Nagas, E., Sahin, C. et al. (2009). Effects of different irrigation regimens on the sealing properties of repaired furcal perforations. *Oral Surg. Oral Med. Oral Pathol. Oral Radiol. Endod.* 107 (3): e91–e95.

104 Aguiar, B.A., Frota, L.M.A., Taguatinga, D.T. et al. (2019). Influence of ultrasonic agitation on bond strength, marginal adaptation, and tooth discoloration provided by three coronary barrier endodontic materials. *Clin. Oral Investig.* 23 (11): 4113–4122.

105 Leiendecker, A.P., Qi, Y.-P., Sawyer, A.N. et al. (2012). Effects of calcium silicate-based materials on collagen matrix integrity of mineralized dentin. *J. Endod.* 38 (6): 829–833.

106 Sawyer, A.N., Nikonov, S.Y., Pancio, A.K. et al. (2012). Effects of calcium silicate-based materials on the flexural properties of dentin. *J. Endod.* 38 (5): 680–683.

107 Yoldaş, S.E., Bani, M., Atabek, D., and Bodur, H. (2016). Comparison of the potential discoloration effect of bioaggregate, biodentine, and white mineral trioxide aggregate on bovine teeth: in vitro research. *J. Endod.* 42 (12): 1815–1818.

108 Vallés, M., Mercadé, M., Durán-Sindreu, F. et al. (2013). Color stability of white mineral trioxide aggregate. *Clin. Oral Investig.* 17 (4): 1155–1159.

109 Vallés, M., Mercadé, M., Durán-Sindreu, F. et al. (2013). Influence of light and oxygen on the color stability of five calcium silicate-based materials. *J. Endod.* 39 (4): 525–528.

110 Pashley, D.H. (1996). Dynamics of the pulpo-dentin complex. *Crit. Rev. Oral Biol. Med.* 7 (2): 104–133.

111 Gronthos, S., Mankani, M., Brahim, J. et al. (2000). Postnatal human dental pulp stem cells (DPSCs) in vitro and in vivo. *Proc. Natl. Acad. Sci. U. S. A.* 97 (25): 13625–13630.

112 Bjørndal, L. and Darvann, T. (1999). A light microscopic study of odontoblastic and non-odontoblastic cells involved in tertiary dentinogenesis in well-defined cavitated carious lesions. *Caries Res.* 33 (1): 50–60.

113 Bjørndal, L. (2008). The caries process and its effect on the pulp: the science is changing and so is our understanding. *J. Endod.* 34 (7 Suppl): S2–S5.

114 Fitzgerald, M., Chiego, D.J., and Heys, D.R. (1990). Autoradiographic analysis of odontoblast replacement following pulp exposure in primate teeth. *Arch. Oral Biol.* 35 (9): 707–715.

115 Magloire, H., Joffre, A., and Bleicher, F. (1996). An in vitro model of human dental pulp repair. *J. Dent. Res.* 75 (12): 1971–1978.

116 Smith, A.J., Cassidy, N., Perry, H. et al. (1995). Reactionary dentinogenesis. *Int. J. Dev. Biol.* 39 (1): 273–280.

117 Simon, S.R.J., Berdal, A., Cooper, P.R. et al. (2011). Dentin–pulp complex regeneration:

from lab to clinic. *Adv. Dent. Res.* 23 (3): 340–345.

118 Graham, L.W., Cooper, P.R., Cassidy, N. et al. (2006). The effect of calcium hydroxide on solubilisation of bio-active dentine matrix components. *Biomaterials* 27 (14): 2865–2873.

119 Komichi, S., Takahashi, Y., Okamoto, M. et al. (2019). Protein S100-A7 derived from digested dentin is a critical molecule for dentin pulp regeneration. *Cells* 8 (9): 1002.

120 Byers, M.R., Schatteman, G.C., and Bothwell, M. (1990). Multiple functions for NGF receptor in developing, aging and injured rat teeth are suggested by epithelial, mesenchymal and neural immunoreactivity. *Development* 109 (2): 461–471.

121 Magloire, H., Romeas, A., Melin, M. et al. (2001). Molecular regulation of odontoblast activity under dentin injury. *Adv. Dent. Res.* 15: 46–50.

122 Nosrat, C.A., Fried, K., Ebendal, T., and Olson, L. (1998). NGF, BDNF, NT3, NT4 and GDNF in tooth development. *Eur. J. Oral Sci.* 106 (Suppl. 1): 94–99.

123 Caviedes-Bucheli, J., Muñoz, H.R., Azuero-Holguín, M.M., and Ulate, E. (2008). Neuropeptides in dental pulp: the silent protagonists. *J. Endod.* 34 (7): 773–788.

124 Karim El, I.A., Linden, G.J., Irwin, C.R., and Lundy, F.T. (2009). Neuropeptides regulate expression of angiogenic growth factors in human dental pulp fibroblasts. *J. Endod.* 35 (6): 829–833.

125 Kline, L.W. and Yu, D.C. (2009). Effects of calcitonin, calcitonin gene-related peptide, human recombinant bone morphogenetic protein-2, and parathyroid hormone-related protein on endodontically treated ferret canines. *J. Endod.* 35 (6): 866–869.

126 Mitsiadis, T.A. and Luukko, K. (1995). Neurotrophins in odontogenesis. *Int. J. Dev. Biol.* 39 (1): 195–202.

127 Amano, O., Bringas, P., Takahashi, I. et al. (1999). Nerve growth factor (NGF) supports tooth morphogenesis in mouse first branchial arch explants. *Dev. Dyn.* 216 (3): 299–310.

128 Arany, S., Koyota, S., and Sugiyama, T. (2009). Nerve growth factor promotes differentiation of odontoblast-like cells. *J. Cell. Biochem.* 106 (4): 539–545.

129 Nosrat, I., Seiger, A., Olson, L., and Nosrat, C.A. (2002). Expression patterns of neurotrophic factor mRNAs in developing human teeth. *Cell Tissue Res.* 310 (2): 177–187.

130 Gale, Z., Cooper, P.R., and Scheven, B.A.A. (2011). Effects of glial cell line-derived neurotrophic factor on dental pulp cells. *J. Dent. Res.* 90 (10): 1240–1245.

131 Farges, J.-C., Alliot-Licht, B., Renard, E. et al. (2015). Dental pulp defence and repair mechanisms in dental caries. *Mediators Inflamm.* 2015 (3): 230251–230216.

132 McLachlan, J.L., Sloan, A.J., Smith, A.J. et al. (2004). S100 and cytokine expression in caries. *Infect. Immun.* 72 (7): 4102–4108.

133 Cooper, P.R., Holder, M.J., and Smith, A.J. (2014). Inflammation and regeneration in the dentin–pulp complex: a double-edged sword. *J. Endod.* 40 (4 Suppl): S46–S51.

134 Veerayutthwilai, O., Byers, M.R., Pham, T.-T.T. et al. (2007). Differential regulation of immune responses by odontoblasts. *Oral Microbiol. Immunol.* 22 (1): 5–13.

135 Wei, L., Liu, M., Xiong, H., and Peng, B. (2018). Up-regulation of IL-23 expression in human dental pulp fibroblasts by IL-17 via activation of the NF-κB and MAPK pathways. *Int. Endod. J.* 51 (6): 622–631.

136 Cooper, P.R., Chicca, I.J., Holder, M.J., and Milward, M.R. (2017). Inflammation and regeneration in the dentin-pulp complex: net gain or net loss? *J. Endod.* 43 (9S): S87–S94.

137 Holder, M.J., Wright, H.J., Couve, E. et al. (2019). Neutrophil extracellular traps exert potential cytotoxic and proinflammatory effects in the dental pulp. *J. Endod.* 45 (5): 513–520.

138 Bergenholtz, G. (1981). Inflammatory response of the dental pulp to bacterial irritation. *J. Endod.* 7 (3): 100–104.

139 Rutherford, R.B. and Gu, K. (2000). Treatment of inflamed ferret dental pulps with recombinant bone morphogenetic protein-7. *Eur. J. Oral Sci.* 108 (3): 202–206.

140 Baumgardner, K.R. and Sulfaro, M.A. (2001). The anti-inflammatory effects of human recombinant copper-zinc superoxide dismutase on pulp inflammation. *J. Endod.* 27 (3): 190–195.

141 Inoue, T. and Shimono, M. (1992). Repair dentinogenesis following transplantation into normal and germ-free animals. *Proc. Finn. Dent. Soc.* 88 (Suppl. 1): 183–194.

142 Yang, J., Yuan, G., and Chen, Z. (2016). Pulp regeneration: current approaches and future challenges. *Front. Physiol.* 7 (99): 58.

143 Di Filippo, G., Sidhu, S.K., and Chong, B.S. (2014). Apical periodontitis and the technical quality of root canal treatment in an adult sub-population in London. *Br. Dent. J.* 216 (10): E22–E22.

144 Ng, Y.-L., Mann, V., and Gulabivala, K. (2011). A prospective study of the factors affecting outcomes of nonsurgical root canal treatment: Part 1: Periapical health. *Int. Endod. J.* 44 (7): 583–609.

145 Shimizu, E., Jong, G., Partridge, N. et al. (2012). Histologic observation of a human immature permanent tooth with irreversible pulpitis after revascularization/regeneration procedure. *J. Endod.* 38 (9): 1293–1297.

146 Peng, C., Zhao, Y., Wang, W. et al. (2017). Histologic findings of a human immature revascularized/regenerated tooth with symptomatic irreversible pulpitis. *J. Endod.* 43 (6): 905–909.

147 Yamamoto, K., Kishida, T., Sato, Y. et al. (2015). Direct conversion of human fibroblasts into functional osteoblasts by defined factors. *Proc. Natl. Acad. Sci. U. S. A.* 112 (19): 6152–6157.

148 Fischbach, G.D. and Fischbach, R.L. (2004). Stem cells: science, policy, and ethics. *J. Clin. Invest.* 114 (10): 1364–1370.

149 Mason, C. and Dunnill, P. (2008). A brief definition of regenerative medicine. *Regen. Med.* 3 (1): 1–5.

150 Bojic, S., Volarevic, V., Ljujic, B., and Stojkovic, M. (2014). Dental stem cells – characteristics and potential. *Histol. Histopathol.* 29 (6): 699–706.

151 Fayazi, S., Takimoto, K., and Diogenes, A.R. (2017). Comparative evaluation of chemotactic factor effect on migration and differentiation of stem cells of the apical papilla. *J. Endod.* 43 (8): 1288–1293.

152 Jeanneau, C., Lundy, F.T., Karim El, I.A., and About, I. (2017). Potential therapeutic strategy of targeting pulp fibroblasts in dentin-pulp regeneration. *J. Endod.* 43 (9S): S17–S24.

153 Piva, E., Silva, A.F., and Nör, J.E. (2014). Functionalized scaffolds to control dental pulp stem cell fate. *J. Endod.* 40 (4 Suppl): S33–S40.

154 Saito, K. and Ohshima, H. (2017). Differentiation capacity and maintenance of dental pulp stem/progenitor cells in the process of pulpal healing following tooth injuries. *J. Oral Biosci.* 59 (2): 63–70.

155 Cooper, P.R., Takahashi, Y., Graham, L.W. et al. (2010). Inflammation-regeneration interplay in the dentine–pulp complex. *J. Dent.* 38 (9): 687–697.

156 Alongi, D.J., Yamaza, T., Song, Y. et al. (2010). Stem/progenitor cells from inflamed human dental pulp retain tissue regeneration potential. *Regen. Med.* 5 (4): 617–631.

157 Sonoyama, W., Liu, Y., Yamaza, T. et al. (2008). Characterization of the apical papilla and its residing stem cells from human immature permanent teeth: a pilot study. *J. Endod.* 34 (2): 166–171.

158 Galler, K.M., Eidt, A., and Schmalz, G. (2014). Cell-free approaches for dental pulp tissue engineering. *J. Endod.* 40 (4 Suppl): S41–S45.

159 Chrepa, V., Pitcher, B., Henry, M.A., and Diogenes, A.R. (2017). Survival of the apical papilla and its resident stem cells in a case of advanced pulpal necrosis and apical periodontitis. *J. Endod.* 43 (4): 561–567.

160 Huang, G.T.-J., Gronthos, S., and Shi, S. (2009). Mesenchymal stem cells derived from dental tissues vs. those from other sources: their biology and role in regenerative medicine. *J. Dent. Res.* 88 (9): 792–806.

161 Ruangsawasdi, N., Zehnder, M., Patcas, R. et al. (2017). Effects of stem cell factor on cell homing during functional pulp regeneration in human immature teeth. *Tissue Eng. Part A* 23 (3–4): 115–123.

162 Hattori, K., Dias, S., Heissig, B. et al. (2001). Vascular endothelial growth factor and angiopoietin-1 stimulate postnatal hematopoiesis by recruitment of vasculogenic and hematopoietic stem cells. *J. Exp. Med.* 193 (9): 1005–1014.

163 Tamma, R. and Ribatti, D. (2017). Bone niches, hematopoietic stem cells, and vessel formation. *Int. J. Mol. Sci.* 18 (1): 151.

164 Asahara, T., Takahashi, T., Masuda, H. et al. (1999). VEGF contributes to postnatal neovascularization by mobilizing bone marrow-derived endothelial progenitor cells. *EMBO J.* 18 (14): 3964–3972.

165 He, G., Dahl, T., Veis, A., and George, A. (2003). Nucleation of apatite crystals in vitro by self-assembled dentin matrix protein 1. *Nat. Mater.* 2 (8): 552–558.

166 Fisher, L.W., Torchia, D.A., Fohr, B. et al. (2001). Flexible structures of SIBLING proteins, bone sialoprotein, and osteopontin. *Biochem. Biophys. Res. Commun.* 280 (2): 460–465.

167 Hunter, G.K. and Goldberg, H.A. (1993). Nucleation of hydroxyapatite by bone sialoprotein. *Proc. Natl. Acad. Sci. U. S. A.* 90 (18): 8562–8565.

168 Goldberg, H.A., Warner, K.J., Stillman, M.J., and Hunter, G.K. (1996). Determination of the hydroxyapatite-nucleating region of bone sialoprotein. *Connect. Tissue Res.* 35 (1–4): 385–392.

169 Butler, W.T., Brunn, J.C., and Qin, C. (2003). Dentin extracellular matrix (ECM) proteins: comparison to bone ECM and contribution to dynamics of dentinogenesis. *Connect. Tissue Res.* 44 (Suppl. 1): 171–178.

170 Butler, W.T. and Ritchie, H. (1995). The nature and functional significance of dentin extracellular matrix proteins. *Int. J. Dev. Biol.* 39 (1): 169–179.

171 Miura, M., Gronthos, S., Zhao, M. et al. (2003). SHED: stem cells from human exfoliated deciduous teeth. *Proc. Natl. Acad. Sci. U. S. A.* 100 (10): 5807–5812.

172 Seo, B.-M., Miura, M., Gronthos, S. et al. (2004). Investigation of multipotent postnatal stem cells from human periodontal ligament. *Lancet* 364 (9429): 149–155.

173 Morsczeck, C., Götz, W., Schierholz, J. et al. (2005). Isolation of precursor cells (PCs) from human dental follicle of wisdom teeth. *Matrix Biol.* 24 (2): 155–165.

174 Chrepa, V., Henry, M.A., Daniel, B.J., and Diogenes, A.R. (2015). Delivery of apical mesenchymal stem cells into root canals of mature teeth. *J. Dent. Res.* 94 (12): 1653–1659.

175 Prescott, R.S., Alsanea, R., Fayad, M.I. et al. (2008). In vivo generation of dental pulp-like tissue by using dental pulp stem cells, a collagen scaffold, and dentin matrix protein 1 after subcutaneous transplantation in mice. *J. Endod.* 34 (4): 421–426.

176 Kim, N.R., Lee, D.H., Chung, P.-H., and Yang, H.-C. (2009). Distinct differentiation properties of human dental pulp cells on collagen, gelatin, and chitosan scaffolds. *Oral Surg. Oral Med. Oral Pathol. Oral Radiol. Endod.* 108 (5): e94–e100.

177 Huang, G.T.-J., Yamaza, T., Shea, L.D. et al. (2010). Stem/progenitor cell-mediated de novo regeneration of dental pulp with newly deposited continuous layer of dentin in an in vivo model. *Tissue Eng. Part A* 16 (2): 605–615.

178 Palma, P.J., Ramos, J.C., Martins, J.B. et al. (2017). Histologic evaluation of regenerative endodontic procedures with the use of chitosan scaffolds in immature dog teeth with apical periodontitis. *J. Endod.* 43 (8): 1279–1287.

179 Galler, K.M., Brandl, F.P., Kirchhof, S. et al. (2018). Suitability of different natural and synthetic biomaterials for dental pulp tissue engineering. *Tissue Eng. Part A* 24 (3–4): 234–244.

180 Galler, K.M., Hartgerink, J.D., Cavender, A.C. et al. (2012). A customized self-assembling peptide hydrogel for dental pulp tissue engineering. *Tissue Eng. Part A* 18 (1–2): 176–184.

181 Wang, S., Hu, Q., Gao, X., and Dong, Y. (2016). Characteristics and effects on dental pulp cells of a polycaprolactone/submicron bioactive glass composite scaffold. *J. Endod.* 42 (7): 1070–1075.

182 Yu, H., Zhang, X., Song, W. et al. (2019). Effects of 3-dimensional bioprinting alginate/gelatin hydrogel scaffold extract on proliferation and differentiation of human dental pulp stem cells. *J. Endod.* 45 (6): 706–715.

183 Ducret, M., Montembault, A., Josse, J. et al. (2019). Design and characterization of a chitosan-enriched fibrin hydrogel for human dental pulp regeneration. *Dent. Mater.* 35 (4): 523–533.

184 Wang, F., Xie, C., Ren, N. et al. (2019). Human freeze-dried dentin matrix as a biologically active scaffold for tooth tissue engineering. *J. Endod.* 45 (11): 1321–1331.

185 Alqahtani, Q., Zaky, S.H., Patil, A. et al. (2018). Decellularized swine dental pulp tissue for regenerative root canal therapy. *J. Dent. Res.* 97 (13): 1460–1467.

186 Song, J.S., Takimoto, K., Jeon, M. et al. (2017). Decellularized human dental pulp as a scaffold for regenerative endodontics. *J. Dent. Res.* 96 (6): 640–646.

187 Howard, C., Murray, P.E., and Namerow, K.N. (2010). Dental pulp stem cell migration. *J. Endod.* 36 (12): 1963–1966.

188 Zhang, W., Walboomers, X.F., and Jansen, J.A. (2008). The formation of tertiary dentin after pulp capping with a calcium phosphate cement, loaded with PLGA microparticles containing TGF-beta1. *J. Biomed. Mater. Res. A* 85 (2): 439–444.

189 Smith, A.J., Murray, P.E., Sloan, A.J. et al. (2001). Trans-dentinal stimulation of tertiary dentinogenesis. *Adv. Dent. Res.* 15 (1): 51–54.

190 Nakashima, M. (1994). Induction of dentin formation on canine amputated pulp by recombinant human bone morphogenetic proteins (BMP)-2 and -4. *J. Dent. Res.* 73 (9): 1515–1522.

191 Iohara, K., Nakashima, M., Ito, M. et al. (2004). Dentin regeneration by dental pulp stem cell therapy with recombinant human bone morphogenetic protein 2. *J. Dent. Res.* 83 (8): 590–595.

192 Six, N., Decup, F., Lasfargues, J.J. et al. (2002). Osteogenic proteins (bone sialoprotein and bone morphogenetic protein-7) and dental pulp mineralization. *J. Mater. Sci. Mater. Med.* 13 (2): 225–232.

193 Almushayt, A., Narayanan, K., Zaki, A.E., and George, A. (2006). Dentin matrix protein 1 induces cytodifferentiation of dental pulp stem cells into odontoblasts. *Gene Ther.* 13 (7): 611–620.

194 Alliot-Licht, B., Bluteau, G., Magne, D. et al. (2005). Dexamethasone stimulates differentiation of odontoblast-like cells in human dental pulp cultures. *Cell Tissue Res.* 321 (3): 391–400.

195 Couble, M.L., Farges, J.-C., Bleicher, F. et al. (2000). Odontoblast differentiation of human dental pulp cells in explant cultures. *Calcif. Tissue Int.* 66 (2): 129–138.

196 Cassidy, N., Fahey, M., Prime, S.S., and Smith, A.J. (1997). Comparative analysis of transforming growth factor-beta isoforms 1-3 in human and rabbit dentine matrices. *Arch. Oral Biol.* 42 (3): 219–223.

197 Smith, A.J. (2003). Vitality of the dentin-pulp complex in health and disease: growth factors as key mediators. *J. Dent. Educ.* 67 (6): 678–689.

198 Mazzoni, A., Tjäderhane, L., Checchi, V. et al. (2015). Role of dentin MMPs in caries progression and bond stability. *J. Dent. Res.* 94 (2): 241–251.

199 Smith, A.J., Duncan, H.F., Diogenes, A.R. et al. (2016). Exploiting the bioactive properties of the dentin–pulp complex in regenerative endodontics. *J. Endod.* 42 (1): 47–56.

200 Dung, S.Z., Gregory, R.L., Li, Y., and Stookey, G.K. (1995). Effect of lactic acid and proteolytic enzymes on the release of organic matrix components from human root dentin. *Caries Res.* 29 (6): 483–489.

201 Charadram, N., Farahani, R.M., Harty, D. et al. (2012). Regulation of reactionary dentin formation by odontoblasts in response to polymicrobial invasion of dentin matrix. *Bone* 50 (1): 265–275.

202 Smith, A.J., Tobias, R.S., Cassidy, N. et al. (1994). Odontoblast stimulation in ferrets by dentine matrix components. *Arch. Oral Biol.* 39 (1): 13–22.

203 Galler, K.M., Widbiller, M., Buchalla, W. et al. (2016). EDTA conditioning of dentine promotes adhesion, migration and differentiation of dental pulp stem cells. *Int. Endod. J.* 49 (6): 581–590.

204 Duncan, H.F., Smith, A.J., Fleming, G.J.P. et al. (2017). Release of bio-active dentine extracellular matrix components by histone deacetylase inhibitors (HDACi). *Int. Endod. J.* 50 (1): 24–38.

205 Ferracane, J.L., Cooper, P.R., and Smith, A.J. (2013). Dentin matrix component solubilization by solutions of pH relevant to self-etching dental adhesives. *J. Adhes. Dent.* 15 (5): 407–412.

206 Smith, A.J., Tobias, R.S., Plant, C.G. et al. (1990). In vivo morphogenetic activity of dentine matrix proteins. *J. Biol. Buccale* 18 (2): 123–129.

207 Martin, D.E., De Almeida, J.F.A., Henry, M.A. et al. (2014). Concentration-dependent effect of sodium hypochlorite on stem cells of apical papilla survival and differentiation. *J. Endod.* 40 (1): 51–55.

208 Dobie, K., Smith, G., Sloan, A.J., and Smith, A.J. (2002). Effects of alginate hydrogels and TGF-beta 1 on human dental pulp repair in vitro. *Connect. Tissue Res.* 43 (2–3): 387–390.

209 McLachlan, J.L., Smith, A.J., Bujalska, I.J., and Cooper, P.R. (2005). Gene expression profiling of pulpal tissue reveals the molecular complexity of dental caries. *Biochim. Biophys. Acta* 1741 (3): 271–281.

210 Cheung, B.M.Y. and Tang, F. (2012). Adrenomedullin: exciting new horizons. *Rec. Pat. Endocr. Metab. Immune Drug Discov.* 6 (1): 4–17.

211 Zudaire, E., Portal-Núñez, S., and Cuttitta, F. (2006). The central role of adrenomedullin in host defense. *J. Leukoc. Biol.* 80 (2): 237–244.

212 Musson, D.S., McLachlan, J.L., Sloan, A.J. et al. (2010). Adrenomedullin is expressed during rodent dental tissue development and promotes cell growth and mineralization. *Biol. Cell* 102 (3): 145–157.

213 Duncan, H.F., Smith, A.J., Fleming, G.J.P., and Cooper, P.R. (2013). Histone deacetylase inhibitors epigenetically promote reparative events in primary dental pulp cells. *Exp. Cell Res.* 319 (10): 1534–1543.

214 Kearney, M., Cooper, P.R., Smith, A.J., and Duncan, H.F. (2018). Epigenetic approaches to the treatment of dental pulp inflammation and repair: opportunities and obstacles. *Front. Genet.* 9: 311.

215 Huang, X. and Chen, K. (2018). Differential expression of long noncoding rnas in normal and inflamed human dental pulp. *J. Endod.* 44 (1): 62–72.

216 Zhong, S., Zhang, S., Bair, E. et al. (2012). Differential expression of microRNAs in normal and inflamed human pulps. *J. Endod.* 38 (6): 746–752.

217 Bird, A. (2002). DNA methylation patterns and epigenetic memory. *Genes Dev.* 16 (1): 6–21.

218 Zhang, D., Li, Q., Rao, L. et al. (2015). Effect of 5-Aza-2′-deoxycytidine on odontogenic differentiation of human dental pulp cells. *J. Endod.* 41 (5): 640–645.

219 Cardoso, F.P., Viana, M.B., Sobrinho, A.P.R. et al. (2010). Methylation pattern of the IFN-gamma gene in human dental pulp. *J. Endod.* 36 (4): 642–646.

220 Wang, X., Feng, Z., Li, Q. et al. (2018). DNA methylcytosine dioxygenase ten-eleven translocation 2 enhances lipopolysaccharide-induced cytokine expression in human dental pulp cells by regulating MyD88 hydroxymethylation. *Cell Tissue Res.* 373 (2): 477–485.

221 Duncan, H.F., Smith, A.J., Fleming, G.J.P., and Cooper, P.R. (2012). Histone deacetylase inhibitors induced differentiation and accelerated mineralization of pulp-derived cells. *J. Endod.* 38 (3): 339–345.

222 Jin, H., Park, J.-Y., Choi, H., and Choung, P.-H. (2013). HDAC inhibitor trichostatin A promotes proliferation and odontoblast differentiation of human dental pulp stem cells. *Tissue Eng. Part A* 19 (5–6): 613–624.

223 Paino, F., La Noce, M., Tirino, V. et al. (2014). Histone deacetylase inhibition with valproic acid downregulates osteocalcin gene expression in human dental pulp stem cells and osteoblasts: evidence for HDAC2 involvement. *Stem Cells* 32 (1): 279–289.

224 Cordeiro, M.M., Dong, Z., Kaneko, T. et al. (2008). Dental pulp tissue engineering with stem cells from exfoliated deciduous teeth. *J. Endod.* 34 (8): 962–969.

225 Iohara, K., Zheng, L., Ito, M. et al. (2009). Regeneration of dental pulp after pulpotomy by transplantation of CD31(−)/CD146(−) side population cells from a canine tooth. *Regen. Med.* 4 (3): 377–385.

226 Nakashima, M. and Iohara, K. (2011). Regeneration of dental pulp by stem cells. *Adv. Dent. Res.* 23 (3): 313–319.

227 Nakashima, M., Iohara, K., Murakami, M. et al. (2017). Pulp regeneration by transplantation of dental pulp stem cells in pulpitis: a pilot clinical study. *Stem Cell Res. Ther.* 8 (1): 61.

228 Xuan, K., Li, B., Guo, H. et al. (2018). Deciduous autologous tooth stem cells regenerate dental pulp after implantation into injured teeth. *Sci. Transl. Med.* 10 (455): eaaf3227.

229 Chen, F.-M., Wu, L.-A., Zhang, M. et al. (2011). Homing of endogenous stem/progenitor cells for in situ tissue regeneration: promises, strategies, and translational perspectives. *Biomaterials* 32 (12): 3189–3209.

230 Fukushima, K.A., Marques, M.M., Tedesco, T.K. et al. (2019). Screening of hydrogel-based scaffolds for dental pulp regeneration – a systematic review. *Arch. Oral Biol.* 98: 182–194.

231 Ahmadian, E., Eftekhari, A., Dizaj, S.M. et al. (2019). The effect of hyaluronic acid hydrogels on dental pulp stem cells behavior. *Int. J. Biol. Macromol.* 140: 245–254.

232 Widbiller, M., Driesen, R.B., Eidt, A. et al. (2018). Cell homing for pulp tissue engineering with endogenous dentin matrix proteins. *J. Endod.* 44 (6): 956–962.e2.

233 He, L., Lin, Y., Hu, X. et al. (2009). A comparative study of platelet-rich fibrin (PRF) and platelet-rich plasma (PRP) on the effect of proliferation and differentiation of rat osteoblasts in vitro. *Oral Surg. Oral Med. Oral Pathol. Oral Radiol. Endod.* 108 (5): 707–713.

234 Torabinejad, M., Faras, H., Corr, R. et al. (2014). Histologic examinations of teeth treated with 2 scaffolds: a pilot animal investigation. *J. Endod.* 40 (4): 515–520.

235 Gomes-Filho, J.E., Duarte, P.C.T., Ervolino, E. et al. (2013). Histologic characterization of engineered tissues in the canal space of closed-apex teeth with apical periodontitis. *J. Endod.* 39 (12): 1549–1556.

236 Lolato, A., Bucchi, C., Taschieri, S. et al. (2016). Platelet concentrates for revitalization of immature necrotic teeth: a systematic review of the clinical studies. *Platelets* 27 (5): 383–392.

237 Nagas, E., Uyanik, M.O., and Cehreli, Z.C. (2018). Revitalization of necrotic mature permanent incisors with apical periodontitis: a case report. *Restor. Dent. Endod.* 43 (3): e31.

238 Saoud, T.M., Martin, G., Chen, Y.-H.M. et al. (2016). Treatment of mature permanent teeth with necrotic pulps and apical periodontitis using regenerative endodontic procedures: a case series. *J. Endod.* 42 (1): 57–65.

239 Arslan, H., Şahin, Y., Topçuoğlu, H.S., and Gündoğdu, B. (2019). Histologic evaluation of regenerated tissues in the pulp spaces of teeth with mature roots at the time of the regenerative endodontic procedures. *J. Endod.* 45 (11): 1384–1389.

4

Endodontic Instruments and Canal Preparation Techniques

Laurence Jordan[1,2,3], Francois Bronnec[4], and Pierre Machtou[5]

[1] *Faculty of Dentistry, Paris University, Paris, France*
[2] *Chimie ParisTech, PSL Research University, Paris, France*
[3] *Rothschild Hospital AP-HP, Paris, France*
[4] *Private practice, Paris, France*
[5] *UFR d'Odontologie, Paris Diderot University, Paris, France*

TABLE OF CONTENTS

Endodontic Materials in Clinical Practice, First Edition. Edited by Josette Camilleri.
© 2021 John Wiley & Sons Ltd. Published 2021 by John Wiley & Sons Ltd.

4.1 Classification and Components of Endodontic Instruments

The aim of shaping is to create space for irrigant delivery in order to clean and disinfect the root canal system, and then for the placement of filling materials. Dedicated endodontic instruments have been manufactured for this purpose. The main problem encountered during shaping is the production of dentine debris, potentially leading to procedural mishaps. This chapter restricts itself to root canal shaping instruments and concepts. Table 4.1 shows a classification of shaping instruments based on ISO 3630-5 [1], whilst Table 4.2 provides a timeline of the key dates in their development.

4.1.1 Brief History

From the second half of the nineteenth century, coarse instruments were created from piano wires in order to allow the removal of

Table 4.1 Classification of shaping and cleaning instruments, based on ISO 3630-5.

Group	Specification	Type
1	Instruments for hand use	Barbed broaches, K-files, H-files
2	Engine-driven – latch	Gates Glidden, Peezo drills
3	Engine-driven – NiTi	Profile, ProTaper, Race
4	Engine-driven – adapting to canal anatomy	SAF, XP-Shaper/Finisher
5	Engine-driven – reciprocating	Wave one, Reciproc
6	Sonic and ultrasonic	

Table 4.2 Timeline of the development of different generations of root canal shaping instruments.

Date	Development	Details
1904	K-Files, Reamers	Kerr's development of the first endodontic instruments
1959	Standardization	
1976	Specification No. 28	American Dental Association
1988	NiTi hand files	
1991	NiTi rotary	Passive radial lands, fixed tapers, single cross-section
1999–2001	NiTi rotary	Active cutting tips, variable tapers, alternating cutting edges
2007	Thermal treatment	M Wire
2008	Generation 2 thermal	Twisted files
		Changing cross-section
		Reciprocation: WaveOne, Reciproc
		Structure change: SAF
2010–2018	Further NiTi development	2rd generation thermal treatment: CM (Coltene), Blue/Gold (Dentsply)
		Electric discharge machining (Coltene)
		Shape Memory (FKG)

tissue remnants from the root canals. But in 1904, Kerr Manufacturing Company (Romulus, MI) manufactured what can be considered the first true endodontic instruments: the K-type files (K-files) and K-type reamers (K-reamers). A third type of root canal instrument is the H-file, shaped like a wood screw and developed in 1940 by the Swedish company Sendoline in collaboration with the Swedish doctor Gustav Hedström. For years, files and reamers were manufactured in carbon steel and numbered from one to six, where each consecutive number was bigger than the preceding one. However, each company had its own way of producing the instruments, and there was no correlation between the different brands.

In 1955, Ingle called for the standardization of endodontic instruments [2], and he officially proposed the idea at the Second Conference of Endodontics held in Philadelphia in 1958 [3]. This standardization set specific dimensions for the tip (D1) and the top of the cutting portion (D2) (Figure 4.1). From the start, despite the reluctance of most other companies, the

Swiss brand Maillefer embraced this project, inventing and manufacturing the first testing machines and quickly becoming the market leader. In 1961, the publication of Ingle's seminal article, 'A Standardized Endodontic Technique Utilizing Newly Designed Instruments and Filling Materials' [4] was a turning point in the endodontics field. Ingle advocated replacing corrodible carbon steel with stainless steel, refined the standardization of instruments with the addition of a 0.08 file and of larger ones from 110 to 140, and implemented a colour-coding system. A new standardized technique was proposed, thanks to the matching of the new standardized shaping instruments and filling materials. It is interesting to note that at that time, more attention was paid to filling than to effective cleaning and disinfection.

In 1976, the Council of Dental Materials and Devices of the American Dental Association (ADA) approved the specification No. 28 [5] for endodontic files and reamers. In this specification were included Hedström files (No. 58), rasps and barbed broaches (No. 63), probes, applicators, condensers, and spreaders (No. 71). The materials used were carbon and stainless steel. Details regarding dimensions, sampling, inspection, and test procedures were given; these included diameter, taper, tip length, resistance to fracture, stiffness, and resistance to corrosion. Later, a group of experts from Fédération Dentaire Internationale (FDI), the World Health Organization (WHO), and the ADA created a committee as part of the International Organization for Standardization (ISO) to elaborate international norms based on the ADA's initial work. Both ADA/ANSI (American National Standards Institute) specification No. 28 and ISO norms are updated on a regular five-year basis. Thus, work is in progress on root canal shaping instruments for the ISO 3630-1; 2019 specification Dentistry – Endodontic Instruments – Part 1 [5], specifying general requirements and tests methods for endodontic instruments and covering general size designations, tolerances for

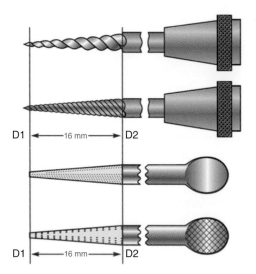

Figure 4.1 Ingle's first standardization proposal. *Source:* Ingle, J.I., Bakland, L.K., Baumgartner, J.C. *Ingle's Endodontics*, 6th ed., chapter 26 C: Svec, T.A.: Instruments for cleaning and shaping, p. 821, 2008, PMPH USA, New Haven, Connecticut, USA.

all design features, colour coding, packaging, and other details [6].

At the end of the 1980s, a promising idea was developed to substitute stainless steel with nickel–titanium (NiTi) alloy in the manufacture of endodontic hand files [7]. These files were supposed to be three times more flexible than their counterparts in stainless steel, and also to be more resistant to torsion [8]. But they turned out to cut much less and to have a tendency to break without warning. It was later realized that, due to their flexibility, the traditional filing motion was a drawback, as was the standardized technique of placing all files sequentially at the working length, which promoted a taper-lock effect. However, it has since become possible to use them as engine-driven instruments, making them more efficient and increasing their taper.

The Quantec and Profile, both featuring radial lands, are good examples of the 1990s era; notably, the Profile system developed by B. Johnson was the first mechanized system to advocate a pure crown-down technique. In 2001, the innovative and patented ProTaper system was designed with sharp edges; this was the first to feature a working portion with variable (i.e. increasing and decreasing) tapers.

Some years later, it became clear that the only way to further improve the behaviour of these instruments was to work on the properties of the NiTi alloy [9]. Thus, in 2007, M-Wire, the first NiTi heat treatment, significantly increased both flexibility and resistance to cyclic fatigue [10]. This was followed by the launch of the Twisted files [11], with a specific heat treatment used to identify the R Phase allowing them to be twisted instead of being ground. Since 2010, several more technological advances have emerged: a new shaping technique using reciprocation with only one instrument (WaveOne and Reciproc, Dentsply Sirona) [12], a self-adjusting file (SAF, ReDent) with an innovative structure [13], and new NiTi alloys – CM wire (Coltene) [14], Blue and Gold heat treatments (Dentsply) [15], Electrical

Discharge Machining (Coltene) [16], and, most recently, NiTi shape memory by FKG (XP Finisher and XP Shaper) [17]. For a review of the new thermomechanically treated NiTi alloys, see Zupanc et al. [18].

4.1.2 Alloys

4.1.2.1 Carbon Steel versus Stainless Steel
Steel is an alloy made of iron and carbon. Carbon steel was the first alloy used to manufacture K-files and K-reamers. Compared to stainless steel, it has a higher carbon content (usually up to 2.1% of its weight), which makes it stronger and harder. Its main shortcoming is it susceptibility to corrosion: it may rust and corrode when exposed to moisture, even moisture vapour in the air. Therefore, it cannot be autoclaved and is prone to rust in contact with sodium hypochlorite. It is also less ductile than stainless steel [19].

Nowadays, the majority of hand instruments are manufactured from stainless steel. Stainless-steel instruments have greater resistance to breakage but less resistance to torque, and therefore tend to become deformed under stress [20]. Gates Glidden and Peeso drills are also manufactured from it.

Stainless steel has a high chromium content, which forms an invisible layer on the steel that prevents corrosion and staining. The chromium layer provides the material's shiny aspect. Austenitic stainless steel is the largest family of stainless steel. Within the 300 series, type 304, which contains 18% chromium, 8–10% nickel, and 0.12% carbon, is mainly used for machining surgical instruments.

4.1.2.2 Nickel–Titanium
NiTi has been shown to be the alloy of choice for the manufacture of engine-driven instruments, although some hand instruments are also made from it. It was first developed between 1959 and 1963 by William Buehler, a mechanical engineer at the United States Naval Ordnance Laboratory, and commercialized

under the trade name Nitinol (which stood for 'NiTi Naval Ordnance Laboratory'). This invention was not related to dentistry, as Buehler was looking for intermetallic compounds for the nose cone of a below-the-surface missile. He serendipitously discovered NiTi's shape-memory properties [21].

In 1972, the orthodontist George Andreasen [22] was the first to introduce NiTi into dentistry, and in 1988, Harmeet Walia [8] thought to use it to substitute stainless steel in endodontic hand instruments. The NiTi alloy composition used in endodontics is close to equiatomic: around 55 wt% Ni and 45 wt% Ti [7]. Since this discovery, these alloys have been used in many different fields: the automotive industry, the aerospace industry, and the medical device industry – particularly in cardiac and orthopaedic surgery [23].

4.1.3 Manufacture and Standardization

K-files and reamers are made from a raw stainless-steel wire which is ground into a 0.02 tapered square, triangular, or rhomboid blank. Locked on one end, the wire is then twisted counter-clockwise to transform the edges of the blank into multiple cutting edges. In contrast, Hedström files are micro-ground from a round stainless-steel blank. Likewise, all NiTi instruments, whether hand-operated or engine-driven, are ground because they cannot be twisted due to the alloy's superelasticity.

4.1.3.1 Standardization of Stainless-Steel Instruments

According to Ingle [4], standardization implies (Figure 4.2):

- A uniform length of the active portion for all instruments from diameter D1 at 1 mm from the tip to diameter D2 at 16 mm.
- Numbering using the metric system to determine instrument size at D1, with a 0.05 mm increase per instrument from size 15 to 60 and a 0.10 mm increase from size 60 to 110. Sizes 0.08 and 0.06 and 110–150 were later added, along with a colour coding.
- A uniform 0.02 taper of the active portion, providing a 0.32 diameter increase at D2.
- A tolerance limit of ±0.02 mm for each diameter on the active portion.
- Colour coding: white, yellow, red, blue, green, and black from size 15 to 40, then

COLOR		ISO Numbering	ISO Numbering	ISO Numbering
PINK		6	——	——
GREY		8	——	——
PURPLE		10	——	——
WHITE		15	45	90
YELLOW		20	50	100
RED		25	55	110
BLUE		30	60	120
GREEN		35	70	130
BLACK		40	80	140

Figure 4.2 Standardization of endodontic instruments: sizing, numbering, and colour-coding.

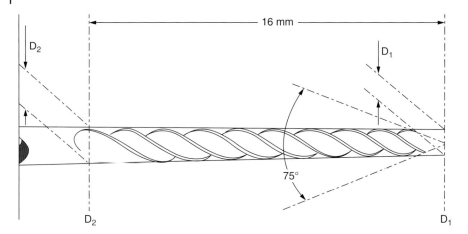

Figure 4.3 Tip modification.

repeating for subsequent instruments. The colours grey and pink were later added for sizes 0.08 and 0.06.

- Standard lengths: 21, 25, and 31 mm.

Two modifications from Ingle's initial proposal have since been implemented [6]:

- An additional measurement at D3, 3 mm from the tip (D1).
- Specification of the shape of the pyramidal tip: for standard instruments, the angulation of the tip is $75 \pm 15°$ (Figure 4.3).

The status of the standardization of endodontic instruments has been investigated [24], and it was found that the dimensions of all files tested were within tolerance limits according to the ISO 3630-1 specification [5]. In 1992, at the second International Federation of Endodontic Associations (IFEA) meeting in Paris, France, Schilder proposed the Profile Serie 29.02 hand files (Tulsa Dental), featuring a constant 29% increase between tip diameters. Instead of the 0.05 classical arithmetical tip size progression between standardized instruments, a geometrical progression provides a gradual increase in tip diameter, resulting in more instruments in small sizes, where they are most needed, and fewer in large ones.

4.1.3.2 Design of Endodontic Instruments: Terms and Definitions

A number of terms and definitions exist pertaining to the design of endodontic instruments. According to the third ISO 3630-1; 2019 specification for Dentistry – Endodontic Instruments – Part 1 [5], general terms and definitions include (Figure 4.4):

- *Standard instrument*: An endodontic instrument having a uniform taper of 0.02 mm/mm length of the working part throughout the range of available sizes.
- *Taper instrument*: An endodontic instrument whose size is determined by the tip size and which has a uniform taper of the working part other than 0.02 mm/mm length.
- *Nontaper instrument*: An endodontic instrument with a cylindrical shape along its long axis.
- *Non-uniform (variable) taper instrument*: An endodontic instrument with more than one taper along its working part.
- *Shape instrument*: An endodontic instrument with a contoured working part with a continuously varying profile.
- *Tip*: The part of an instrument intended as its point, the shape of which is at the discretion of the manufacturer.
- *Working part*: The part of an instrument with a cutting surface.

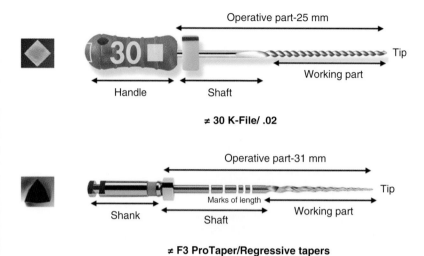

≠ 30 K-File/ .02

≠ F3 ProTaper/Regressive tapers

Figure 4.4 Instrument components. *Source:* Courtesy Dentsply Sirona/Maillefer.

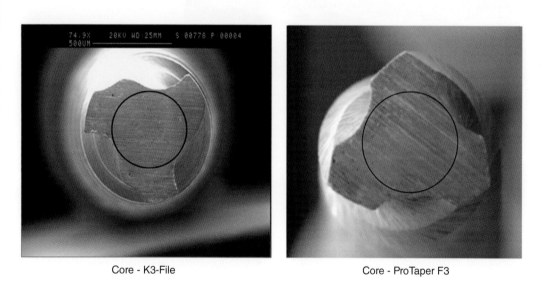

Core - K3-File   Core - ProTaper F3

Figure 4.5 Cores. *Source:* Courtesy Kerr Endo and Dentsply Sirona/Maillefer.

- *Shaft*: The part of an instrument between the handle or shank and the working part.
- *Shank*: The part of a rotary, oscillating, or reciprocating instrument designed to fit into the chuck of a handpiece.
- *Operative part*: The part of an instrument running from the tip to the handle or shank. Endodontic instruments are available in 21, 25, and 31 mm lengths.

Other definitions have been proposed [25] for the other components of an endodontic instrument:

- *Core*: The cylindrical central part of the file, the circumference of which is outlined and bordered by the depth of the flutes (Figure 4.5).
- *Flute*: The groove in the working surface of an instrument used to collect debris (soft

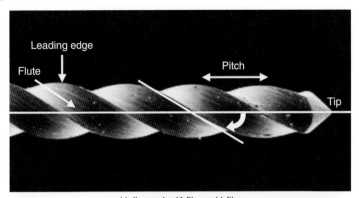

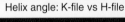

Helix angle: K-file vs H-file

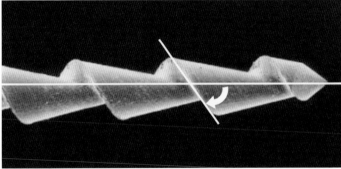

Figure 4.6 Flute, edge, pitch, and helix angle. *Source:* Courtesy Dentsply Sirona/ Maillefer.

tissue and dentine chips removed from the canal walls). Its depth, width, and surface aspect can vary according to the particular instrument (Figure 4.6).

- *Land*: The peripheral portion of a rotary instrument, kept flat and smooth in order to centre the instrument in the canal space. Its planning action limits operator aggressiveness and provides peripheral resistance to the instrument (Figure 4.7).
- *Cutting or leading edge or blade*: The area with the greatest diameter that follows the groove (Figure 4.8).
- *Pitch*: The distance between a point on the leading edge and the corresponding point on the adjacent leading edge along the working surface. The smaller the pitch, the tighter the spirals and the greater the helix angle. Most files have a variable pitch that changes along the active surface (Figure 4.6).
- *Helix angle*: The angle formed by the cutting edge (the blade) and the long axis of the file.

It helps augur debris from the flutes. The helix angle can be fixed or can change along the active portion; in the latter case, we speak of a 'variable pitch' (Figure 4.6).

- *Rake angle*: The angle formed by the leading edge and the radius of the file when the file is cut perpendicular to its long axis (Figure 4.7).
- *Cutting angle (or effective rake angle)*: The angle formed from the cutting edge (leading edge) and the radius of the file when the file is cut perpendicular to the cutting edge. It is the best indication of the cutting ability of a file. It can be positive, neutral or negative (Figure 4.7).
- *Tip design*: The pyramidal distal end of the active part of a file. A pyramidal tip provides excellent cutting efficiency but may be too aggressive (Figure 4.8) [26]. Tips have been described as cutting, noncutting, or semicutting, but no clear distinction exists between the three. In 1985, in a seminal article on the

Figure 4.7 Radial land, rake, and cutting angles. *Source:* Courtesy Dentsply Sirona/Maillefer.

Rake angle

Cutting angle

Radial Land

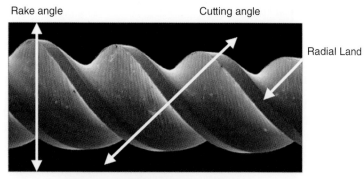

Radial Landed Instrument : ProFile

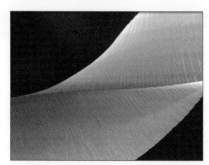

Sharp Cutting Instrument: Protaper

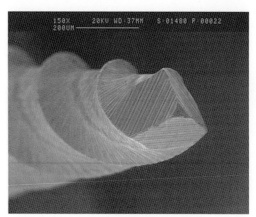

Active Tip
(Protaper Retreatment D1)

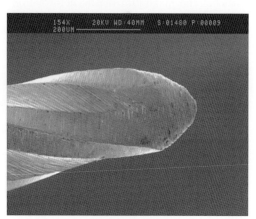

Non Active Tip
(Protaper Universal F3)

Figure 4.8 Active tip (ProTaper Retreatment D1) and non-active tip (ProTaper F3). *Source:* Courtesy Dentsply Sirona/Maillefer.

balanced-force technique, Roane et al. [27] proposed a modification of the tip for the purpose of eliminating the transition angle between it and the first blade (Figure 4.8), thereby avoiding canal ledging and transportation. A comparison of three different hand techniques and one mechanized technique demonstrated that canal preparation with a modified tip was significantly better than that using a traditional (unmodified) tip [28].

4.1.3.3 Physical Properties of Endodontic Instruments: Terms and Definitions

A number of definitions also exist for the physical properties of endodontic instruments:

- *Stress*: The resisting force (expressed in N/mm^2) per unit area of a material against deformation when external force is applied on it.
- *Tensile strength*: The capacity of a material or structure to withstand loads tending to elongate it.
- *Yield strength*: The stress which a material can withstand without permanent deformation.
- *Strain*: The change of original dimension (deformation) of a material under stress or load.
- *Elastic limit*: The greatest stress that an elastic solid can sustain without undergoing permanent deformation.
- *Plastic deformation*: The state of permanent deformation that pertains when a load is removed that exceeds a material's elastic limit.
- *Plastic limit*: The point at which a material reaches the maximum plastic deformation and breaks (the breaking point).

- *Superelasticity*: An elastic (reversible) response to an applied stress, caused by a phase transformation between the austenitic and martensitic phases of a crystal. It is exhibited in shape-memory alloys.
- *Shape memory alloys (SMAs)*: A class of alloys than can recover apparent permanent strains when heated above a certain temperature.

4.1.4 Cleaning and Shaping Instruments

Cleaning and shaping instruments are divided into six groups according to their material of manufacture, mode of action, and shape (Table 4.1).

4.1.4.1 Group 1: Instruments for Hand Use (K-Files, H-Files, Barbed Broaches, Rasps)

4.1.4.1.1 K-Files (ANSI/ADA Specification No. 28)
Stainless-steel K-files (Figure 4.9) are the most commonly used instruments for root canal shaping [20]. Conventionally, they are manufactured by twisting a 0.02 taper square

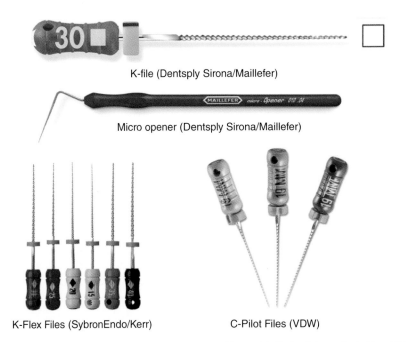

K-file (Dentsply Sirona/Maillefer)

Micro opener (Dentsply Sirona/Maillefer)

K-Flex Files (SybronEndo/Kerr)   C-Pilot Files (VDW)

Figure 4.9 K-files. *Source:* Courtesy Dentsply Sirona/Maillefer, Sybron Endo/Kerr, VDW.

stainless-steel wire, but from sizes 30–140, a triangular cross-section is generally used for better flexibility and cutting efficiency. This action creates tight and almost parallel cutting flutes; such a short pitch gives the instruments both strength and flexibility. Indeed, small-sized K-files resist buckling and therefore are considered the best instruments for penetration and initial negotiation of narrow canals [29, 30]. The most widely taught technique for scouting canals involves using a watch-winding movement. The inward pressure of this motion has a tendency to block canals, and care should be taken to use a light touch with frequent irrigation. For canal negotiation, a watch-winding/pull motion allowing a more careful apical progression should be preferred. West advocated precurving a small K-file and letting it follow the canal pathway with a very light touch to the first light resistance [31]. At this stage, an envelope of motion (i.e. a 360° rotation) on withdrawal of the file is implemented to cut canal interferences [32]. On reinsertion, the file usually moves passively deeper.

For canal shaping, K-files are mainly used with a rasping action and a push/pull motion. This in-and-out motion cuts debris from the canal walls, which can become packed in front of the instrument, leading to canal blockage. In large canals, a circumferential filing motion is usually advocated. K-files can also be used with a reaming motion but, due to their negative rake angle, they are less efficient than reamers [33]. In this situation, care should be taken not to lock the file, because a counter-clockwise rotation to unlock it again increases the risk of a quick instrument fracture [34].

The K-file square cross-section has been modified into a triangular one on Flexofiles (Dentsply-Sirona/Maillefer) and a rhomboid one on K-Flex (Sybron Endo/Kerr Dental) (Figure 4.9). Both are more flexible and have a better cutting efficiency. The obtuse angles of the rhomboid cross-section of K-Flex allow space for auguring debris, whilst the Batt tip of Flexofiles makes them well suited for the balanced-force technique [35]. Flexicut files (VDW) are similar to Flexofiles.

The K Flexofile-Golden Medium file series features intermediate sizes, providing a more gradual increase between instruments – especially smaller ones. With a triangular cross-section and a Batt tip, they represent an alternative to the Profile Serie 29.02 (Tulsa Dental) mentioned previously. They are available in assorted packs of sizes 12–37 at 21, 25, and 31 mm. Dentsply Sirona/Maillefer offers stainless-steel instruments in sterile blisters (Ready Steel Range) and with an ergonomic and comfortable silicone handle (Senseus Range).

C+ Files (Dentsply Sirona/Maillefer) are dedicated instruments for the location of canal orifices and negotiation of calcified canals. They are available in ISO sizes 06, 08, 10, and 15 with a pyramidal tip and a 4% taper on the last apical 3 mm, which provides an increased resistance to buckling [29, 30], and a 0.02 taper on the rest of the active portion. Well-polished C+ Files are very aggressive instruments; their use should be restricted to retreatment cases.

Senseus Profinders are stainless-steel K-files featuring a decreasing taper .02 from the tip to the end of the active part 0.01. They are intended to be used during initial scouting of narrow root canals. They have an ergonomic silicone handle for finger comfort and a 65° tip, and are available in two lengths (21 and 25 mm) and three tip diameters (10, 13, and 15 mm).

C Pilot files (VDW) (Figure 4.9) are the best suited instruments for initial negotiation of narrow canals. They are regular K-files which have undergone a specific hardening process to make them more resistant to buckling [30]. They are available in sizes 06, 08, 12.5, and 15 and three lengths (19, 21, and 25 mm), with measuring marks at 18, 19, 20, and 22 mm. The C-Files (Dentsply Sirona/Maillefer) are similar to C-Pilot files but are available only in 06, 08, and 10 sizes, without length marks.

Micro Openers (Dentsply-Maillefer) (Figure 4.9) are stainless-steel K-files bent at 200° and connected to a long silicone handle. They are available in ISO sizes 10/04, 10/06, and 15/04 and are designed to be used under microscope vision control without finger obstruction to help locate and penetrate hidden or calcified canals.

4.1.4.1.2 K-Reamers (ANSI/ADA Specification No. 28)
Stainless-steel reamers (Figure 4.10) have a triangular cross-section with sharp edges. Their manufacturing process is the same as that for K-files, but with much less twists of the blank. This creates fewer spirals (approximately half as many as with a file), and hence a longer pitch and shorter helix angle: 20° compared to 40° for K-files. Reamers are used with a reaming action to cut dentine (i.e. penetration to get in contact with the canal walls), a one-quarter to one-half rotation clockwise to engage the dentine, and then cutting on withdrawal [20]. A different mode of use is described in Schilder's serial shaping technique, where precurved reamers were used on withdrawal in a series of recapitulations in order to create tapered canal preparations [32].

4.1.4.1.3 Hedström Files (ANSI/ADA Specification No. 58)
H-files (Figure 4.10) have a single-helix teardrop cross-sectional shape [36]. They look like wood crews and are micromilled from a stainless-steel round 0.02 taper wire. This blank rotates on a lathe machine that cuts a continuous spiral along its length. As a result, the core of an H-file is much smaller that its external diameter, making it a fragile instrument. Due to their positive rake angle, H-files are very effective in traction with pull strokes [33], but they should never be rotated at the risk of being locked and fractured (Figures 4.7 and 4.10). The Safety Hedström (Sybron Endo/Kerr, Romulus, MI, USA) proposed by Buchanan is a modification of the conventional H-file. It has a flattened edge design with a noncutting, safe-ended tip to help prevent ledging and stripping of the furcal region in curved and flat root canals.

Micro-debriders (Dentsply-Maillefer) have a 16 mm-long working portion on a 200° bent H-type file with a long silicone handle (Figure 4.10). They are available in sizes 20/0.02 and 30/0.02. Like micro-openers, they are intended to be used under the microscope to help remove pulpal residues and remnants of paste or filling materials in retreatment cases, employing a pulling or circumferential action.

4.1.4.1.4 Machined K-Type and H-Type Files
The Flex-R file (Miltex) is a machined stainless-steel K-file with a modified rounded tip intended to be used with the balanced-force

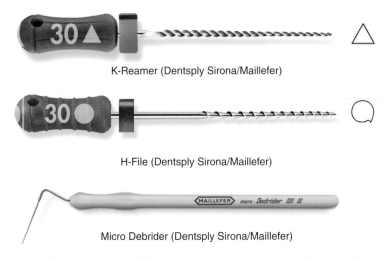

K-Reamer (Dentsply Sirona/Maillefer)

H-File (Dentsply Sirona/Maillefer)

Micro Debrider (Dentsply Sirona/Maillefer)

Figure 4.10 K-reamer and H-files. *Source:* Courtesy Dentsply Sirona/Maillefer.

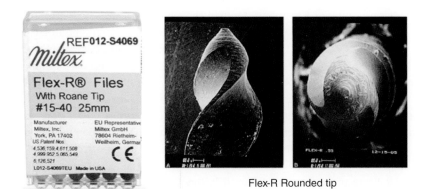

Flex-R Rounded tip

Flex-R files (Miltex, USA)

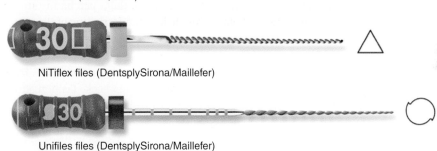

NiTiflex files (DentsplySirona/Maillefer)

Unifiles files (DentsplySirona/Maillefer)

Figure 4.11 Flex-R files (Miltex), with their rounded patented tips. *Source:* Reproduced from Ingle, J.I., Bakland, L.K., Baumgartner, J.C. *Ingle's Endodontics*, 6th ed., chapter 26 C: Svec, T.A.: Instruments for cleaning and shaping, p. 821, 2008, BC Decker Inc., Hamilton, Ontario; Nitiflex file and Unifile file (Courtesy Dentsply Sirona/Maillefer).

technique (Figure 4.11). The transition angle between the tip and the first blade is removed to reduce the risk of canal transportation [28]. On the active portion, the flutes have less depth in small sizes, in order to give more strength and more depth in the larger ones so as to improve flexibility.

MMC and MME (Micro Mega-Coltene) are machined stainless-steel K-files and H-files mainly dedicated to initial canal negotiation and subsequent enlargement.

Nitiflex or Sureflex files (Dentsply-Maillefer) are NiTi machined K-type files available from sizes 15 to 60 in 21 and 25 mm lengths. The special core geometry and cross-section change progressively throughout the range of sizes, giving Nitiflex/SureFlex files their unique linear flexibility, which is practically constant throughout the range. The special alloy, special design, and special machining procedures give them

outstanding long-term sharpness fatigue and fatigue strength [37]. The large sizes are well suited for the balanced-force technique [38].

The Unifile (DentsplySirona/Maillefer), first designed by McSpadden, was the first modification of H-files. It is a double H-file design available in 21 and 25 mm lengths and sizes 10–80 following the ISO standards. It is machined with the same grinding process as H-files, but the flutes are less deep and the core is more important. It is a robust instrument that can be used with either pull strokes or a reaming action. Mounted on the Giromatic handpiece, the Dynatrak system is a mechanized version [25].

The S-file (Sendoline) has an S cross-section with double edges, giving it excellent cutting efficiency. Unlike the Unifile, the S-file has a thin cylindrical core, resulting from an increasing depth of the flutes along the active portion.

It can be used with either a rasping or a reaming action. There is a NiTi version named the NiTi S-file.

4.1.4.1.5 Barbed Broaches and Rasps (ANSI/ADA Specification No. 63) Barbed broaches

(Figure 4.12) represent the oldest endodontic instruments, manufactured as early as the mid-nineteenth century. They are made from a nontapered round blank of soft steel. A chisel is used to cut barbs at a definite angle along the long axis, which are then elevated. They serve mainly to extirpate the pulp tissue, but should be used carefully. They must never be used in curved or narrow canals, and only in the coronal two-thirds of straight and large ones. They are first rotated to engage the pulp and then pulled out in order to remove it in one piece. They may also be used to remove cotton pellets or paper points. Rasps, or 'rat tail files', are no longer used today. They were historically employed to enlarge the root canal, applying a longitudinal rasping action to the walls. Compared to barbed broaches, their barbs are shorter and blunter.

4.1.4.2 Group 2: Engine-Driven Latch-Type Instruments

The various instrument types in this group are shown in Figure 4.12. These include Gates Glidden drills and Peeso reamers, which are run at slow speed.

Gates Glidden drills are safe side-cutting instruments. They have an American

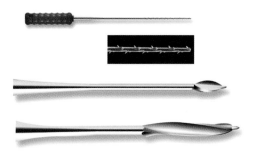

Figure 4.12 Barbed broach, Gates Glidden drill, and Peeso drill. *Source:* Courtesy Dentsply Sirona/Maillefer.

football-shaped cutting head with a U-shaped cross-section and radial lands mounted on a long, smooth, and flexible shaft attached to a latch-type shank. Six instruments numbered from 1 to 6 with sizes 0.5, 0.7, 0.9, 1.1, 1.3, and 1.5 mm, respectively, are available in 32 or 28 mm length. They are used at slow speed (between 800 and 1.200 rpm), mainly to relocate canal orifices and create straight-line access to the root canal. They should only be used in the straight portion of curved canals, and always on the outstroke. Another indication is the removal of gutta-percha in retreatment cases. A safety feature breaks the shaft of the drill close to the shank when too much force is applied or in case of a poor angle of incidence to the root canal. They can be used in a step-back fashion from small to big or in a crown-down approach from big to small.

Compared to Gates Glidden drills, Peeso drills or reamers have a long side-cutting portion but the same cross-section and the same safe, noncutting tip. They are available in six sizes of 0.7, 0.9, 1.1, 1.3, 1.5, and 1.7 mm and are mainly used for post-space preparation.

4.1.4.3 Group 3: Engine-Driven NiTi Rotary Instruments

These instruments are shown in Figures 4.13–4.15. Only those with some innovative features will be described here. Thanks to the introduction of NiTi alloys, the early 1990s saw the rebirth of mechanized instrumentation in endodontics. The first NiTi rotary instruments were the Quantec and ProFile systems. Launched by McSpadden, the Quantec system was the first to feature a 25/0.06, 17 mm-long orifice opener and a series of NiTi files with different tip sizes and tapers. Unfortunately, at that time, the mode of use advocated a conventional shaping technique, with the placement of all instruments (from small to large) at the working length (see sequence in Figure 4.13, Figure 4.14). In contrast, W.B. Johnson's Profile system featured a pure crown-down technique and fewer instruments.

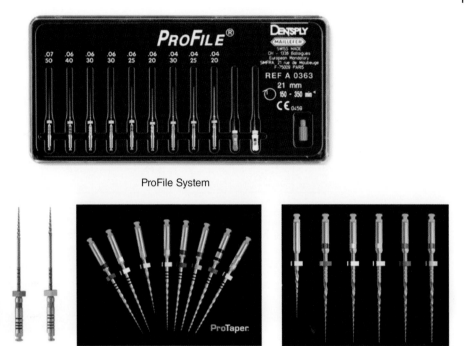

ProFile System

GT File System
20 Series

ProTaper Universal

ProTaperGold

Figure 4.13 Dentsply Sirona/Maillefer systems.

4.1.4.3.1 Profile .04 .06 Taper Series (Densply Sirona/Maillefer)

Introduced in 1994, Profile instruments quickly became a reference in NiTi shaping instrumentation (Figure 4.13). Their main characteristic is a U-shape cross-section with radial lands. This type of cross-section gives the file excellent flexibility, and the radial lands are supposed to increase the peripheral resistance, maintain the file centred in the canal, and decrease the screwing effect. Due to the radial lands, the instruments work with a planing action. Available with Orifice Shapers (OSs) in sizes 20–80 and with tapers of 5–8%, a crown-down sequence with short pecking actions is advocated: one OS in the coronal portion of the canal, Profile 06 in the middle, and ProFile 04 and 02 in the apical region.

4.1.4.3.2 Quantec System (Sybron Endo/Kerr)

This system offers a wide range of tapers and tip sizes (Figure 4.14). The cross-section has a double-helical flute design with large radial lands and a relief area behind the blade to reduce friction. A slightly positive cutting angle provides efficiency. As already described, the Quantec system was initially launched with a traditional sequence, which was later stage substituted by a crown-down one.

4.1.4.3.3 K3 NiTi Rotary Endo File System (Sybron Endo/Kerr)

This system was introduced in 2002 (Figure 4.14). Unlike Quantec files, the K3 system has a three-blade cross-section with positive cutting angle and land reliefs behind the blades. Tapers from 0.12 to 0.02 are used with a crown-down technique.

4.1.4.3.4 Lightspeed System

Developed by Senia in the early 1990s, the Lightspeed System has a unique design that looks like a Gates Glidden drill. A very short active portion (0.25–2 mm in length) with a noncutting tip has a U-shaped cross-section and is followed

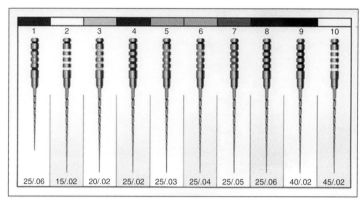

Quantec Files

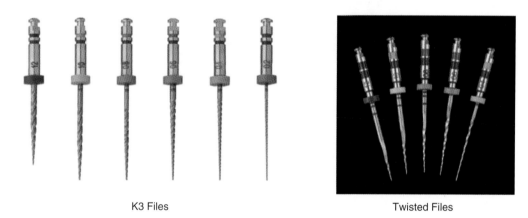

K3 Files

Twisted Files

Figure 4.14 Sybron Endo/Kerr systems.

by a long, parallel-sided nonactive flexible shaft. A big range of instruments from size 20 to 160 makes the shaping procedure time-consuming and tedious. The advocated speed of 750–2500 rpm is considerably higher than that of other rotary system. The Lightspeed instruments are well suited to gauging apical foramen size.

4.1.4.3.5 GT File Rotary System (DentsplySirona/Maillefer)
This system, developed by Buchanan, was very innovative when introduced on to the market in 1996. It features four instruments with 0.04, 0.06, 0.08, and 0.10 tapers, a constant tip size of 20, and a variable length of the active portion: short on the biggest file and increasing regularly towards the smallest. It is interesting to note

that the maximum flute diameter (MFD) was the same (1 mm) on all instruments, making the GT system the first to maximize dentine preservation in the coronal third of the root canal. GT files were used with a straightforward crown-down technique. In 2007, alongside the initial Series 20, the ProSystem GT file was manufactured in M-wire and supplemented by the addition of a 30 Series, a 40 Series, and three accessory files. A GT hand file series is also available, which can be used in a reverse balanced-force technique.

4.1.4.3.6 ProTaper System (DentsplySirona/Maillefer)
Due to its innovative features, the ProTaper System has been the leading product on the market since its introduction in 2001. It was the first system to implement cutting

edges on NiTi instruments and to feature dedicated files for shaping and finishing, with variable progressive and regressive tapers on their working portion. Whatever the clinical situation, the shaping sequence remained the same, with a reduced number of files. In 2006, minor changes occurred in the ProTaper Universal system with the addition of two finishing files (F4 and F5) and a modification of the initial triangular convex cross-section to improve flexibility on finishers F3, F4, and F5. Hand ProTaper files featuring the six instruments from the initial set are available as well as three retreatment rotary files: D1, D2, and D3. In 2015, a gold alloy replaced the original NiTi. Manual plastic handles can be clipped on to the rotary files so they can be used as hand instruments.

4.1.4.3.7 Race (FKG)
Race instruments (Figure 4.15) are machined with a triangular cross-section and alternative cutting edges to eliminate the screwing effect. They are electropolished to improve resistance to fatigue and corrosion, and their tip is rounded for

safety. A limitation of this system is its large number of files, with several complex sequences that must be selected between according to the clinical case.

4.1.4.3.8 Twisted File (Sybron/Endo-Kerr, Romulus, MI, USA)
These files (Figure 4.14) are not ground but twisted, as their name suggests. Through a complex heating and cooling process, the R Phase – the intermediate phase between austenite and martensite – is identified, allowing the file to be twisted in a soft state. A second complex heating and cooling process then brings it back to austenite. Compared to other NiTi files, the twisted files are more flexible and more resistant to cyclic fatigue and torsion [11], but they are still too soft.

4.1.4.3.9 Pathfiles (DentsplySirona/Maillefer)
These files are pathfinding NiTi rotary instruments used to create a sufficient and indispensable glide path prior to NiTi rotary shaping. They are 0.02 taper instruments with progressive tip sizes 0.13, 0.16, and 0.19. Today, all NiTi systems offer their own

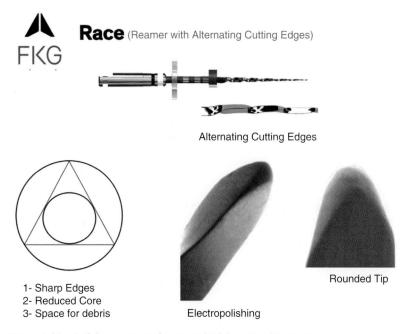

Race (Reamer with Alternating Cutting Edges)

Alternating Cutting Edges

1- Sharp Edges
2- Reduced Core
3- Space for debris

Electropolishing

Rounded Tip

Figure 4.15 FKG Race system. *Source:* © FKG Dentaire SA, all rights reserved.

pathfinding instruments, sometimes with two or three files. Dentsply Sirona/Maillefer was the first company to launch a pathfile in the form of the Proglider, a single glide-path instrument in M-wire with progressive tapers on the working portion. The same option was adopted on the WaveOneGold Glider, for use before reciprocation shaping.

4.1.4.3.10 Heat-Treated Files: M-Wire, CM-Wire, Blue and Gold Wire

At the end of the 2000s, after testing, combining, and implementing all possible design parameters on endodontic NiTi files with the aim of creating better instruments, it became apparent that the only way to improve their behaviour was to exploit the properties of the NiTi alloy. In 2008, Dentsply carried out the first heat treatment of the raw material prior to machining, giving the M-wire [10]. The second generation was the R phase treatment [39] of twisted files (see earlier). Finally, the third generation of thermal treatments was recently carried out in order to optimize the mechanical properties of NiTi (flexibility and resistance to cyclic fatigue), giving the CM-wire [14], Blue wire [15], and Gold wire [40]. Hyflex EDM

(Coltene) is manufactured from CM-wire, but with an electrical-discharge machining process [16] to improve resistance to fracture and provide a better cutting action. Unlike with CM-wire, the Gold heat treatment is done after machining, with an increase of the Af temperature to provide higher flexibility and resistance to cyclic fatigue whilst maintaining torsional strength. For a literature review on the new thermomechanically treated alloys, see Zupanc et al. [18].

4.1.4.4 Group 4: Engine-Driven Instruments that Adapt Themselves to the Root Canal Anatomy

These instruments are shown in Figure 4.16. They include the self-adjusting file (SAF), XP Shaper, and XP Finisher.

4.1.4.4.1 Self-Adjusting File (ReDent NOVA)

The SAF is different from all other available endodontic shaping instruments. It is a hollow cylinder (i.e. without a central core) made of a fine peripheral NiTi lattice that can be compressed during use [13]. It has an asymetrical tip and is available in 1.5 and 2.0 mm diameters. The 1.5 mm-diameter file

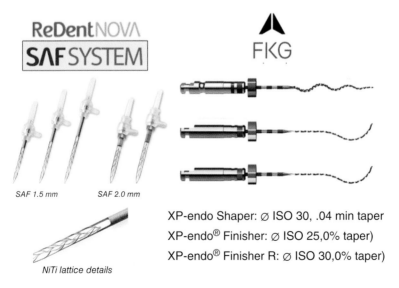

SAF 1.5 mm   SAF 2.0 mm

NiTi lattice details

XP-endo Shaper: ⌀ ISO 30, .04 min taper
XP-endo® Finisher: ⌀ ISO 25,0% taper)
XP-endo® Finisher R: ⌀ ISO 30,0% taper)

Figure 4.16   SAF system, XP Shaper, and XP Finishers. *Source:* ReDent Nova; © FKG Dentaire SA, all rights reserved.

may be compressed to the dimensions of a size-20 K-file, and the 2.0 mm one to the dimensions of a size-35 K-file. The file is attached to a rotary and vibrating handpiece connected to a pump that delivers irrigant. The solution flows through the hollow file, providing true intracanal irrigation. The SAF is not a cutting instrument but has an abrading action. Extensively studied, it may be suited for large canals but has shown limitations in narrow ones, where a glide path must be created with a size-20 K-file minimum.

4.1.4.4.2 XP Shaper and XP Finisher (FKG)

These are made of Max Wire, another proprietary thermomechanically treated NiTi alloy. They are the only NiTi endodontic instruments whose use is based on the NiTi shape-memory property.

The XP Finisher is a single-use instrument with 0 taper and a 25 or 30 tip size. Straight and soft in the martensitic phase at room temperature, it expands and becomes curved and stiff at body temperature when moving to the austenitic phase. The XP Endo Finisher ø 25 is efficient at the end of the shaping step in agitating irrigants, and the XP Finisher ø 30 in retreatment cases in removing remnants of filling materials [41]; it is used at 1.000 rpm and 1 N/cm torque.

The XP Shaper is a one-file shaping instrument with a 1% taper and a 30 tip size [42]. Like the XP Finisher, it works on the same shape-memory principle [43]. It can reach a 30/04 minimum taper at body temperature. The recommended speed is 1000 rpm with 1 N/cm torque.

4.1.4.5 Group 5: Engine-Driven Reciprocating Instruments

In 1998, Yared proposed using a single instrument to completely shape root canals. This procedure necessitates the use of a specific reciprocating motion with unequal angulations set on a preprogrammed motor and handpiece. Initially tested with a F2 ProTaper, Dentsply simultaneously launched the reciprocating files, WaveOne (Dentsply Sirona/Maillefer) and Reciproc (VDW), in 2011. Both are single-use instruments manufactured in M-wire, and both work by a reverse cutting action. The WaveOne system [44] features a convex triangular cross-section and three instruments: the Primary (25/0.08), the Small (20/0.06), and the Large (40/08). The Reciproc system, on the other hand, features one Primary (25/0.08) and two Large (40/0.06 and 50/0.05) files. In 2016, new heat treatments were incorporated into the manufacturing process of both systems, resulting in distinctive colours for WaveOne Gold (WOG) [45] and Reciproc Blue instruments depending on the thickness of the oxide deposit [46]. However, whilst the design of Reciproc remained unchanged, there was a complete overhaul of the WaveOne system, which now comprised four instruments: in addition to the Primary (25/0.07), Small (20/0.07), and Large (45/0.05), there was now an additional intermediate instrument called the Medium (35/0.06). Regarding the systems' mechanical properties, the WOG Primary (25/0.07) instrument shows a higher flexibility and cyclic fatigue resistance when compared to the WaveOne Primary and a higher flexibility compared to the Reciproc R25. It also generates a significantly lower maximum torque [47]. A WaveOneGold Glider, used in reciprocation, completes the WOG series. Similarly, at VDW, an R-Pilot (12.5/0.4) has been added (Figure 4.17).

4.1.4.6 Group 6: Sonic and Ultrasonic Instruments

In 1979, attempts were made to use ultrasonic instrumentation for canal shaping. Howard Martin filed a patent in which a file was mounted on a magnetostriction ultrasonic handpiece. This 'ultrasonic synergistic system of endodontics' consisted of special diamond and machined stainless-steel files that were energized by a Cavitron ultrasound magnetostriction generator with simultaneous activation of irrigant flowing around the

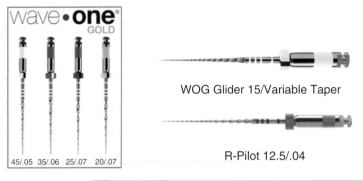
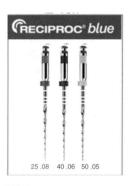

WOG Glider 15/Variable Taper

R-Pilot 12.5/.04

	Reciproc	**WO**	**WOG**
Cross-Cutting	3	3	1 et 2
Alloy	Blue wire	M-wire	Gold Wire
Taper	Variable	Variable	Variable
Files & ∅ Sizes	R25 025 R40 040 R50 050	Small 019 Primary 025 Large 040	Small 020 Primary 025 Medium 035 Large 045
Apical Taper	R25 8% R40 6% R50 5%	Small 6% Primary 8% Large 8%	Small 7% Primary 7% Medium 6% Large 5%
ABS Ring	Yes	Yes	Yes
Lengths	21, 25, 31	21, 25, 31 mm	21, 25, 31 mm

Figure 4.17 Parameter comparison between WaveOne and Reciproc: WOG Glider and R-Pilot. *Source:* © 2007–2019 WOG Group; © 2020 VDW GmbH, Munich; Dentsply Sirona.

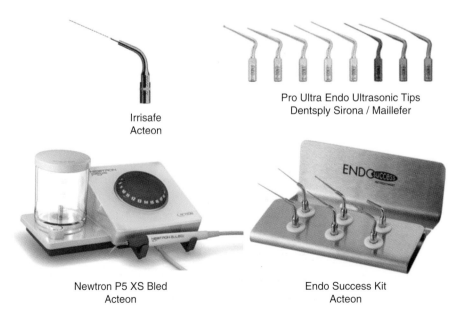

Irrisafe
Acteon

Pro Ultra Endo Ultrasonic Tips
Dentsply Sirona / Maillefer

Newtron P5 XS Bled
Acteon

Endo Success Kit
Acteon

Figure 4.18 Irrisafe tip (Acteon) and ultrasonic endo tips: ProUltra (Dentsply Sirona/Maillefer), Endo success kit (Acteon), Newtron P5 XS Bled Ultrasonic generator (Acteon). *Source:* Acteon; Dentsply Sirona/Maillefer.

file [48]. Whilst ultrasonic activation of irrigants (Irrisafe needle ø 20 and 25, Acteon) is still used with benefit today, albeit with piezoelectricity (Figure 4.18) instead of magnetostriction, the ultrasonic shaping devices soon proved disappointing and were abandoned. Currently, ultrasonic tips (ProUltra: Dentsply Sirona/Maillefer, Endo Success: Acteon) are mainly dedicated to refining access cavities and removing broken instruments (Figure 4.18).

The MM1500 Sonic Air Endo handpiece and Rispi Sonic files (MicroMega) tested by Lumley [49] never met with success in endodontics and are no longer in use today.

The use of ultrasonic systems for root canal irrigation is discussed in Chapter 5.

4.2 Properties of NiTi Alloys and Improvements by Thermomechanical Treatments

The introduction of NiTi alloy to the manufacture of endodontic instruments was done in order to overcome the limitations of conventional stainless steel, as well as the limitations of the taper defined by the ISO. The use of these alloys increased in recent years because they are not only three times more elastic than stainless steel but also have unique pseudoelastic properties (superelasticity and shape memory), which gives them very important flexibility. This makes NiTi files less rigid, allowing better access to the root canal paths and avoiding the problems encountered with stainless-steel instruments [50]. When marketing the first endodontic NiTi files, many studies showed their benefits compared with stainless steel, including:

- Less foraminal displacement in situations of significant root canal curvature [51].
- Less risk of deviation from the root canal, avoiding blockages and tears of the apical foramen [52].

The same flexibility is also observed on large-diameter and largely tapered instruments. Indeed, the increase in flexural rigidity as a function of diameter is not exponential as for ordinary alloys. Thus, it becomes possible to instrument curved root canals with large diameters without the risk of deviating from the original path. NiTi files have today become an indispensable complement to traditional instrumentation during endodontic treatments, both in the quality of the preparations induced and in the time they save. These instruments make it possible to respect the canal morphology whilst reducing the risks of apical transportation, and offer improved safety to the practitioner. Since the introduction of endodontic NiTi files in the 1990s, at least five generations of instruments have been produced [53]. Indeed, new manufacturing processes have been developed with a dual objective: to make files both more flexible and more resistant to cyclic fatigue fracture through thermomechanical treatments.

The pseudoelastic properties of NiTi alloys, which give them their very high flexibility, depend on a reversible solid-state phase transformation known as martensitic transformation occurring during temperature changes. This transformation is reversible [8]. Thus, these NiTi alloys have various crystallographic forms:

- Austenite at high temperature (cubic or B2 structure).
- Martensite at low temperature (monoclinic or B19 structure).
- R-phase at intermediate temperatures (hexagonal lattice with rhombohedral symmetry).

4.2.1 Martensitic Transformation

A martensitic transformation can be defined as a 'first-order displacive structural transition with homogeneous crystallographic lattice deformation, essentially by shear-like mechanism' [54]. The term 'displacive' means that during the transformation, the relative coordinated displacements of the atoms are weak (of the order of one-tenth of the interatomic distance). The absence of diffusion (without long displacements of atoms) makes the martensitic transformation almost instantaneous. The term 'homogeneous', meanwhile, means that during the transformation, there is no variation in the chemical composition and degree of atomic order, since the motion of the atoms is cooperative (i.e. each atom moves to its new position by moving its neighbouring atoms). The transformation is homogeneous because all of the transformed volume is affected by these shears [55]. The martensite generated causes only elastic and therefore reversible deformations, and this transformation has a character of reversibility not only in the chemical sense but also for the microstructures.

In order to relax internal stresses during to the martensitic transformation, the martensite is organized in microstructures called martensite variants (Figure 4.19), forming a self-accommodating group (cooperative rearrangement of atoms). These variants correspond to equivalent shears oriented in different equiprobable directions [56]. Without external stress, the different variants are equiprobable and compensate one another (twinned martensite). Thus, during the martensitic transformation, no change of form is observed.

Two types of phase transformations exist in NiTi:

- austenitic phase ⇔ martensitic phase
- austenitic phase ⇔ R-phase ⇔ martensitic phase

Theses transformations can be induced by temperature (1) or stress (2), or by a combination of the two (Figure 4.20). The structural transformation is responsible for the NiTi alloy's pseudoelastic properties, including shape memory and superelasticity. The R-phase can be stress induced and has the same pseudoelastic properties as thermoelastic martensite.

4.2.2 Pseudoelastic Properties

When the martensitic transformation is induced mechanically by stress (stress-induced martensite, SIM), this property is the superelasticity. The material is deformed in the direction of the applied stress by a process known as detwinning (detwinned martensite, 2 in Figure 4.20); in clinical practice, this can be observed at the level of a root canal curvature that induces the bending of austenitic file. When the file comes out of the root canal, it resumes its original straight shape and becomes austenitic again (3 in Figure 4.20).

Under stress (Figure 4.21), at a temperature where the austenite is stable, the file first deforms elastically (1) like any alloy: the stress is proportional to the strain. Then, on the stress

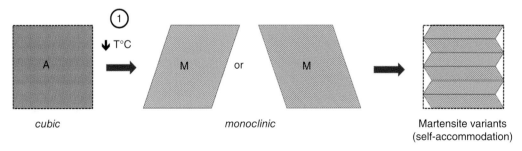

Figure 4.19 Transformation from austenite (A) to martensite (M) by temperature and formation of martensite variants (twinned martensite).

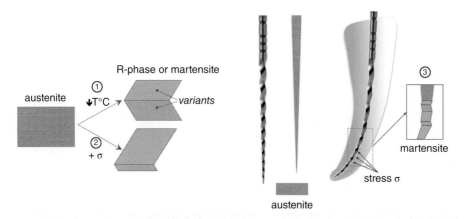

Figure 4.20 Martensitic transformation: 1) induced by temperature; 2) stress-induced martensite (SIM); 3) SIM in a root canal curvature (superelasticity). *Source:* Laurence Jordan.

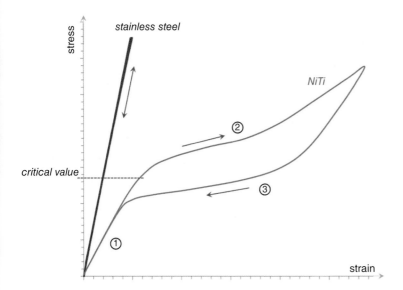

Figure 4.21 Superelasticity.

reaching a critical value (σc), martensite is induced (2). The martensite variants induced are directly orientated in the direction of the strain; the sample deforms significantly. When the stress is removed, there is total reversion towards austenite (3), and no residual deformation remains as the martensite is not stable in this temperature range [57].

This important possibility of reversible deformity is the main property used in endodontics; a file must be capable of deforming easily in order to negotiate the curves of a root canal. Superelasticity gives the NiTi alloys extraordinary flexibility, even in instruments of large diameter and taper, and makes their precurvature unnecessary [58] – unlike stainless steel, which, at equal deformation, undergoes permanent deformation (plastic deformation) [59].

The application of a stress on an already martensitic file (induced by a lowering of temperature) will cause the growth of martensite variants orientated in the direction of the deformation, with a decrease or even the disappearance of the variants in the opposite direction (Figure 4.22) upon the reorientation of the variants. When the stress ceases, the material covers a small part of its original shape, which corresponds to a partial return of intervariant interfaces. There will be permanent deformation if the file remains at a temperature at which martensite is stable. If the file is then heated to a temperature that allows it to reverse to austenite, it will resume its original shape – this is the shape-memory effect [54, 58].

The physical origin of these particular pseudoelastic properties is related to the existence of interfaces between martensite variants. The possibility of reversible deformation thus reaches 6–8%, whereas the usual mechanism of the elastic deformation of metals (minimal displacement of the atoms around their equilibrium position) is very limited, reaching at most 1% [7].

4.2.3 Transformation Temperatures

The properties of NiTi alloys depend on transformation temperature ranges. Indeed, the martensitic transformation does not take place at a constant temperature, but is characterized by several (Figure 4.23): it starts cooling at temperature Ms (martensite start) and is complete at temperature Mf (martensite finish); between the two, there is a coexistence of the two phases. With increasing temperature, the reverse transformation occurs at temperature As (austenite start), to be completed at temperature Af (austenite finish) – which is higher than Ms. The difference between the two temperatures induces the existence of a hysteresis [60].

Similarly, the transformation inducing the R-phase is also characterized by four transformation temperatures: Rs and Rf at cooling and Rs' and Rf' at heating. These are obtained experimentally by the measurement of any property sensitive to the structure (electrical resistivity, dilatometry) or, more commonly, by differential scanning calorimetry (DSC).

DSC is a thermal-analysis technique used to determine the transformation temperature ranges of NiTi. In order to correctly interpret its results, it is important that the temperature scanning is wide enough (high and low temperatures) that all transformations are clearly visible. The signal will show peaks

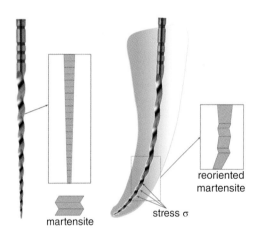

Figure 4.22 Detwinned or reorientated martensite. *Source:* Laurence Jordan.

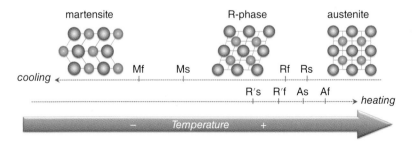

Figure 4.23 Transformation temperature ranges.

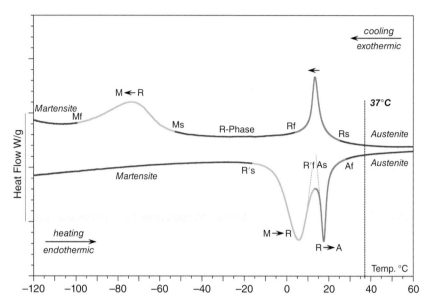

Figure 4.24 Example of a NiTi alloy DSC diagram: orange, A ⇔ R; blue, R ⇔ M.

characteristic of the phase transformations (Figure 4.24). During cooling, two transformations occur: the austenite transforms into R-phase (orange), which then transforms into martensite (blue). These transformations produce a release of heat (exothermic reaction). During heating, the martensite reverses into R-phase (blue), which then transforms into austenite (orange). These reactions absorb heat (endothermic reaction). The height and area of the peaks reflect the enthalpy of transformation. Thus, the more the peaks are marked, the more the transformations are facilitated. The direct and reverse transformation temperature ranges A⇔R are narrow compared to R⇔M. It is important to identify the transformation temperature ranges in relation to the clinical temperature of the files, which is close to 37 °C. The crystallographic structure present at that temperature helps explain the mechanical behaviour of endodontic instruments. In our example, the file is fully austenitic at 37 °C, and the superelasticity is probably operable.

These transformation temperature ranges depend on the chemical composition (nickel/titanium ratio, NiTiX ternary alloys) and the microstructure of the instruments – and thus on the manufacturing processes. For many medical devices, the temperature at which martensite reverses completely into austenite (Af) is the most important transformation temperature, because it dictates the transition between shape memory and superelasticity. It can be adjusted using thermomechanical treatments in order to optimize the performance of the device. These temperatures allow us to understand the mechanical behaviours of different files currently on the market [61].

4.2.4 Manufacturing Processes

Usually, the NiTi endodontic files are 'machined' from a NiTi wire and contain approximately 55.8 wt.% nickel, with titanium accounting for the balance [10, 62]. The wire drawing and the machining of NiTi alloys into endodontic instruments promote work hardening (high density of dislocations) and create surface defects, which weaken the instrument; literature in the 2000s often reported 'premature' failures of endodontic files [63]. The machining process also generates an irregular surface characterized by grooves and cracks [63], the frequency of which increases with increasing taper [64]. This causes a major alteration in the instrument's resistance to fatigue. Manufacturers have sought to improve the mechanical properties of files by controlling cold-working thermal treatments before and after machining and by reducing surface irregularities (electropolishing), allowing subsequent generations of endodontic instruments to be less brittle and more flexible. This polishing eliminates the milling striations and microcracks present on instrument surfaces, leading to a significant improvement in fatigue resistance during bending and torsion [65, 66]. In recent years, a new shaping process has been developed, involving the use of electroerosion; this is known as electric discharge machining (EDM). With EDM, the material is removed or eroded from the work piece by the energy produced by a series of electric discharges generated between the tool electrode and the work-piece electrode. The piece is then 'machined' by melting and evaporation. The advantages of this process are its high precision (micron), stable machining parameters, and limitation of stress to the instrument surface [56, 67].

Meanwhile, new thermomechanical treatments have been developed with a dual objective: to obtain instruments that are both more resistant to cyclic fatigue and more flexible, whilst at the same time maintaining cutting efficiency [15, 18, 67–72]. These new file manufacturing processes combine machined procedures with thermal treatments. Each company uses its own vocabulary when referring to them, including 'M-wire', 'R phase', 'CM-wire', 'Gold', and 'Blue' (Table 4.3).

Each new thermomechanical treatment changes the NiTi alloy; at a given temperature, the proportions of the phases (A, M, or R) are different because the transformation temperature ranges evolve. For a number of these different instruments, the ranges are increased (compared to conventional instruments) so that at the clinical operating temperature (37 °C), the material is preferably in R-phase

(and not only the 'R phase' process). Indeed, this phase is less sensitive to cyclic fatigue and has a greater flexibility than martensite [73, 74]. This point may explain much of the increased flexibility of these new instruments [14, 75].

All brands of endodontic instruments have their own, very specific design process. In DSC, each file therefore has a spectrum of its own (Figure 4.25), with well-defined transformation temperatures. The higher these are (and the closer to 37 °C), the lower the load required to bend the file and the lower the maximum torque required to twist it – and therefore the more flexible the file [76].

At ambient temperature (22 °C), the majority of files are in R-phase, and it is very easy to distort them; often, however, some remain deformed at this temperature. This is not a permanent deformation as it is sufficient to heat the instrument above Af to resume its original shape. Indeed, SIM can exist at this temperature, and it is only above Af that it will transform back into austenite (shape memory). Thus, strictly speaking, there are no martensitic endodontic files at the oral temperature. Studies that perform tests (torsion and cyclic fatigue) at room temperature should be interpreted with caution because this does not at all reflect the phases present (and therefore the mechanical behaviours) in endodontic files at 37 °C. In Figure 4.25, all instruments present the three phases of transformation: austenite ⇔ R-phase ⇔ martensite. The phase transformation temperatures of ProTaper Universal are significantly lower than those of the other two files. These transformation temperatures are very dependent on the nickel composition and can be finely adjusted by thermal treatment. As with most medical applications using superelasticity, the NiTi alloy used in endodontics is enriched in nickel and generally consists of 50.8 atomic% and 49.2% titanium [77]. Indeed, this composition of 50.8 atomic% allows a precipitation of Ni_4Ti_3 in the austenite as a result of appropriate thermal treatments at around 400 °C disrupting the composition of

Table 4.3 Examples of current endodontic instruments: A, austenite; M, martensite; R, R-phase.

Instrument	Manufacturer	Kinematics	Manufacturing process	Specific treatment	Phase at 22 °C	Phase at 37 °C
ProTaper Universal (2006)	Dentsply Sirona, Ballaigues, Switzerland	Rotary centric	Micromilling	Conventionnal	A	A
ProTaper Next (2013)	Dentsply Sirona, Ballaigues, Switzerland	Rotary centric	Micromilling	M-wire	R>A	A>R
WaveOne (2011)	Dentsply Sirona, Ballaigues, Switzerland	Reciprocating	Micromilling	M-wire	R>A	A>R
Reciproc (2011)	VDW, Münich, Germany	Reciprocating	Micromilling	M-wire		
TF (2008)	SybronEndo, Orange, CA, USA	Rotary centric	Twisted under heat	R-phase	A>>R	A
TF adaptative (2013)	SybronEndo, Orange, CA, USA	Rotary and reciprocating	Twisted under heat	R-phase	A	A
K3XF (2011)	SybronEndo, Orange, CA, USA	Rotary centric	Micromilling	R-phase	A>>R	A
Hyflex CM (2011)	Coltene, Altstätten, Switzerland	Rotary centric	Micromilling	CM-wire	A>>R	A
Hyflex EDM (2016)	Coltene, Altstätten, Switzerland	Rotary centric	Electrodischarge machining	CM-wire	R	R>A
Neoniti (2013)	Neolix, Châtres-la-Forêt, France	Rotary centric	Electrodischarge machining	CM-wire	R	R>A
ProTaper Gold (2013)	Dentsply Sirona, Ballaigues, Switzerland	Rotary centric	Micromilling	Gold treatment	R>A	A>R
WaveOne Gold (2015)	Dentsply Sirona, Ballaigues, Switzerland	Reciprocating	Micromilling	Gold treatment	R>A	A>R
Reciproc Blue (2016)	VDW, Münich, Germany	Reciprocating	Micromilling	Blue treatment	R	A
XP finisher or shaper (2015)	FKG Dentaire, La Chaux-de-Fonds, Switzerland	Rotary eccentric	Micromilling	Maxwire	R	A
2Shape 4% or 6% (2017)	MicroMega, Besançon, France	Rotary centric	Micromilling	T-wire	A	A
One Curve (2017)	MicroMega, Besançon, France	Rotary centric	Micromilling	C-wire	R	A>R

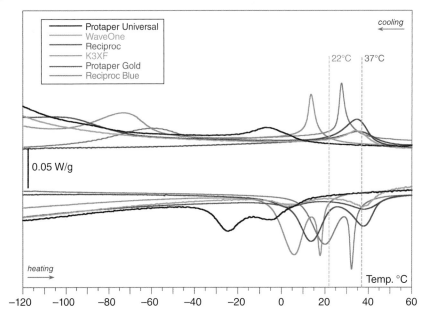

Figure 4.25 DSC diagram of several endodontic instruments.

the matrix [78]. It is this strategy that manufacturers have used in recent years to increase transformation temperature ranges – especially those of the R-phase, so that at 37 °C the instrument has a high proportion of this phase.

Moreover, this precipitation and its effects on the chemical composition (nickel depletion) of the matrix have been disputed in a number of publications [7, 75, 79, 80]. Two parameters must be taken into consideration here:

- The various thermomechanical processes of each industrial procedure do not cause the same density of precipitates; the chemical composition of the matrix may introduce great variability.
- During a chemical quantification, the composition may vary depending on the measurement site (matrix area close to a precipitate or precipitate).

Figure 4.26 shows the variation of the nickel concentration around a precipitate of a nickel-rich alloy of composition 51.8 atomic% Ni [81]. These precipitates consume nickel present in

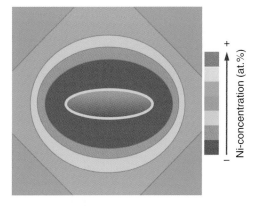

Figure 4.26 Variation in nickel concentration close to a Ni_4Ti_3 precipitate (according to Haikel et al. [50]).

the matrix. Consequently, the more precipitate, the more the percentage of nickel in the matrix decreases and the transformation temperature ranges increases [82]. In recent years, new treatments have been carried out during manufacture in order to create this precipitation, which is the origin of the increase in transformation temperature ranges and thus of the improved flexibility seen.

4.2.5 Flexibility

To simulate the bending of files in the root canal curvature, a bending bench can be used. This includes a device capable of immobilizing a file at 45° to a 20 N-load cell. The set is placed in a bath filled with water whose temperature is controlled by a thermostat and set at 37 °C, in order to approximate the oral temperature. The file is bent on its last 5 mm at a rate of 5 mm/min.

The results of several instrument (25/0.08, 25 mm length) bending tests are shown in Figure 4.27. The ordinate in Newtons (N) is the force required for the deflection (mm) imposed (abscissa). The slope of the curves provides information on the flexibility of the instruments. This depends on both the file design (shape of the section and taper) and the rigidity of the alloy. Thus, the steeper the slope, the less flexible the instrument. It can be seen that all of the new thermomechanical processes ('M-wire', 'R phase', 'Gold' or 'Blue' treatment) increase the flexibility of files when compared with ProTaper Universal, with ProTaper Gold the most flexible. These results are in agreement with the transformation temperature ranges of these instruments (Figure 4.25), as ProTaper Universal has the lowest range and

ProTaper Gold the highest (R-phase at the level of 37 °C). Both instruments have exactly the same design. With equal deformation in the same root canal, the force applied is twice as high at the curvature for ProTaper Universal as for ProTaper Gold (1.1 versus 0.5 N for 2 mm of deflection). Thus, the 'Gold' thermomechanical process is not only a marketing asset but a real treatment capable of improving flexibility. On the other hand, the 'Blue' treatment slightly reduces the transformation temperature range of Reciproc Blue compared with Reciproc, resulting in a better flexibility for the latter. The differences in mechanical behaviour in bending and the DSC results for ProTaper Universal, WaveOne, and ProTaper Gold are shown in Figures 4.28.

On cooling, both R-phase and martensite transformations can be seen with ProTaper Gold (Figure 4.28a, Table 4.4). For ProTaper Universal and WaveOne, the R→M transformation peak is virtually invisible and appears to extend over a wide temperature range. However, it does exist, since a reverse transformation peak heating is identified. On heating, the two peaks of transformations M→R and R→A are clearly visible for the three files studied (Figure 4.28a, Table 4.5). When the

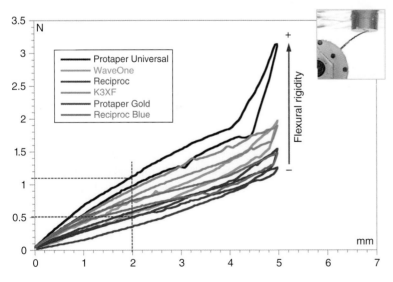

Figure 4.27 Bending curves of several endodontic instruments at 37 °C. *Source:* Laurence Jordan.

(a)

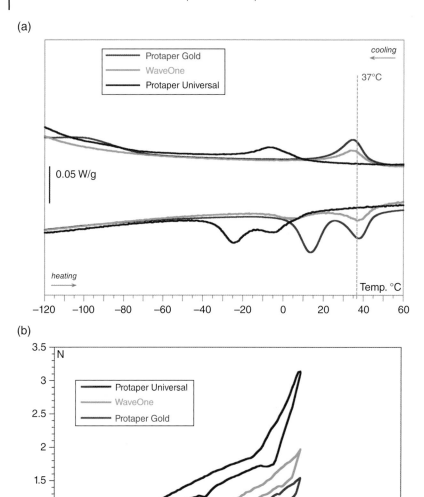

(b)

Figure 4.28 (a) DSC results and (b) bending curves for ProTaper Universal, WaveOne, and ProTaper Gold files.

transformation peaks overlap, this means that there is a small temperature range at which the three phases can coexist. The first martensite transformation in R-phase is not yet complete, as some R-phase variants are already transforming into austenite.

Thus, at oral temperature (37 °C), ProTaper Universal benefits from the superelasticity of the NiTi alloy, a property associated with the presence of austenite. When the instrument is constrained in the root canal, the martensitic transformation occurs and it can more easily bend at the canal curvature. Upon removal from the canal, the file returns to its original shape. WaveOne Gold and ProTaper Gold have both the R-phase and austenite phase; the

Table 4.4 DSC characteristics of endodontic files on cooling.

	A → R		R → M	
	Peak (°C)	Peak characteristics	Peak (°C)	Peak characteristics
ProTaper Universal	−6	Modest Wide base	—	No visible Extended base
WaveOne	35	Modest Wide base	—	No visible Extended base
ProTaper Gold	35	Significant Wide base	−98	Very modest Wide base

Table 4.5 DSC characteristics of endodontic files on heating.

	M → R		R → A	
	Peak (°C)	Peak characteristics	Peak (°C)	Peak characteristics
ProTaper Universal	−24	Significant Wide base	−5	Modest Wide base
WaveOne	3	Modest Wide base	37	Modest Wide base
ProTaper Gold	14	Very significant Wide base	37	Significant Wide base

presence of phase-R, with its opportunities for auto-accommodations, is responsible for the flexibility of these instruments. Under the stress effect, R-phase variants are aligned in the same direction and turn into martensite. The austenite, due to the same stress, can also be transformed (SIM).

Correlation with the bending test (Figure 4.28b) shows the first part of the bending curves corresponding to the conventional elastic deformation and therefore depends on the modulus of elasticity of the phases present at the test temperature (37 °C). Austenite has the highest modulus ($E_A \approx 70\,GPa$), followed by martensite ($E_M \approx 35\,GPa$), and then the R-phase ($E_R \approx 20\,GPa$) [67]. Thus, the beginning of the bending curve of the ProTaper Universal (Figure 4.28b) shows a high rigidity, which corresponds to the austenite modulus. The slopes of the WaveOne Gold and ProTaper

Gold curves are less steep because they correspond to the elastic deformation of a biphasic material (austenite and R-phase) and a martensitic transformation facilitated for ProTaper Gold (significant peaks on DSC).

Different studies have compared these endodontic files, concluding as follows:

- Compared with conventional NiTi instruments, the 'M-wire' technology has mechanical properties that improve flexibility and cyclic fatigue resistance [10, 83, 84].
- ProTaper Gold is significantly more flexible and resistant to cyclic fatigue than ProTaper Universal [40, 85].
- ProTaper Gold has the greatest cyclic fatigue resistance, followed by ProTaper Next, and then finally ProTaper Universal [86].

Thus, bending behaviour depends on both the phases present at the clinical-use

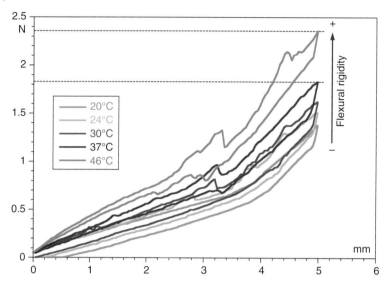

Figure 4.29 Impact of temperature on the bending behaviour of a ProTaper Next file.

temperature and the possibility of martensitic transformation (superelasticity linked to the R-phase and martensite), and therefore on what thermal treatments an instrument has undergone.

4.2.6 Clinical Implications

In recent years, the use of hypochlorite heated during shaping has sometimes been recommended. Heating 1% sodium hypochlorite to 45 °C renders the irrigating solution more effective than at 20 °C, not only in terms of dissolution of the pulp tissue, but also in its antibacterial action (100 times higher) [87, 88]. It therefore seems interesting – and without contraindication – to use less concentrated solutions heated extemporaneously at 45 or 60 °C in order to reduce their toxicity without limiting their effectiveness [87]. However, the increase in the intracanal temperature affects the properties of NiTi files: the same instrument becomes more rigid when the temperature of clinical use is increased, as this changes the temperatures of its transformations. Figure 4.29 shows that bending the last 5 mm of a file at 37 °C requires a force of 1.8 N, whilst

doing so at 46 °C requires a force of 2.4 N – a nearly 33% increase. This corresponds to less martensitic transformation and therefore less superelasticity to accommodate the bending stresses – which explains the decrease in cyclic fatigue resistance described by several authors [55, 89, 90]. In order to reconcile the effectiveness of heated hypochlorite (dissolution and antibacterial effect) and the efficiency of NiTi files (superelasticity), it may be wise to use hypochlorite at room temperature or even slightly below it during shaping and to reserve its heated use for the final rinse [91].

4.3 Concepts in Root Canal Shaping

Shaping of root canals encompasses mechanical debridement of the canal contents and enlargement of the canal itself to create a suitable space for irrigant delivery and adaptation of filling materials. The main benefit of instrument standardization [2] is to provide tools for shaping canals in a systematized manner. This results in the proposal of instrumentation techniques relying on various therapeutic concepts. Instrument standardization and the root canal shaping methodology lead to a specific canal shape and size.

4.3.1 Instrument Motions

The traditional description of the motion of a hand instrument involved engagement of the tip in rotation or an active push–pull. Due to the aggressiveness of active tips and the inward manual pressure used for instrument advancement, it was common to observe mishaps such as canal wall alteration in the form of a ledge, blockage of the canal path by dentine debris, and instrument separation. Motions like a half- or quarter-turn followed by pulling are no longer recommended; nor is the indiscriminate use of push–pull.

Whilst some manufacturers and their key opinion leaders claim that no hand instrumentation is necessary anymore, even for glide path management, this is not the belief of the authors.

NiTi rotary files definitely surpass hand instrumentation in terms of canal enlargement during shaping, but they also present some limitations. Tactile feedback is grossly impaired whilst holding a handpiece, as the number of revs per min is quite high, mishaps arise fast, and NiTi instruments tend to follow the easiest pathway and cannot avoid some of the pitfalls routinely found in the root canal system, especially in its apical third (abrupt canal curvature, canal confluence or bifidity). Mastering manual motions is thus still the cornerstone of clinical excellence in two main clinical stages: before implementation of rotary instrumentation and when faced with apical impediments.

Exploration of the coronal two-thirds of any given canal should proceed with a gradually precurved #10 K-file in reciprocating clockwise then counterclockwise motions. This merely passive and random kinematics carries the instrument deeper into the canal. Progression should stop before the instrument stalls, whether due to coronal or apical constraints. Whilst initially known as 'watch-winding', this repetitive movement is best described as 'follow' – a term coined by West [92] – as no pressure is needed, and the instrument simply follows the natural canal path, guided by its curved tip.

The curved instrument is then removed in a backward precession movement. First described for reamers as the 'envelope of motion' in the seminal article by Schilder [32], this kind of movement performs well with any gradually precured K-style instrument. It releases coronal constraints through minute enlargement and allows for further deeper and passive insertions.

Exploration of the apical third deserves a gentle touch and specific attention in order to preserve the spatial position of the apical foramen and its dimensions. A new #10 K-file is curved in its last 3 mm and acts as a blind cane to scout the more delicate and unpredictable anatomy. Watch-winding pull of lesser amplitude when approaching the foramen translates into a simple rocking followed by increasing back-and-forth filling motions once patency has been obtained [31]. Before considering rotary instrumentation, it is important to verify that the canal path will accept the passive insertion of at least a straight #15 K-file.

When faced with an abrupt apical curvature or bifidity, it is wise to consider manual instrumentation to complete the case. Flexofile (Dentsply-Sirona), Triple-Flex (Sybron Endo, Kerr), and Flex-R (Miltex) instruments are best suited for the balanced-force technique [27, 93]. This requires appropriate enlargement of the body of the canal to alleviate any coronal constraint, as well as apical canal patency. The modified K-style instrument is inserted straight into the canal and made to progress by watch-winding motions until it binds. It is then rotated 90° (or less with the smaller-sized instruments) *without any pressure* on the handle; this makes the tip engage the dentine walls and progress apically. The second step is to cut the dentine by rotating the file more than 120° whilst *maintaining the pressure* on the handle so that it will withstand unscrewing. This step may be repeated to release the instrument. The third step is to remove the instrument in a clockwise rotation in order to hold debris. A series of three or four instruments used in step-back is usually sufficient to shape the apical curvature in a conical form.

4.3.2 Canal Management Strategies

As early as 1961, Ingle proposed a standardized technique [4] for filling the apical third of the root canals, initially with a silver point and later with a gutta-percha point corresponding to the exact diameter of the last instrument used at the working length. In this technique, increasing sizes of reamers were used successively at the same working length in a rotational movement. This cylindrical apical preparation had two objectives: to involve the whole canal cross-section through an important widening of the canal lumen in the apical third and to create both a resistance and a retention form in order to confine the filling material inside the root. Shaping of the coronal two-thirds of the canal was then performed using Hedström files with a circumferential rasping motion (Figure 4.30). This technique, initially developed by Washington University, was quickly adopted by a large number of dental schools, including the Scandinavian ones [94, 95], to the point of being considered as the reference technique for many years [96]. Its main limitations lay in the apical enlargement necessary to fulfil its objectives and in the difficulty of its clinical implementation, particularly when treating the more delicate canals of curved roots. The restoring force of the steel instruments and their use at the same length whatever their diameter caused frequent and dramatic alterations of the canal anatomy [97], including internal transportation (ledges and perforation; Figure 4.31) and external transportation (zipping or tearing of the apical foramen; Figure 4.32).

Even more problematic was the risk of fracture inherent to the method of use of these

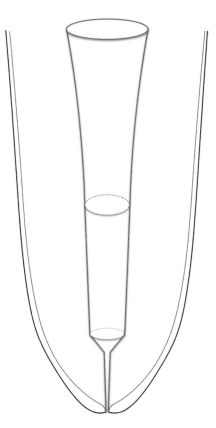

Figure 4.30 Standardized preparation. An apical is box is established 1–2 mm short of the radiographic apex. Enlargement should result in a round preparation capable of accommodating a single cone. Coronal and straight portions are flared to instrument ovoid and irregular canals.

instruments. To be effective, reamers must engage the walls with each of their cutting flutes and rotate at least 180° to make the cut and allow disengagement. Consequently, there is a tendency to screw rather than cut, resulting in an increasing engagement as the instrument progresses in an apical direction. Since they were made by twisting a steel wire counter-clockwise, if the tip was locked in the walls and rotation was forced beyond the elastic limit of the alloy, the first coronal flutes would plastically deform, resulting in unwinding. It then became dangerous to attempt unscrewing because of over-winding followed by fracture (Figure 4.33).

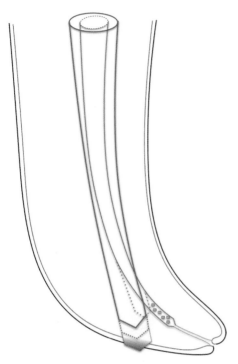

Figure 4.31 Mechanism of internal transportation. If larger and stiffer instruments are carried in the canal to the same working length, this results in deviation from the natural path and creates a ledge in the wall opposite to the curvature. As the apical segment is clogged with debris, attempts to regain the working length will further aggravate the transportation and ultimately cause perforation.

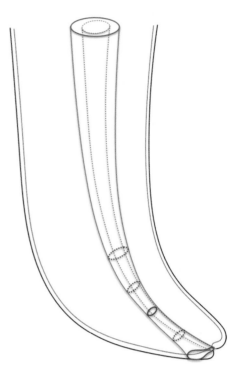

Figure 4.32 Mechanism of external transportation. As larger and stiffer instruments are worked past the foramen, the foramen is deviated from its natural position and its size is increased. This results in a teardrop outline form of the orifice and an hourglass shape of the apical preparation.

In order to overcome these drawbacks, various authors proposed a 'backward' preparation: the so-called telescopic or step-back technique [98–101]. After determination of the working length and a limited apical enlargement, the apical third is shaped with instruments of increasing size, each instrument being used successively shorter from the previous one, with intervals set at 0.5–1 mm depending on the severity of the canal curvature. The recommended instruments are K-files, used with a quarter-turn motion followed by withdrawal; the rest of the canal is then shaped with Gates Glidden drills. The manual files are precurved at their tip to accommodate the curvature of the canal and are moved in with a watch-winding motion until resistance to

progression is felt. The tip of the instrument is then locked with a quarter-turn clockwise rotation to engage the walls and cut dentine whilst retracted. This kinematic tends to gouge the walls, resulting in steps that need to be smoothed at the end of the preparation. Shaping the coronal two-thirds of the canals with Gates Glidden burs gives the prepared canals a characteristic 'Coke bottle' appearance (Figure 4.34) and dangerously predisposes to strip perforation (Figure 4.35).

It was also at this time that Herbert Schilder proposed his concept of cleaning and shaping the root canals. This is based on pre-enlargement and passive apical instrumentation, with recapitulations of series of increasingly larger reamers set back from one another. Permanent verification of the foramen patency is achieved

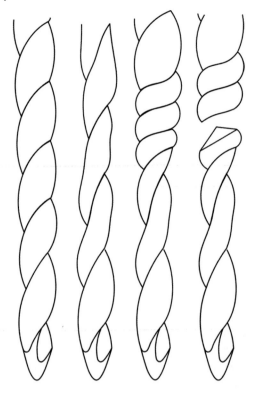

Figure 4.33 From left to right: sequences of events during plastic deformation of stainless-steel instruments subjected to rotation when the tip is blocked.

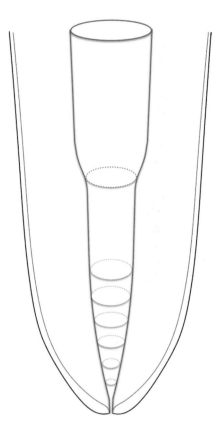

Figure 4.34 Step-back preparation.

with a precurved thin file. Best known as the 'serial technique' [32], this, like the standardized technique, is a global concept – almost a philosophy of treatment. The canal shaping must meet mechanical objectives and is based on a close relation between shaping and obturation [102]. The objectives advocated by Schilder include:

1) To develop a continuously tapered canal preparation.
2) To keep the canal narrow apically, with the narrowest cross-sectional diameter at its terminus.
3) To have the conical preparation exist in multiple planes, not only in ones where a geometric cone can be described.
4) To leave the apical foramen in its original position spatially.
5) To keep the apical foramen as small as is practical.

Within a series, each instrument use facilitates the placement of the following larger one behind it, and its passive work. Each series used in sequence facilitates the apical progression of the next in recapitulations. The instruments employed for this technique are reamers with a gradual curvature, used in a recessed rotary movement. Thus, cutting is done not by the tip but by the body of the instrument, at any level of the envelope of motion during rotation and withdrawal (Figure 4.36). The successive use of these instruments results in a tapered shape. Two conditions must be respected, for safety reasons: patency of the segment of the canal initially accessible without undue force using pre-bent K-files, and early coronary enlargement achieved by reamers (passive apical instrumentation) and Gates Glidden drills (used in wall brushing on

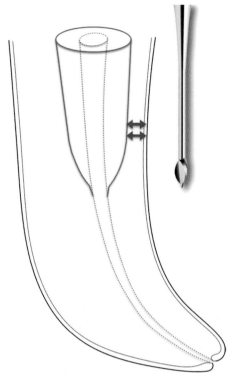

Figure 4.35 Overzealous use of Gates Glidden drills predispose to furcal perforation of the inner wall of the root when a curve is present.

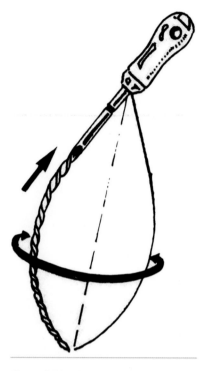

Figure 4.36 Envelope of motion of reamers in Schilder's technique.

withdrawal) [103]. Apical finishing and the connection of the different root segments give the prepared canal a continuously conical shape from the orifice to the apex (Figure 4.37). The major innovation of Schilder's technique was that it released the instruments from constraint (suppression of the sheath and tip effect) and allowed a real three-dimensional preparation of the canal. It remained little used, however, because of its steep learning curve and the dogmatic oppositions to it that prevailed at the time.

At the turn of the 1980s, Marshall and Papin [104] proposed an original technique of corono-apical preparation, but this was quickly abandoned because of the iatrogenic errors it repeatedly generated. The technique was rediscovered in the 1990s, however, with the introduction of NiTi. In the original crown-down technique [105], straight instruments were used from largest to smallest in a rotational movement (twice 360° without apical pressure). This was a brand-new concept in that the canal was shaped and cleaned from the orifice to the apex. The preferred instrument was a Kerr's K-Flex file with a rhomboid section; this modification of shape increases the flexibility of the instrument, especially after the 30/100 diameter, and decreases the risk of ledging.

Abou-Rass et al. [106] with the anticurvature filling technique recommended the early use of rotating instruments in a parietal outstroke brushing of the wall opposite to the furcation (the danger zone). The goal was to limit the risk of strip perforation and of deflection of the tip of a hand file during negotiation of the apical part. Goerig et al. [107] proposed a hybrid technique called step-down in which the coronal two-thirds were prepared first using H-files and Gates Glidden drills, before performing a step-back preparation of the apical third. Variants of

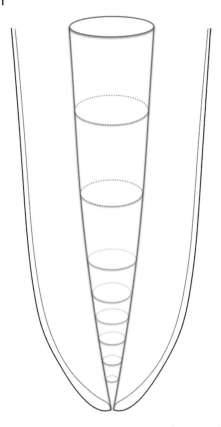

Figure 4.37 Continuously tapered preparation.

files (Union Broach, Miltex), Triple-Flex files (Sybron Endo/Kerr), and Flexofiles (Dentsply Sirona/Maillefer). It was also the subject of a long controversy, until the reciprocation movement rehabilitated it definitively, by resuming its mode of operation. Today, it remains the reference technique for the management of an abrupt curvature in the apical third [109].

With the introduction of NiTi by Walia et al. [8] in 1988, a number of instruments were introduced on the market. Initially, these were manual, but they had very little success because, compared with their steel counterparts, they had a much lower cutting efficiency and, unexpectedly, broke more frequently, without warning. Apparently, the clinical causes of these failures were not understood at the time, as shown by the evolution of NiTi file design in the years that followed. Indeed, from 1989 to 1994, all possible types of file were tested to compensate for these deficiencies, without reaching success. In fact, NiTi files were being used in the same way as stainless-steel files, with the traditional vertical back-and-forth rasping motion; their great flexibility combined with this kinematic reduced their cutting capacity. Even more problematic was the increased risk of fracture, which occurred due to the willingness of most dentists to go straight to the working length with the first instrument and to stay there with all subsequent ones. Doing so encouraged locking of the tip, and values of stress in torsion were well above the elastic limit of the alloy when dentists tried to rotate the instrument to disengage it. Based on this observation, two lessons were learnt:

this technique were then introduced as the 'double flare technique' [108].

Following experimental work on the cause of fracture of instruments used in rotation [93], Roane et al. [27] described a new technique for the use of hand instruments. The concept of balanced force is based on the restoration of the force stored in the instrument when it is disengaged under pressure after being screwed into dentinal walls (Figure 4.38). The cutting work is done immediately behind the tip of the instrument, at the first two or three flutes. To operate correctly, three conditions must be respected: patency of the apical pathway, elimination of the transition angle at the tip of the file, and sufficient shaping of the body of the canal to eliminate coronal constraint. If these are not met, ledging and file fracture ensue. The balanced-force technique led to the development of the Flex-R

1) NiTi files must be used in a corono-apical sequence and not in step-back, in order to reduce engagement and thus limit the risk of fracture.
2) NiTi files must be used in continuous rotation at low torque (with a light-touch vertical back-and-forth motion) in order to improve their cutting efficiency and reduce file engagement.

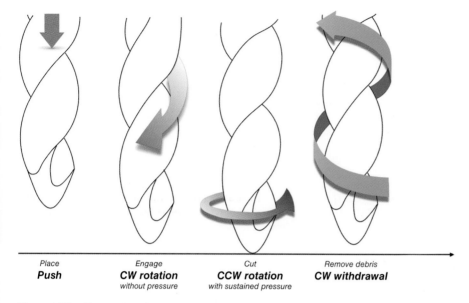

Place	Engage	Cut	Remove debris
Push	**CW rotation**	**CCW rotation**	**CW withdrawal**
	without pressure	*with sustained pressure*	

Figure 4.38 Kinematics of the balanced-force technique.

Dentists – especially general practitioners – quickly adopted continuous rotation because of the time it saved and the improvements it made in the quality of preparations. Specialists were slow to perceive the benefits of this technical shift, mainly out of fear of the potential consequences of an instrumental fracture [110, 111]. Electric motors with torque control soon appeared, however, allowing for safer and more efficient use of rotary NiTi files. Further, in order to reduce the contact area with the canal walls, instruments with taper >2% became available and made possible by the greater flexibility of the NiTi alloy.

Since the introduction of NiTi rotary instrumentation, most systems have advocated the crown-down technique (Figure 4.39) in order to reduce file engagement due to taper lock. Complex sequences are used, with numerous recapitulations before they reach the working length. Larger and more tapered files are used first, allowing thinner and less tapered – and thus more flexible – ones to progress deeper into the canal, whilst reducing the risk of instrument separation by cyclic fatigue in curved canals. Semi-active tips have replaced the notoriously dangerous active ones, rounding the pointed end and eliminating the transition angle. The canal path has had to be enlarged to at least the size of the tip of the first rotary file in order to reduce tip engagement and torsional stress, which can lead to fracture in constricted canals.

The core section has a greater influence on the fracture resistance of NiTi rotary instruments than their size or taper [112]:

- When an instrument operates in rotation in a curved portion, it bends and alternates cycles of tension on the outer side and compression on the inner side of the curve [113]. Repetition of these bending deformations leads to stress accumulation, which can end in fracture by cyclic fatigue. The more important the mass of the instrument, the more stress is induced, and so the more it is prone to fracture in flexion.
- When any portion of an instrument engages the walls on two diametrically opposed points, it binds. Continued rotation will then result in torsional stress, leading to twisting deformation of the instrument [114]. If an

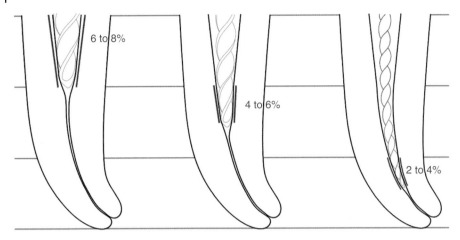

Figure 4.39 Crown-down technique applied to NiTi rotary instrumentation. Larger or more tapered instruments are used before thinner or less tapered ones. They engage the walls at the tip or – even better – at the first millimetres coronal to the tip in order to limit taper lock.

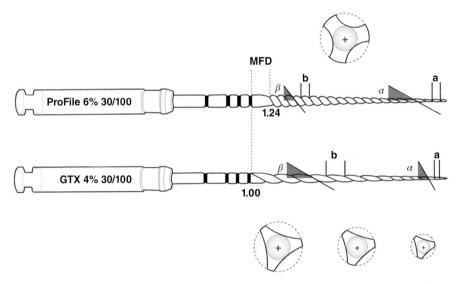

Figure 4.40 Modification of the flute's pitch and helical angle from the ProFile to the GTX rotary instruments.

instrument cannot cut the dentine before reaching the elastic limit of the alloy, it will plastically deform before fracturing. Thinner parts are more prone to catastrophic torsional load. Almost every modification of design was field-tested within the space of a decade. Manufacture of NiTi rotary instruments by grinding instead of twisting allowed for the conception and fabrication of instruments with a variety of section designs. Whilst improvement most often translated to limitation in one way or another, some major innovations did lead to changes in the way instruments were used (Figures 4.40–4.42).

- Today, most instruments feature a variable helical angle and flute's pitch in order to reduce the screwing effect. This also leads to

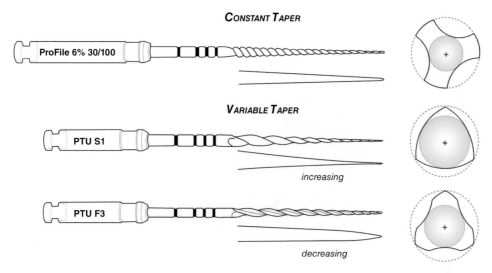

Figure 4.41 Distinctive tapers along the active parts of different instruments.

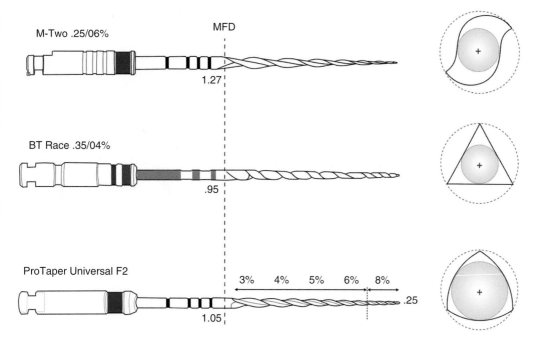

Figure 4.42 Cross-sections and maximal flute diameters (MFDs) of different finishing instruments.

increased flexibility near the tip and improved removal of debris coronally.

- Radial lands thought to produce a centric preparation and positive rake angle predisposing to excessive file engagement were abandoned in favour of neutral or even negative rake angles.

- Almost all file systems on the market use instruments with a fixed >2% taper. However, some feature variable tapers (increasing or decreasing) along their active portion.

Whilst older systems used a pecking motion or fed the blades into the canal walls during

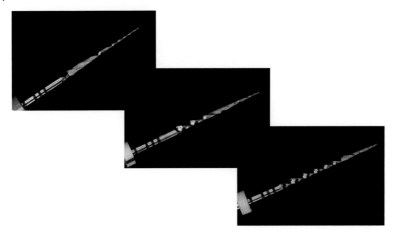

Figure 4.43 Accumulation of debris in the flutes of ProTaper instruments according to specific cutting locations. *Source:* Laurence Jordan.

insertion and then moved to a less tapered instrument when the present one stalled, more modern systems use an active-side brushing action on withdrawal following passive insertion into the canal.

Launched in 2001, the ProTaper system (Dentsply Sirona/Maillefer) still stands apart [115] in employing a universal instrument sequence whatever the clinical situation and in its unique variable taper design on the instruments active portion. Above all, it is distinguished by its method of use. Rather than needing to employ a crown-down technique, ProTaper instruments may be used one after another at the same working length. The cutting action occurs on the oustroke, each path of the shaping instrument facilitating its deeper and passive placement, resuming the work of a series of reamer in the original Schilder's technique. The finishing instruments can then be used in a single-path insertion to produce the so-called deep shape and blend the apical third with the already enlarged coronal two-thirds (Figures 4.43 and 4.44).

A few years later, a major step forward in the evolution of the preparation technique was represented by the use of reciprocating instruments in a single-instrument technique, either by alternative rotations (WaveOne, Dentsply-Maillefer; Reciproc, VDW) [12] or by

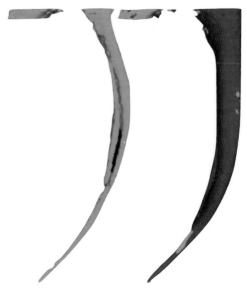

Figure 4.44 Pre- and post-instrumentation microCT reconstructions of canals, showing the continuously tapered preparation obtained with ProTaper rotary files. *Source:* Unpublished data reprinted with the permission of P. Lambrecht and L. Bergmans.

up-and-down vibrations (SAF, ReDent Nova) [13]. Unfortunately, these modifications of kinematics could not be considered a universal solution. If the alternative rotation improved safety regarding the risk of instrument separation and canal transportation, especially in the hands of beginners [116], it did not lead to a

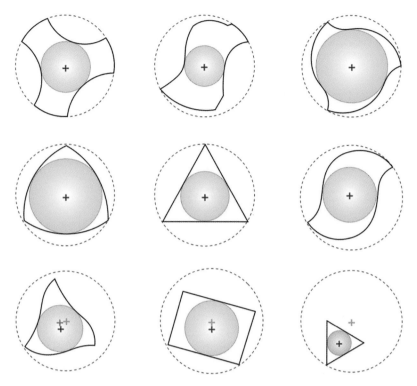

Figure 4.45 Evolution of cross-section designs over the years. Top: 1990s – ProFile, Quantec, HeRo. Middle: 2000s – ProTaper, RaCE, M-Two. Bottom: 2010s – RevoS, ProTaper Next, XP-endo Shaper.

major improvement in terms of cleaning results with regards to the variety of root canal dimensions, whilst at the same time increasing the amount of apically extruded debris [117]. The unpredictability of canal shape obtained during the expansion of the instrument and the need for a specific motor to operate it limited the general acceptance of the SAF, even if the results in terms of surface instrumentation and cleanliness were promising [118, 119].

Since then, research and development efforts have been focused towards two points: limiting the central mass of the instrument with respect to its outer section and minimizing wall engagement by reducing the surface of the blades. Improvements made in the micromilling process have allowed the manufacture of ever more sophisticated cross-section designs: offset mass of rotation, asymmetric core design, recessed blades, and alternative cutting edges (Figures 4.45–4.47).

Single use of instruments and thermomechanical treatment of the alloy (both pre- and post-machining), which drastically improves both flexibility and resistance to fracture [9, 76], are the two main factors which explain why safety is no longer an issue, even when attempting to shape severely curved canals. All instruments remain well centred in the canal [120, 121], and fractures only occur where there is a lack of respect for procedures.

Marketing-driven propositions for new instrument systems continue to be launched every year, often before being properly tested. Instrumental sequences are simplified to the extreme, and the time required to shape a canal has shortened so much that questions can be raised about the effectiveness of these mechanized preparations in terms of cleaning and disinfection [122–124]. Indeed, where shaping is centred in the canal, more than a

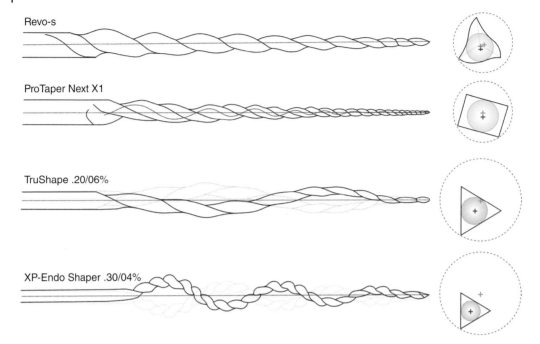

Figure 4.46 Different presentations of off-centred cross-section designs.

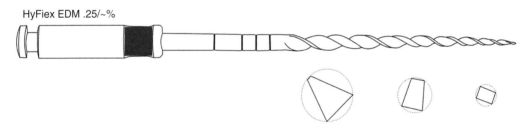

Figure 4.47 Example of an instrument with variable cross-sections along its active part.

third of the canal wall surfaces remain uninstrumented [125, 126], whilst debris and smear layers are allowed to accumulate [118]. The goal of shaping should not be to instrument the canal *per se* [127], but to facilitate its cleaning (and possibly disinfection) and to seal it as tightly as possible! The conceptual revolution is yet to come: instrumentation should be kept to a minimum, and new irrigation devices and smart sealers used to effectively clean and seal the canal space.

4.4 Conclusion

Whilst advances in the biological sciences hold the promise for a regeneration of the pulp tissue in the near future, endodontic treatment of the irreversibly diseased pulp still relies on methodical root canal debridement and disinfection, followed by the placement of an impervious seal to prevent reinfection of the immunologically deprived root canal system. Thus, appropriate root canal enlargement by shaping with root canal instrumentation should be considered the best way to facilitate cleaning and disinfection by irrigating solutions and obturation by filling materials. Although progress is being made in the manufacture of safer and better instruments, the fundamental role of shaping in the success of endodontic treatment must not be minimized, as biological prognosis is closely related to achievement of the technical objectives of root canal preparation.

Root canal instrumentation will thus continue to be the accepted means of restoring or maintaining the health of an endodontically compromised tooth, for the time being at least.

References

1 ISO/DIS 3630-5 (2019). Dentistry – endodontic instruments — Part 5: Shaping and cleaning instruments.

2 Ingle, J.I. (1955). The need for endodontic instrument standardization. *Oral Surg. Oral Med. Oral Pathol.* 8 (11): 1211–1213.

3 Ingle, J.I. and Levine, M. (1958). The need for uniformity of endodontic instruments, equipment and filling materials. In: *Transactions of the Second International Conference on Endodontics* (ed. L.I. Grossman), 123–140. Philadelphia, PA: University of Pennsylvania Printing Office.

4 Ingle, J.I. (1961). A standardized endodontic technique utilizing newly designed instruments and filling materials. *Oral Surg. Oral Med. Oral Pathol.* 14 (1): 83–91.

5 ISO/DIS 3630-1 (2019). Dentistry – endodontic instruments — Part 1: General requirements.

6 Council on Dental Materials, Instruments, and Equipment (1989). Revised ANSI/ADA specifications no. 28 for root canal files and reamers, type K, and No. 58 for root canal files, type H (Hedstrom). *J. Am. Dent. Assoc.* 118 (2): 239–240.

7 Thompson, S.A. (2000). An overview of nickel–titanium alloys used in dentistry. *Int. Endod. J.* 33 (4): 297–310.

8 Walia, H.M., Brantley, W.A., and Gerstein, H. (1988). An initial investigation of the bending and torsional properties of nitinol root canal files. *J. Endod.* 14 (7): 346–351.

9 Kuhn, G. and Jordan, L. (2002). Fatigue and mechanical properties of nickel–titanium endodontic instruments. *J. Endod.* 28 (10): 716–720.

10 Johnson, E., Lloyd, A., Kuttler, S., and Namerow, K. (2008). Comparison between a novel nickel–titanium alloy and 508 nitinol on the cyclic fatigue life of ProFile 25/.04 rotary instruments. *J. Endod.* 34 (11): 1406–1409.

11 Gambarini, G., Grande, N.M., Plotino, G. et al. (2008). Fatigue resistance of engine-driven rotary nickel–titanium instruments produced by new manufacturing methods. *J. Endod.* 34 (8): 1003–1005.

12 Yared, G. (2008). Canal preparation using only one Ni-Ti rotary instrument: preliminary observations. *Int. Endod. J.* 41 (4): 339–344.

13 Metzger, Z., Teperovich, E., Zary, R. et al. (2010). The self-adjusting file (SAF). Part 1: Respecting the root canal anatomy – a new concept of endodontic files and its implementation. *J. Endod.* 36 (4): 679–690.

14 Zhou, H.M., Shen, Y., Zheng, W. et al. (2012). Mechanical properties of controlled memory and superelastic nickel–titanium wires used in the manufacture of rotary endodontic instruments. *J. Endod.* 38 (11): 1535–1540.

15 Plotino, G., Grande, N.M., Cotti, E. et al. (2014). Blue treatment enhances cyclic fatigue resistance of vortex nickel–titanium rotary files. *J. Endod.* 40 (9): 1451–1453.

16 Pirani, C., Iacono, F., Generali, L. et al. (2016). HyFlex EDM: superficial features, metallurgical analysis and fatigue resistance of innovative electro discharge machined NiTi rotary instruments. *Int. Endod. J.* 49 (5): 483–493.

17 Elnaghy, A. and Elsaka, S. (2018). Cyclic fatigue resistance of XP-endo Shaper compared with different nickel–titanium alloy instruments. *Clin. Oral Investig.* 22 (3): 1433–1437.

18 Zupanc, J., Vahdat-Pajouh, N., and Schafer, E. (2018). New thermomechanically treated NiTi alloys – a review. *Int. Endod. J.* 51 (10): 1088–1103.

19 Oliet, S. and Sorin, S.M. (1978). Inhibition of the corrosive effect of sodium hypochlorite on carbon steel endodontic instruments. *J. Endod.* 4 (1): 12–16.

20 Craig, R.G. and Peyton, F.A. (1963). Physical properties of stainless steel endodontic files and reamers. *Oral Surg. Oral Med. Oral Pathol.* 16 (2): 206–217.

21 Kauffmann, G.B. and Mayo, I. (1997). The story of nitinol: the serendipitous discovery of the memory metal and its applications. *Chem. Educ.* 2 (2): 1–21.

22 Andreasen, G.F. and Brady, P.R. (1972). A use hypothesis for 55 nitinol wire for orthodontics. *Angle Orthod.* 42 (2): 172–177.

23 Duering, T., Pelton, A., and Stockel, D. (1999). An overview of nitinol medical applications. *Mater. Sci. Eng. A* 273–275: 149–160.

24 Zinelis, S., Magnissalis, E.A., Margelos, J., and Lambrianidis, T. (2002). Clinical relevance of standardization of endodontic files dimensions according to the ISO 3630-1 specification. *J. Endod.* 28 (5): 367–370.

25 McSpadden, J.T. (2007). Mastering endodontic instrumentation. Cloudland Institute.

26 Miserendino, L.J., Moser, J.B., Heuer, M.A., and Osetek, E.M. (1985). Cutting efficiency of endodontic instruments. Part 1: A quantitative comparison of the tip and fluted regions. *J. Endod.* 11 (10): 435–441.

27 Roane, J.B., Sabala, C.L., and Duncanson, M.G. Jr. (1985). The 'balanced force' concept for instrumentation of curved canals. *J. Endod.* 11 (5): 203–211.

28 Powell, S.E., Simon, J.H., and Maze, B.B. (1986). A comparison of the effect of modified and nonmodified instrument tips on apical canal configuration. *J. Endod.* 12 (7): 293–300.

29 Lopes, H.P., Elias, C.N., Mangelli, M. et al. (2012a). Buckling resistance of pathfinding endodontic instruments. *J. Endod.* 38 (3): 402–404.

30 Lopes, H.P., Elias, C.N., Siqueira, J.F. Jr. et al. (2012b). Mechanical behavior of pathfinding endodontic instruments. *J. Endod.* 38 (10): 1417–1421.

31 West, J.D. (2010). The endodontic glide path: 'secret to rotary safety'. *Dent. Today* 29 (9): 86, 88, 90–93.

32 Schilder, H. (1974). Cleaning and shaping the root canal. *Dent. Clin. N. Am.* 18 (2): 269–296.

33 Tepel, J. and Schäfer, E. (1997). Endodontic hand instruments: cutting efficiency, instrumentation of curved canals, bending and torsional properties. *Endod. Dent. Traumatol.* 13 (5): 201–210.

34 Lautenschlager, E.P., Jacobs, J.J., Marshall, G.W. Jr., and Heuer, M.A. (1977). Brittle and ductile torsional failures of endodontic instruments. *J. Endod.* 3 (5): 175–178.

35 Bishop, K. and Dummer, P.M. (1997). A comparison of stainless steel Flexofiles and nickel–titanium NiTiFlex files during the shaping of simulated canals. *Int. Endod. J.* 30 (1): 25–34.

36 Stenman, E. and Spangberg, L.S. (1990). Machining efficiency of endodontic K files and Hedstrom files. *J. Endod.* 16 (8): 375–382.

37 Elliott, L.M., Curtis, R.V., and Pitt Ford, T.R. (1998). Cutting pattern of nickel–titanium files using two preparation techniques. *Endod. Dent. Traumatol.* 14 (1): 10–15.

38 Royal, J.R. and Donnelly, J.C. (1995). A comparison of maintenance of canal curvature using balanced-force instrumentation with three different file types. *J. Endod.* 21 (6): 300–304.

39 Hou, X., Yahata, Y., Hayashi, Y. et al. (2011). Phase transformation behaviour and bending property of twisted nickel–titanium endodontic instruments. *Int. Endod. J.* 44 (3): 253–258.

40 Hieawy, A., Haapasalo, M., Zhou, H. et al. (2015). Phase transformation behavior and resistance to bending and cyclic fatigue of ProTaper Gold and ProTaper Universal instruments. *J. Endod.* 41 (7): 1134–1138.

41 Kolli, S., Balasubramanian, S.K., Kittappa, K., and Mahalaxmi, S. (2018). Efficacy of XP-endo finisher file in endodontics. *Aust. Endod. J.* 44 (1): 71–72.

42 Azim, A.A., Piasecki, L., da Silva Neto, U.X. et al. (2017). XP shaper, a novel adaptive core rotary instrument: micro-computed tomographic analysis of its shaping abilities. *J. Endod.* 43 (9): 1532–1538.

43 Velozo, C. and Albuquerque, D. (2019). Microcomputed tomography studies of the effectiveness of XP-endo Shaper in root canal preparation: a review of the literature. *Sci. World J.* 2019: 3570870.

44 Ruddle, C.J., Machtou, P., and West, J.D. (2014). Endodontic canal preparation: innovations in glide path management and shaping canals. *Dent. Today* 33 (7): 118–123.

45 Ruddle, C.J. (2016). Single-file shaping technique: achieving a gold medal result. *Dent. Today* 35 (1): 98, 100, 102–103.

46 De-Deus, G., Silva, E.J., Vieira, V.T. et al. (2017). Blue thermomechanical treatment optimizes fatigue resistance and flexibility of the Reciproc files. *J. Endod.* 43 (3): 462–466.

47 Fangli, T., Maki, K., Kimura, S. et al. (2019). Assessment of mechanical properties of WaveOne Gold Primary reciprocating instruments. *Dent. Mater. J.* 38 (3): 490–495.

48 Martin, H. and Cunningham, W. (1985). Endosonics – the ultrasonic synergistic system of endodontics. *Endod. Dent. Traumatol.* 1 (6): 201–206.

49 Lumley, P.J. (1997). Cutting ability of Heliosonic, Rispisonic, and Shaper files. *J. Endod.* 23 (4): 221–224.

50 Haikel, Y., Serfaty, R., Wilson, P. et al. (1998). Mechanical properties of nickel–titanium endodontic instruments and the effect of

sodium hypochlorite treatment. *J. Endod.* 24 (11): 731–735.

51 Glosson, C.R., Haller, R.H., Dove, S.B., and Del Rio, C.E. (1995). A comparison of root canal preparations using NiTi hand, NiTi engine-drivenn K-flex endodontic instruments. *J. Endod.* 21 (3): 146–151.

52 Kavanagh, D. and Lumley, P.J. (1998). An in vitro evaluation of canal preparation using profile .04 and .06 taper instruments. *Endod. Dent. Traumatol.* 14: 16–20.

53 Haapasalo, M. and Shen, Y. (2013). Evolution of nickel–titanium instruments: from past to future. *Endod. Top.* 29 (1): 3–17.

54 Guenin, G. (1996). Alliages à mémoire de forme. Tech Ing – Matér Act Intell. M530.

55 Keles, A., Ozyurek, E.U., Uyanik, M.O., and Nagas, E. (2019). Effect of temperature of sodium hypochlorite on cyclic fatigue resistance of heat-treated reciprocating files. *J. Endod.* 45 (2): 205–208.

56 Uslu, G., Özyürek, T., and Yilmaz, K. (2018). Comparison of alterations in the surface topographies of HyFlex CM and HyFlex EDM nickel–titanium files after root canal preparation: a three-dimensional optical profilometry study. *J. Endod.* 44 (1): 115–119.

57 Jordan, L., Vermaut, P., Prima, F., and Portier, R. (2013). Un point sur no. 18: les alliages à mémoire de forme. *Actual. Chim.* 371–372: 119–120.

58 Peters, O.A. (2004). Current challenges and concepts in the preparation of root canal systems: a review. *J. Endod.* 30 (8): 559–567.

59 Schäfer, E., Schulz-Bongert, U., and Tulus, G. (2004). Comparison of hand stainless steel and nickel titanium rotary instrumentation: a clinical study. *J. Endod.* 30: 432–438.

60 Gotthard, R. and Lehnert, T. (2001). Alliages à mémoire de forme. In: *Traité des matériaux no. 19: Matériaux émergents* (eds. C. Janot and B. Ilschner), 81–105. Lausanne: Presses polytechniques et universitaires romandes.

61 Jordan, L., Sultan, A., and Vermaut, P. (2015). Microstructural and mechanical characterizations of new Ni-Ti endodontic instruments. *MATEC Web Conf.* 33: 3005.

62 Pelton, A.R., Russell, S.M., and DiCello, J. (2003). The physical metallurgy of nitinol for medical applications. *JOM* 55 (5): 33–37.

63 Kuhn, G., Tavernier, B., and Jordan, L. (2001). Influence of structure on nickel–titanium endodontic instruments failure. *J. Endod.* 27 (8): 516–520.

64 Valois, C.R., Silva, L.P., and Azevedo, R.B. (2005). Atomic force microscopy study of stainless-steel and nickel–titanium files. *J. Endod.* 31: 882–885.

65 Anderson, M.E., Price, J.W., and Parahos, P. (2007). Fracture resistance of electropolished rotary nickel–titanium endodontic instruments. *J. Endod.* 33: 1212–1216.

66 Lopes, H.P., Elias, C.N., Vieira, V.T.L. et al. (2010). Effects of electropolishing surface treatment on the cyclic fatigue resistance of BioRace nickel–titanium rotary instruments. *J. Endod.* 36: 1653–1657.

67 Pedullà, E., Lo Savio, F., Boninelli, S. et al. (2016). Torsional and cyclic fatigue resistance of a new nickel–titanium instrument manufactured by electrical discharge machining. *J. Endod.* 21 (1): 156–159.

68 Adiguzel, M. and Capar, I.D. (2017). Comparaison of cyclic fatigue resistance of wave one and wave one gold small, primary, and large instruments. *J. Endod.* 43 (4): 623–627.

69 AlShwaimi, S.A. (2000). An overview of nickel–titanium alloys used in dentistry. *Int. Endod. J.* 33 (4): 297–310.

70 Capar, I.D., Ertas, H., and Arslan, H. (2015). Comparison of cyclic fatigue resistance of novel nickel–titanium rotary instruments: cyclic fatigue of novel instruments. *Aust. Endod. J.* 41 (1): 24–28.

71 Goo, H.-J., Kwak, S.W., Ha, J.-H. et al. (2017). Mechanical properties of various heat-treated nickel–titanium rotary instruments. *J. Endod.* 43 (11): 1872–1877.

72 Shen, Y., Qian, W., Abtin, H. et al. (2012). Effect of environment on fatigue failure of controlled memory wire nickel–titanium rotary instruments. *J. Endod.* 38 (3): 376–380.

73 Tobushi, H., Yamada, S., Hachisuka, T. et al. (1996). Thermomechanical properties due to martensitic and R-phase transformations of TiNi shape memory alloy subjected to cyclic loadings. *Smart Mater. Struct.* 5 (6): 788–795.

74 Wang, X.B., Verlinden, B., and Van Humbeeck, J. (2014). R-phase transformation in NiTi alloys. *Mater. Sci. Technol.* 30 (13): 1517–1529.

75 Pereira, E.S.J., Peixoto, I.F.C., Viana, A.C.D. et al. (2012). Physical and mechanical properties of a thermomechanically treated NiTi wire used in the manufacture of rotary endodontic instruments. *Int. Endod. J.* 45 (5): 469–474.

76 Miyai, K., Ebihara, A., Hayashi, Y. et al. (2006). Influence of phase transformation on the torsional and bending properties of nickel–titanium rotary endodontic instruments. *Int. Endod. J.* 39 (2): 119–126.

77 Elahinia, M.H., Hashemi, M., Tabesh, M., and Bhaduri, S.B. (2012). Manufacturing and processing of NiTi implants: a review. *Prog. Mater. Sci.* 57: 911–946.

78 Wang, X., Kustov, S., Li, K. et al. (2015). Effect of nanoprecipitates on the transformation behavior and functional properties of a Ti–50.8 at.% Ni alloy with micron-sized grains. *Acta Mater.* 82: 224–233.

79 Bahia, M.G.A., Martins, R.C., Gonzalez, B.M., and Buono, V.T.L. (2005). Physical and mechanical characterization and the influence of cyclic loading on the behaviour of nickel–titanium wires employed in the manufacture of rotary endodontic instruments. *Int. Endod. J.* 38 (11): 795–801.

80 Zinelis, S., Eliades, T., and Eliades, G. (2010). A metallurgical characterization of ten endodontic Ni-Ti instruments: assessing the clinical relevance of shape memory and superelastic properties of Ni-Ti endodontic instruments. *Int. Endod. J.* 43 (2): 125–134.

81 Ke, C.B., Cao, S., and Zhang, X.P. (2015). Phase field modeling of Ni-concentration distribution behavior around Ni4Ti3 precipitates in NiTi alloys. *Comput. Mater. Sci.* 105: 55–65.

82 Zayed, A.A.T. (2013). Investigation of fatigue life characteristics of micropatterned freestanding NiTi thin films. Thesis. Kiel: Christian-Albrechts-Universität.

83 Al-Hadlaq, S.M.S., AlJarbou, F.A., and AlThumairy, R.I. (2010). Evaluation of cyclic flexural fatigue of M-wire nickel–titanium rotary instruments. *J. Endod.* 36 (2): 305–307.

84 Gao, Y., Shotton, V., Wilkinson, K. et al. (2010). Effects of raw material and rotational speed on the cyclic fatigue of ProFile vortex rotary instruments. *J. Endod.* 36 (7): 1205–1209.

85 Elnaghy, A.M. and Elsaka, S.E. (2016). Mechanical properties of ProTaper Gold nickel–titanium rotary instruments. *Int. Endod. J.* 49 (11): 1073–1078.

86 Uygun, A.D., Kol, E., Topcu, M.K.C. et al. (2016). Variations in cyclic fatigue resistance among ProTaper Gold, ProTaper Next and ProTaper Universal instruments at different levels. *Int. Endod. J.* 49 (5): 494 9.

87 Simon, S., Machtou, P., and Pertot, W.-J. (2012). Endodontie. CDP (JPIO).

88 Sirtes, G., Waltimo, T., Schaetzle, M., and Zehnder, M. (2005). The effects of temperature on sodium hypochlorite short-term stability, pulp dissolution capacity, and antimicrobial efficacy. *J. Endod.* 31 (9): 669–671.

89 Alfawaz, H., Alqedairi, A., Alsharekh, H. et al. (2018). Effects of sodium hypochlorite concentration and temperature on the cyclic fatigue resistance of heat-treated nickel–titanium rotary instruments. *J. Endod.* 44 (10): 1563–1566.

90 Peters, O.A., Roehlike, J.O., and Baumann, M.A. (2007). Effect of immersion in sodium hypochlorite on torque and fatigue resistance of nickel–titanium instruments. *J. Endod.* 33 (5): 589–593.

91 Shen, Y., Huang, X., Wang, Z. et al. (2018). Low environmental temperature influences the fatigue resistance of nickel–titanium files. *J. Endod.* 44 (4): 626–629.

92 West, J.D. (2018). Restraint: the lost art of endodontics. *Dent. Today* 39 (5).

93 Roane, J.B. and Sabala, C. (1984). Clockwise or counterclockwise. *J. Endod.* 10 (8): 349–353.

94 Byström, A. and Sundqvist, G. (1983). Bacteriologic evaluation of the effect of 0.5 percent sodium hypochlorite in endodontic therapy. *Oral Surg. Oral Med. Oral Pathol.* 55 (3): 307–312.

95 Kerekes, K. and Tronstad, L. (1979). Long-term results of endodontic treatment performed with a standardized technique. *J. Endod.* 5 (3): 83–90.

96 Baugh, D. and Wallace, J. (2005). The role of apical instrumentation in root canal treatment: a review of the literature. *J. Endod.* 31 (5): 333–340.

97 Weine, F.S., Kelly, R.F., and Lio, P.J. (1975). The effect of preparation procedures on original canal shape and on apical foramen shape. *J. Endod.* 1 (8): 255–262.

98 Clem, W.H. (1969). Endodontics: the adolescent patient. *Dent. Clin. N. Am.* 13 (2): 482–493.

99 Martin, H. (1974). A telescopic technique for endodontics. *J. District Columbia Dent. Soc.* 49: 12.

100 Mullaney, T.P. (1979). Instrumentation of finely curved canals. *Dent. Clin. N. Am.* 23 (4): 575–592.

101 Walton, R. (1976). Histologic evaluation of different methods of enlarging the pulp canal space. *J. Endod.* 2 (10): 304–311.

102 Schilder, H. (1967). Filling root canals in three dimensions. *Dent. Clin. N. Am.*: 723–744.

103 Yu, D.C., Tam, A., and Schilder, H. (2009). Patency and envelope of motion – two essential procedures for cleaning and shaping the root canal systems. *Gen. Dent.* 57 (6): 616–621.

104 Marshall, F.J. and Papin, J. (1980). A Crown-Down Pressureless Preparation Root Canal Enlargement Technique. Technique manual. Portland, OR: Oregon Health Sciences University.

105 Morgan, L.F. and Montgomery, S. (1984). An evaluation of the crown-down

pressureless technique. *J. Endod.* 10 (10): 491–498.

106 Abou-Rass, M., Frank, A.L., and Glick, D.H. (1980). The anticurvature filing method to prepare the curved root canal. *J. Am. Dent. Assoc.* 101 (5): 792–794.

107 Goerig, A.C., Michelich, R.J., and Schultz, H.H. (1982). Instrumentation of root canals in molar using the step-down technique. *J. Endod.* 8 (12): 550–554.

108 Fava, L.R. (1983 Feb). The double-flared technique: an alternative for biomechanical preparation. *J. Endod.* 9 (2): 76–80.

109 Buchanan, L.S. (1996). The art of endodontics: files of greater taper. *Dent. Today* 15 (2): 42, 44–46, 48–49.

110 Parashos, P. and Messer, H.H. (2006). Rotary NiTi instrument fracture and its consequences. *J. Endod.* 32 (11): 1031–1043.

111 Spili, P., Parashos, P., and Messer, H.H. (2005). The impact of instrument fracture on outcome of endodontic treatment. *J. Endod.* 31 (12): 845–850.

112 Zhang, E.W., Cheung, G.S., and Zheng, Y.F. (2010). Influence of cross-sectional design and dimension on mechanical behavior of nickel–titanium instruments under torsion and bending: a numerical analysis. *J. Endod.* 36 (8): 1394–1398.

113 Pruett, J.P., Clement, D.J., and Carnes, D.L. Jr. (1997). Cyclic fatigue testing of nickel–titanium endodontic instruments. *J. Endod.* 23 (2): 77–85.

114 Sattapan, B., Palamara, J.E., and Messer, H.H. (2000). Torque during canal instrumentation using rotary nickel–titanium files. *J. Endod.* 26 (3): 156–160.

115 Machtou, P. and Ruddle, C.J. (2004). Advancements in the design of endodontic instruments for root canal preparation. *Alpha Omegan* 97 (4): 8–15.

116 Yang, Y., Shen, Y., Ma, J. et al. (2016). A micro-computed tomographic assessment of the influence of operator's experience on the quality of WaveOne instrumentation. *J. Endod.* 42 (8): 1258–1262.

117 Caviedes-Bucheli, J., Castellanos, F., Vasquez, N. et al. (2016). The influence of two reciprocating single-file and two rotary-file systems on the apical extrusion of debris and its biological relationship with symptomatic apical periodontitis. A systematic review and meta-analysis. *Int. Endod. J.* 49 (3): 255–270.

118 Paqué, F., Al-Jadaa, A., and Kfir, A. (2012). Hard-tissue debris accumulation created by conventional rotary versus self-adjusting file instrumentation in mesial root canal systems of mandibular molars. *Int. Endod. J.* 45 (5): 413–418.

119 Peters, O.A., Boessler, C., and Paqué, F. (2010). Root canal preparation with a novel nickel–titanium instrument evaluated with micro-computed tomography: canal surface preparation over time. *J. Endod.* 36 (6): 1068–1072.

120 Gagliardi, J., Versiani, M.A., de Sousa-Neto, M.D. et al. (2015). Evaluation of the shaping characteristics of ProTaper Gold, ProTaper NEXT, and ProTaper Universal in curved canals. *J. Endod.* 41 (10): 1718–1724.

121 Zhao, D., Shen, Y., Peng, B., and Haapasalo, M. (2014). Root canal preparation of mandibular molars with 3 nickel–titanium rotary instruments: a micro-computed tomographic study. *J. Endod.* 40 (11): 1860–1864.

122 Card, S.J., Sigurdsson, A., Orstavik, D., and Trope, M. (2002). The effectiveness of increased apical enlargement in reducing intracanal bacteria. *J. Endod.* 28 (11): 779–783.

123 Dalton, B.C., Orstavik, D., Phillips, C. et al. (1998). Bacterial reduction with nickel–titanium rotary instrumentation. *J. Endod.* 24 (11): 763–767.

124 Gazzaneo, I., Vieira, G.C.S., Pérez, A.R. et al. (2019). Root canal disinfection by single- and multiple-instrument systems: effects of sodium hypochlorite volume, concentration, and retention time. *J. Endod.* 45 (6): 736–741.

125 Almeida, B.M., Provenzano, J.C., Marceliano-Alves, M.F. et al. (2019). Matching the dimensions of currently available instruments with the apical diameters of mandibular molar mesial root canals obtained by micro-computed tomography. *J. Endod.* 45 (6): 756–760.

126 Peters, O.A., Schönenberger, K., and Laib, A. (2001). Effects of four Ni-Ti preparation techniques on root canal geometry assessed by micro computed tomography. *Int. Endod. J.* 34 (3): 221–230.

127 Spangberg, L. (2001). The wonderful world of rotary root canal preparation. *Oral Surg. Oral Med. Oral Pathol. Oral Radiol. Endod.* 92 (5): 479.

5

Irrigating Solutions, Devices, and Techniques

Christos Boutsioukis[1] and Maria Teresa Arias-Moliz[2]

[1] Department of Endodontology, Academic Centre for Dentistry Amsterdam (ACTA), University of Amsterdam and Vrije Universiteit Amsterdam, Amsterdam, The Netherlands
[2] Department of Microbiology, Faculty of Dentistry, University of Granada, Granada, Spain

---

TABLE OF CONTENTS

Endodontic Materials in Clinical Practice, First Edition. Edited by Josette Camilleri.
© 2021 John Wiley & Sons Ltd. Published 2021 by John Wiley & Sons Ltd.

5.1 Introduction

Irrigation plays a pivotal role in root canal treatment [1, 2]. A considerable part of the root canal system is beyond the reach of instruments [3], so their main role is to provide radicular access in order to facilitate irrigant delivery [1]. Irrigating solutions are therefore expected to kill microorganisms and disrupt the biofilm in most of the root canal system (Figure 5.1), inactivate virulence factors such as endotoxin, dissolve pulp-tissue remnants, remove hard-tissue debris and the smear layer created during instrumentation or prevent their formation, provide lubrication for instruments, and be biocompatible and easily available at low cost [1, 2, 4]. Amongst all these requirements, the strong antimicrobial effect is arguably the most important. However, even the best irrigating solution will not fulfil these goals if it cannot reach bacteria and tissue remnants inside the root canal system in sufficient amounts. Therefore, effective irrigant delivery and activation/agitation techniques are equally important, in order to ensure that the solutions are delivered throughout the root canal system and adequately refreshed so that a high concentration of their active components is maintained. Irrigation techniques must also create a flow that carries bacteria, biofilm fragments, and tissue remnants out of the root canal; this can contribute to the mechanical cleaning. Finally, the action of irrigating solutions should be limited within the constraints of the root canal system [5].

In order to reach all these goals, a wide variety of solutions and techniques have been proposed for root canal irrigation, and new ones are constantly being introduced. Not all solutions and techniques are equally effective or popular, however, so this chapter will focus only on the most commonly used or known ones. Furthermore, where possible, these will be compared to the current clinical standards, with which most readers are expected to have some experience; that is, sodium hypochlorite (NaOCl), ethylenediamine tetraacetic acid (EDTA), syringe irrigation, and ultrasonic activation.

5.2 Irrigating Solutions

5.2.1 Sodium Hypochlorite

NaOCl is the most popular irrigating solution in use today, and is considered the primary irrigant of choice during chemomechanical preparation [6]. Its active chemical compound is the free available chlorine, consisting of the hypochlorite ion (OCl^-) and hypochlorous acid (HOCl) [7]. The hypochlorite ion prevails in alkaline solutions (pH > 7.6) and has a powerful oxidative effect which is responsible for a tissue-dissolving activity, whereas the hypochlorous acid predominates in more acidic solutions (pH < 7.6) and has a stronger bactericidal effect, possibly because it is a smaller uncharged molecule that easily penetrates the bacterial membrane and disrupts proteins [8]. Lowering the pH renders the solution more unstable without a clear benefit in terms of antimicrobial activity, whilst maintaining a stable high pH can increase the proteolytic action of the solution and improve the chemical debridement of the root canal [9, 10].

NaOCl possesses several of the properties of an ideal root canal irrigant [2]. Due to the free

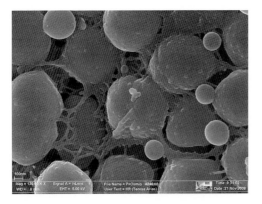

Figure 5.1 Scanning electron microscope photograph of a 24-hour bacterial biofilm grown on dentine. A characteristic network of polysaccharides covering the bacteria is starting to be formed. *Source:* Maria Teresa Arias-Moliz.

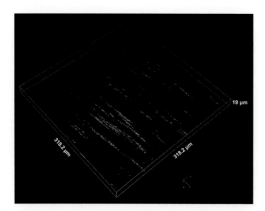

Figure 5.2 Dentinal tubules contaminated with *Enterococcus faecalis* after treatment with 2.5% NaOCl for three minutes. Red-coloured bacteria are cells with damaged membranes, whilst green-coloured bacteria are cells with intact membranes viewed under a confocal laser scanning microscope following LIVE/DEAD staining (BacLight; Invitrogen, Eugene, OR, USA). The pulpal side is at the upper left side of the specimen. *Source:* Maria Teresa Arias-Moliz.

available chlorine, it exerts a strong antimicrobial effect against both planktonic and biofilm bacteria (Figure 5.2) [11–16], and it can also dissolve pulp-tissue remnants [17–19]. In addition, it reduces bacterial virulence factors related to periapical inflammation and clinical symptoms, such as endotoxins and lipoteichoic acids [20]. The main disadvantages of NaOCl are that it cannot dissolve hard-tissue debris and the inorganic components of the smear layer, and it is caustic to soft tissues, leading to rapid haemolysis, ulceration, inhibition of neutrophil migration, and destruction of endothelial and fibroblast cells [21]. Thus, inadvertent extrusion towards the periapical tissues through the apical foramen or a perforation may result in a *NaOCl accident* [22, 23]. Accidental ingestion of small amounts of NaOCl during root canal treatment due to insufficient isolation is unlikely to have any clinically significant effect, but it should nevertheless be prevented [24]. Prolonged skin contact may cause irritation or dermal hypersensitivity [24], whilst contact with the eye may cause a chemical burn [25, 26]. Moreover,

NaOCl is a very reactive solution; in addition to bacteria and pulp-tissue remnants [27–29], it reacts strongly with the proteins in the dentine matrix, possibly altering the mechanical properties of the latter [30], and also with most other irrigants, so the available chlorine is rapidly consumed in the root canal [31–33]. Therefore, it has a strong but short-term effect and is not suitable for use as an inter-appointment medicament.

Concentrations ranging from 0.5 to 6% have been proposed for use during root canal treatment. The desirable effects of NaOCl are concentration-dependent, becoming stronger with increasing concentration [11, 34] – but so too are its undesirable effects [30, 35, 36]. In order to compensate for the rapid consumption of the free available chlorine in the root canal, frequent exchange with large volumes of fresh irrigant is advocated [27-29, 37]. To date, however, there are no specific guidelines concerning the optimum concentration, volume, and contact time, arguably because of the highly variable clinical situation with regard to the microbial load, anatomy, amount of pulp-tissue remnants, and so on.

In order to improve the effectiveness of NaOCl without increasing its concentration, preheating of the solution to 50–60 °C prior to irrigation has been suggested [38]. The temperature increase seems to amplify its antimicrobial activity [18, 39], as well as its ability to dissolve pulp tissue [18, 34, 40] and the organic component of the smear layer [41]. However, the clinical relevance of this additional step is questionable, since the temperature of the solution drops to 37 °C very soon after intracanal delivery *in vivo* [42]. Heating of NaOCl *in situ* (inside the root canal) has been proposed as an alternative to extraoral preheating [43, 44], but the efficacy and the potential side effects of this method have not yet been fully evaluated.

Finally, NaOCl is inexpensive and widely available. The amount of free available chlorine in solutions obtained from domestic sources is unpredictable, so professional sources should be preferred [45]. Even though it has demonstrated an acceptable shelf-life [46], stored NaOCl solutions become unstable when in contact with organic matter, light, and other chemicals, which accelerates the loss of free available chlorine [31, 47]. Storage in opaque nonreactive bottles with air-tight caps placed in a cool, dark place is therefore crucial [48].

5.2.2 Chlorhexidine

Chlorhexidine gluconate (CHX) is a cationic bisbiguanide with an antimicrobial activity against bacteria, yeast, and fungi, particularly *Candida albicans* [15, 49, 50]. The CHX molecule has the ability to bind to the negatively charged microbial cell walls, thereby altering their osmotic equilibrium [51]. At low concentrations, it exerts a bacteriostatic effect, leaking low-molecular-weight substances out of the microorganisms, whereas at higher concentrations it has a bactericidal one, due to precipitation or coagulation of the bacterial cytoplasm components [52, 53].

CHX has been proposed for root canal irrigation at a concentration of 2% [2, 54, 55]. Its antimicrobial activity is stronger against planktonic bacteria than biofilms, probably because of its interaction with the biofilm exopolymeric matrix, which hinders the molecules' diffusion towards the microbial cells [56, 57]. It is generally considered less effective than NaOCl [15, 58, 59], although a systematic review of clinical studies found some controversy on this matter [60]. It can reduce the endotoxin levels in infected root canals after chemomechanical preparation, although this effect is also lower than with NaOCl [61]. In addition, it exerts no dissolution effect against either soft or hard tissues [17, 62]. These disadvantages are the main reasons why NaOCl is preferred as the primary irrigant during root canal treatment [2], except in cases of hypersensitivity to NaOCl [63].

Nevertheless, CHX has some important advantages. For instance, it can be adsorbed to negatively charged surfaces such as the dentine matrix and slowly released back into the root canal, thereby maintaining antimicrobial activity for several hours up to a few weeks [64–69]. This property is known as *substantivity* and is claimed to be CHX's main advantage over NaOCl [66, 67, 70]. It appears to last longest when the application time of CHX is prolonged [64, 69, 71] or when dentine collagen is exposed in the root canal during application [68]. However, it should be noted that many of the studies on this topic have not examined substantivity under clinically realistic conditions.

Another advantage is that CHX does not react with the collagen in the dentine matrix and consequently does not affect its structure, in contrast to NaOCl [72]. Moreover, it inhibits the bacteria-related activation of dentine matrix metalloproteinases (MMPs), enzymes involved in collagen-network degradation within the hybrid layer [73, 74], so it can prolong the integrity and durability of the resin–dentine bond [67]. Finally, CHX has not been associated with adverse side effects when used as a root canal irrigant [53], although it is cytotoxic to human fibroblasts and stem cells of the apical papilla [75, 76] – perhaps even to a greater degree than NaOCl [75, 77]. In addition, it reacts with residual NaOCl in the root canal and forms an orange-brown precipitate [32, 78].

5.2.3 Ethylenediamine Tetraacetic Acid

EDTA is a chelating agent that binds metal ions, such as Ca^{++}, and forms soluble complexes [79]. Chelation is a self-limited process, so that when all the available ions have been bound, equilibrium is reached and no more chelation occurs [80]. EDTA is available in the form of various salts, such as disodium and tetrasodium EDTA [79]. The disodium salt at a concentration 15–17% has a neutral or slightly alkaline pH (~7–8), is a strong chelator, and is the most widely used form for root canal irrigation [6, 81]. It can dissolve hard-tissue debris

(a) (b) (c)

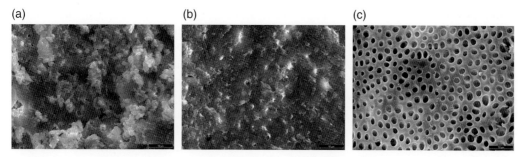

Figure 5.3 Scanning electron microscope photograph of a contaminated smear layer on dentine (a) before and (b) after treatment with 2.5% NaOCl or (c) after 2.5% NaOCl followed by a final flush with 17% EDTA. *Source:* Maria Teresa Arias-Moliz.

formed during root canal instrumentation and the inorganic components of the smear layer [82]. The solution is applied for one to five minutes [82–84], within which time it can demineralize dentine to a depth of 20–30 μm [85]. Prolonged contact with dentine can cause excessive demineralization and reduce its microhardness [85, 86].

Since EDTA acts only on the inorganic component of debris and the smear layer, it must be combined with NaOCl in order to remove them completely (Figure 5.3) [87, 88]. However, when NaOCl is used after EDTA, it attacks the exposed dentine collagen, causing erosion [89], which appears to be unfavourable for bonding [90, 91]. Moreover, EDTA reacts with NaOCl, causing a rapid loss of the free available chlorine [31, 32, 54, 92]. Consequently, the alternating use of NaOCl and EDTA during instrumentation [93], whether in a liquid or a gel form, is contraindicated. Moreover, gels containing EDTA or other chelators that are used in combination with rotary instruments do not reduce the stress applied to the instruments during root canal preparation, and in some cases may even increase it [94, 95]. Aqueous solutions are far more effective lubricants [94, 95], and this effect is mostly independent of the presence of EDTA [94], so NaOCl is currently considered a sufficient lubricant during rotary instrumentation [96]. Nevertheless, EDTA-containing gels may still be useful during the initial negotiation of calcified root canals.

EDTA has little or no antimicrobial activity [11, 97, 98], but its chelating action alters the outer membrane of Gram-negative bacteria [99] and destabilizes the biofilm matrix [57]. It also promotes the detachment of the biofilm [100] and the removal of bacteria present in the smear layer [101]. Some studies have further reported an antifungal action [102, 103]. EDTA exerts a very limited tissue-dissolving effect [104, 105]. It is less cytotoxic than NaOCl and CHX [75], and it lacks genotoxicity [106], but it affects the function and viability of macrophages [106, 107]. Moreover, it is inexpensive and widely available [108].

In contrast to disodium EDTA, the tetrasodium salt (Na_4EDTA) has a higher pH and is a weaker chelator [109]. Thus, when mixed with NaOCl, it does not consume the free available chlorine as rapidly as the disodium salt, and the mixture maintains the properties of both solutions in the short term [105, 110]. However, it should be used immediately, because of the gradual loss of available chlorine over time [105, 111]. Heating of the mixture must be avoided as it accelerates the chlorine loss [112].

5.2.4 Citric Acid

Citric acid (CA) is a weak tricarboxylic acid that can be used instead of EDTA for smear layer removal [113–115]. It sequesters Ca^{++} ions, forming a soluble chelate. Proposed concentrations range between 1 and 50%, although the most commonly used is 10% (pH 1.1–1.9) [116]. CA is more biocompatible and less cytotoxic than EDTA [117, 118]. It is also widely available and inexpensive. Nevertheless, it leaves precipitated crystals on the root canal wall, which may interfere with the filling [113]; it reduces dentine microhardness, although to a lesser extent than EDTA [119]; it causes more dentine erosion than EDTA and other chelators [89]; and it reacts with NaOCl, thereby rapidly consuming the available chlorine [31]. It has shown some antimicrobial activity against planktonic bacteria [97], which may derive from the alteration of cell membrane permeability due to a decrease in the internal pH of the microbial cells [120]. However, the effect against biofilms is very low [11]. Finally, CA lacks the ability to dissolve pulp tissue [17].

5.2.5 Etidronic Acid

1-Hydroxyethane 1,1-diphosphonic acid (HEDP), also known as etidronic acid or etidronate, is a mild chelating agent that has traditionally been used in water treatment [121] and the treatment of patients suffering from osteoporosis or Paget's disease [122, 123]. It is as effective as EDTA in removing the smear layer, but it requires longer application times (five versus one minute) [84]. It was the first weak chelating agent proposed for use in a mixture with NaOCl during root canal preparation under the concept of *continuous chelation*, in order to simplify the irrigation protocol [31]. The mixture maintains the desired properties of both compounds in the short term [12, 31, 59, 104, 111, 124–126], so it reduces smear-layer formation and hard-tissue debris accumulation [124, 125], dissolves pulp-tissue remnants [104, 126], and exerts a strong antimicrobial effect against biofilms on the dentine surface [59] and inside dentinal tubules [12], even in the presence of hard-tissue debris or a smear layer [19, 127, 128]. This antimicrobial effect appears to be at least

similar to that of a protocol including NaOCl followed by a final rinse with EDTA [16].

HEDP can be obtained in a pure form from various chemical producers, but it is also marketed specifically for root canal irrigation in the form of capsules to be mixed with NaOCl solutions (Dual Rinse HEDP; Medcem GmbH, Vienna, Austria). The mixture remains active for one hour at room temperature [111, 129], but storage at lower temperature maintains the free available chlorine for seven hours; heating has the opposite effect [129]. The presence of HEDP in a mixture does not increase its cytotoxicity [130], and no adverse effects have been observed so far during its clinical use [131]. Nevertheless, other weak chelators that can be used for continuous chelation are also under evaluation and may prove to perform better than it [132, 133].

5.2.6 Maleic Acid

Maleic acid (MA), a mild dicarboxylic acid, has also been proposed as an alternative to EDTA, given its capacity to remove the smear layer [134–137]. It is more biocompatible than EDTA [138, 139] and exerts a greater antimicrobial activity than either EDTA or CA against planktonic bacteria and biofilm [140, 141]. Its antimicrobial effect is also related to the internal pH reduction as a consequence of its low pH (~1.05) [120]. The concentration of choice for root canal irrigation is 7% [138], since higher concentrations can cause intertubular dentine damage [142].

5.2.7 Ozonated Water

Ozone (O_3) is a very reactive gas that is normally found in the atmosphere but can also be produced by a generator [143]. In the presence of water, it forms oxygen radicals, which penetrate the cell membranes, disturbing the osmotic balance and promoting the oxidation of aminoacids and nucleic acids [144]. Thus, ozonated water exerts an antimicrobial effect against bacteria, fungi, protozoa, and viruses, which motivates its use in water processing [145], the food industry [146], and the treatment of some diseases [147, 148]. However, its effectiveness against root canal infections is limited. A number of studies have shown that ozonated water is clearly less effective than NaOCl against both planktonic bacteria and biofilms [143, 149-151]. Moreover, it cannot neutralize endotoxin [152]. A recent systematic review concluded that, despite its low toxicity, ozonated water is not indicated for use as a root canal irrigant, whether as a replacement or an adjunct to NaOCl [153].

5.2.8 Electrochemically Activated Water

Electrochemically activated water (EAW) is produced by electrolysis of tap water or low-concentration salt solutions, such as saline, in special devices – a process similar to that used for large-scale production of NaOCl [154]. Two types of solutions are produced: an anolyte and a catholyte. The anolyte seems to contain HOCl and OCl$^-$, and its bactericidal potential is largely attributed to the presence of free available chlorine [155]. However, its concentration is typically much lower than that of NaOCl solutions [156]. The catholyte is alkaline and is claimed to have a cleaning or detergent effect [155, 157]. The antimicrobial effect of EAW against biofilms may be similar to that of NaOCl in the absence of dentine [158], but it is clearly inferior to it inside root canals [154, 159, 160]. In addition, EAW cannot dissolve pulp tissue [161].

5.2.9 Saline

Physiologic saline (0.9% NaCl) is an inert solution with no direct antimicrobial effect and no ability to dissolve pulp-tissue remnants or hard-tissue debris [2, 17]. It is often used as a control solution in experiments. Despite its lack of chemical activity, it can still exert a mechanical cleaning effect when flowing inside the root canal system [162, 163], and it

can act as a lubricant for rotary instruments [94, 95]. Nevertheless, it should not be used as a primary irrigant, only for intermediate flushing to prevent contact between two irrigants that react with each other (e.g. NaOCl and CHX) [164] or where there is a temporary need for an inert irrigant (e.g. after a NaOCl accident) [165].

5.2.10 Mixtures of Irrigating Solutions

None of the available irrigating solutions can satisfy all the requirements outlined at the beginning of this chapter, so mixtures containing more than one have been developed. Many of these include an antimicrobial or a chelating agent together with one or more surfactants, the latter being added in order to reduce the surface tension. Examples include Chlor-XTRa (Vista Dental, Racine, WI, USA), which contains 6% NaOCl, CHX-Plus (Vista Dental, Racine, WI, USA), which contains up to 2% CHX, and SmearClear (SybronEndo, Orange, CA, USA), which contains EDTA. A common misconception amongst dentists is that a reduction of the surface tension can improve the penetration of the mixture in the root canal system [166–169]. However, a decrease in the surface tension of an irrigant does not provide any clinically-relevant advantage. Surface tension only acts on interfaces between immiscible fluids, and there are no such interfaces limiting irrigant penetration in the root canal *in vivo* [170]. Nonetheless, several surfactants exert some direct antimicrobial effect independent of the surface tension reduction. Cetrimide (CTR), for example – a cationic surfactant widely used in mixtures with common irrigants – is known to be bactericidal and also decreases a biofilm's mechanical stability by weakening the cohesive forces within the exopolymeric matrix [171]. This additional effect may not be detectable in mixtures with strong antimicrobial solutions (e.g. NaOCl at high concentration), but it does seem to improve the antimicrobial action of weaker ones (e.g. CHX, EDTA, CA, MA) [15, 68, 141, 172, 173]. Its mixtures with chelators also seem to have a long residual effect [174, 175].

The literature shows that the addition of surfactants does not enhance the antimicrobial effect of NaOCl at high concentrations [172, 176, 177], nor its tissue-dissolution capacity [178–180]. To the contrary, it may actually accelerate the loss of free available chlorine [181]. The combination of 2% CHX with surfactants (CHX-Plus; Vista Dental) appears to have a stronger effect against biofilm than CHX alone [172, 182], but this is likely due to the additional antimicrobial effect of the surfactants [172]. Removal of calcium from dentine and removal of the smear layer also seem to be unaffected by the addition of surfactants to EDTA [183–185]. The same rationale applies to other mixtures containing surfactants together with antimicrobials and chelators (see later).

5.2.10.1 BioPure MTAD

BioPure MTAD (Denstply Sirona, Charlotte, NC, USA) is a mixture of 3% doxycycline, 4.25% CA, and 0.5% surfactant (Tween 80) [186]. It has been recommended for a final five-minute rinse (instead of EDTA) following chemomechanical preparation with 1.3% NaOCl in order to remove the smear layer [186] and supplement the disinfection of the root canal system [187, 188]. The removal of the smear layer has been attributed to the CA and doxycycline, but also to the low pH of the mixture (~2) [116, 187, 189]. Although some studies found that it caused only minimal changes in the dentinal tubule structure [187] and limited erosion [190], others reported that it demineralized dentine more aggressively than EDTA [191].

The antimicrobial activity of MTAD stems from the doxycycline, which has a bacteriostatic effect as well as a residual antimicrobial one over time (substantivity) [192, 193]. However, there is some controversy regarding the magnitude of these effects. Some studies – especially the earlier ones – reported very effective elimination of root canal bacteria [188, 194–197], but several others could not detect any advantage over commonly used irrigants such as NaOCl [98, 198–205]. It was also shown that irrigation with NaOCl prior to MTAD could reduce its substantivity considerably [201].

MTAD cannot dissolve pulp-tissue remnants [205]. Moreover, despite its good biocompatibility [206], it may cause tooth discolouration [207]. It is contraindicated during pregnancy, in children under eight years of age, and in patients with an allergy to doxycycline. It is also more expensive and has a shorter shelf-life than other commonly used root canal irrigants [208].

5.2.10.2 Tetraclean

Tetraclean (TC) (Ogna Laboratori Farmaceutici, Muggiò, Italy) is a mixture similar to MTAD but with a lower concentration of doxycycline (1%), a higher concentration of CA (10%), and two different surfactants: propylene glycol and cetrimide [168, 209–213]. It has also been proposed for a final five-minute rinse after NaOCl [209, 210] because it can remove the smear layer [168, 211] and it exerts an antimicrobial effect against the residual bacteria in the root canal [168, 209, 211]. This antimicrobial effect seems to be stronger than that of MTAD – probably because of the CTR in its composition [209, 210] – but still weaker than that of NaOCl [209]. Its substantivity appears to be greater than that of MTAD [212, 213], but it is decreases by a prior irrigation with NaOCl [214]. It has no tissue-dissolving capacity [209, 210].

The presence of doxycycline in the mixture can lead to similar problems to those of MTAD, such as tooth staining, bacterial resistance, and hypersensitivity [189, 207]. In order to overcome these, a modified mixture without any antibiotic was developed (Tetraclean NA; Ogna Laboratori Farmaceutici). Despite the absence of tetracycline, the modified mixture appears to exert a stronger antimicrobial effect against bacteria inside dentinal tubules compared to MTAD [203].

5.2.10.3 QMix

QMix (Denstply Sirona, Charlotte, NC, USA) is a mixture of 2% CHX, 17% EDTA, and CTR. It has a slightly alkaline pH and has been recommended as a final irrigating solution applied for two to five minutes after NaOCl in order to remove the smear layer and kill the remaining bacteria [205, 215]. It is as effective as EDTA in regard to chelation [205, 215]. It reduces the microhardness of dentine but doesn't seem to cause erosion [89]. It is more effective against biofilms than CHX and MTAD [205, 216], but less so than NaOCl [217–219]. It has also demonstrated a prolonged substantivity because of the presence of CHX in its composition [220], as well as good biocompatibility [221, 222].

5.2.11 Suggested Irrigation Protocol

In the absence of a single solution possessing all the characteristics of an ideal irrigant, it is necessary to use at least two in order to accomplish all the aims of root canal irrigation. There is a wide consensus that NaOCl should be used as the primary irrigant during access and chemomechanical preparation of the root canal [1, 2, 4, 6]. Frequent exchange with copious amounts of fresh irrigant and an extended application time may be required for the effective diffusion of the solution, its antimicrobial action against bacteria organized in biofilms, and the dissolution of pulp-tissue remnants and of the organic components of the smear layer. NaOCl is also considered an excellent means of lubrication for rotary instruments [94, 95]. Although hard-tissue debris packed in uninstrumented parts of the root canal system and the inorganic components of the smear layer also need to be removed, the alternating use of NaOCl and strong chelators during instrumentation is contraindicated, as already explained [31, 92, 132].

A chelator such as EDTA can be applied for a short time after instrumentation to achieve these goals and to partially disrupt the biofilm [57, 82, 100], but this step should not be considered a final rinse. Hard-tissue debris and the smear layer need to be removed mainly in order to allow NaOCl to penetrate deeper into uninstrumented areas and inside dentinal tubules, and NaOCl should always be reapplied after their removal in order to maximize its antimicrobial effect. Alternatively, a mixture of NaOCl and a weak chelator (e.g. HEDP) could be used throughout chemomechanical preparation for continuous chelation [16, 31, 132], but more evidence is needed regarding its performance and possible adverse effects.

It should be emphasized that the final irrigation protocol determines the condition of the dentine surface immediately prior to obturation, so it should take into account the requirements of the obturation materials. For instance, a final rinse with NaOCl seems to dissolve the exposed dentine collagen, which may be detrimental for certain types of root canal sealers that bind to these collagen fibres [90, 223, 224]. However, opposing views have also been expressed [225, 226]. A possible workaround could be to irrigate again with a chelator as a final step before root canal filling in order to expose a new layer of collagen.

5.3 Irrigation Techniques

Rather than categorizing irrigation techniques as either 'manual' or 'mechanically assisted' – a distinction that has very little practical use – it is more reasonable to categorize them as either 'irrigant delivery' or 'irrigant activation/agitation', because these two types of techniques serve different purposes. Delivery techniques aim to transport large amounts of irrigant primarily into the main root canal, whilst activation/agitation techniques aim to distribute an irrigant into the rest of the root canal system and to enhance cleaning and disinfection.

There seems also to be some confusion in the literature regarding the terms 'activation' and 'agitation', which are often used interchangeably. Several irrigation techniques are able to agitate an irrigant inside the root canal, albeit with varying degrees of effectiveness, but not all of them can actually activate one in a chemical way. Therefore, in this chapter, the term 'activation' will be reserved for those techniques that can produce transient cavitation bubbles which, upon collapse, may accelerate chemical reactions in their vicinity [227, 228]. All the irrigants described in the previous section may be transported with any of the delivery techniques described here, and most can be agitated/activated without problems; some notable exceptions are detailed later.

5.3.1 Irrigant Delivery Techniques

5.3.1.1 Syringe Irrigation

Syringe irrigation is a widely used technique for the delivery of irrigants inside root canals. It remains the most popular technique amongst both endodontists and general dentists [6, 81, 229, 230], possibly due to its simplicity and low cost and the wide availability of syringes and needles. Thus, it can be considered the current clinical standard. During syringe irrigation, an irrigant is transferred from the syringe to the root canal through a needle. The irrigant flows inside the root canal from the apical third towards the coronal third and normally exits through the root canal orifice, where it is usually evacuated by an aspirator tip. The cause of the flow is the pressure built up inside the syringe barrel due to the force applied to the plunger by the clinician. The positive pressure drives the irrigant through the needle, for which reason syringe irrigation is categorized as a *positive-pressure* irrigation method [231, 232].

5.3.1.1.1 Syringes Syringes used for root canal irrigation have a capacity between 1 and 20 ml (Figure 5.4) [233–240]. Apart from practical considerations such as the frequency of refilling, the choice of the syringe also depends on the strength of the clinician, the size and length of the needle, and the desired flow rate [170]. A larger syringe, a finer or longer needle, and a higher desired flow rate

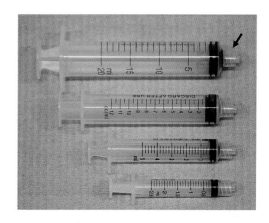

Figure 5.4 Syringes used for root canal irrigation. From top to bottom: 20, 12, 5, and 2.5 ml. All have a Luer-Lock threaded fitting (arrow). *Source:* Reprinted with permission from Springer. Boutsioukis, C., van der Sluis, L.W.M. Syringe irrigation: blending Endodontics and Fluid Dynamics. Chapter 3. In Basrani, B. ed. *Endodontic Irrigation: Chemical Disinfection of the Root Canal System.* New York, NY, USA: Springer, 2015:45–64.

all require a stronger force to be applied by the clinician on the syringe plunger during irrigation [170]. Syringes with a capacity of 5–10 ml appear to be a reasonable compromise. Battery-operated automated syringes have appeared on the market lately and may facilitate irrigation at a stable flow rate, but there are no studies as yet confirming this potential advantage. A secure Luer-Lock threaded fitting is necessary for all syringes and needles used for root canal irrigation, due to the high pressure inside the syringe barrel [241] which could lead to accidental detachment during irrigation [26].

5.3.1.1.2 Needles A wide variety of needles have been suggested for irrigant delivery during root canal treatment [235, 237, 242– 247]. These are typically made of stainless steel (Figure 5.5), but NiTi [248] and, more recently, plastic (Figure 5.6) have also been used in order to increase flexibility and facilitate irrigation in curved root canals. The diameter or size of a needle is often reported in 'gauge' units [248, 249]; a larger gauge number corresponds to a finer needle (Table 5.1). There

(a)   (b)   (c)   (d)   (e)

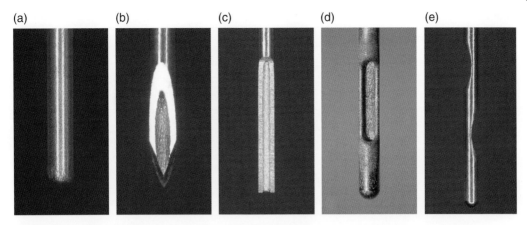

Figure 5.5   Various types of 30G stainless-steel needles used for root canal irrigation. Open-ended needles: (a) flat; (b) bevelled; (c) notched. Closed-ended needles: (d) side-vented; (e) double side-vented. Variable views and magnifications have been used to highlight differences in tip design. *Source:* Reprinted and modified with permission from Elsevier. Boutsioukis, C., Verhaagen, B., Versluis, M., Kastrinakis, E., Wesselink, P., van der Sluis, L.W.M. Evaluation of irrigant flow in the root canal using different needle types by an unsteady Computational Fluid Dynamics model. *J. Endod.* 2010;36:875–9.

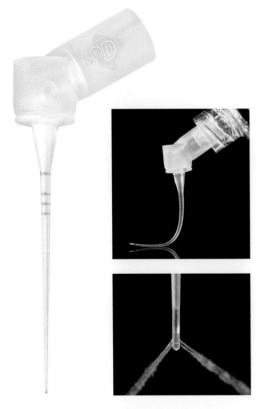

Figure 5.6   Flexible 30G double side-vented Irriflex needle made of plastic. *Source:* Courtesy Produits Dentaires SA, Vevey, Switzerland.

is still no universally accepted colour coding for needles [248], and each manufacturer is free to decide whether their colour represents their size, length, or even type. Large needles (21–25G) were commonly employed in the past for syringe irrigation [236, 250–254]. Evidently, these could only be inserted in the pulp chamber and the coronal third even in wide root canals, so the irrigant was only delivered to these areas and very small amounts actually reached the apical third of the root canals, either carried by instruments or as a result of diffusion [170].

Nowadays, the importance of irrigant delivery to the full extent of the root canal has been recognized, and the use of smaller needles (27–31G) that can reach farther is widely advocated [2, 255–259]. At present, the 30G needle could be considered the standard, but slightly larger and smaller ones are also in use. The main disadvantage of smaller needles is that they require a much stronger force to be applied on the syringe plunger during irrigation to reach the same flow rate; even a minor decrease in the diameter of a needle leads to a substantial increase in the force required [170]. Still, given the current trends in root canal

Table 5.1 Medical needle specifications according to ISO 9626:1991/Amd.1:2001 [249] and corresponding sizes of root canal instruments (non-existent instrument sizes rounded up to the next available size).

Gauge size	Metric size (mm)	Ext. diameter (mm)		Corresponding instrument size
		Min	Max	
21	0.80	0.800	0.830	90
23	0.60	0.600	0.673	70
25	0.50	0.500	0.530	55
26	0.45	0.440	0.470	50
27	0.40	0.400	0.420	45
28	0.36	0.349	0.370	40
29	0.33	0.324	0.351	35
30	0.30	0.298	0.320	35
31	0.25	0.254	0.267	30

Source: Modified from ISO 9626. Stainless Steel Needle Tubing for Manufacture of Medical Devices. Amendment 1. Geneva, Switzerland: International Organization for Standardization, 2001:1–5.

instrumentation [260], finer needles (>30G) may become the standard in the future.

Irrigation needles generally belong to one of two categories: needles that allow the irrigant to flow straight through their tip irrespective of its particular shape (*open-ended*) and needles with a closed tip that prevents the direct outflow of the irrigant, so that it flows through one or more side vents (*closed-ended*) (Figure 5.5) [247]. Open-ended needles create an intense jet of irrigant, which penetrates apically (Figure 5.7) [247, 261]. The penetration depends on the apical size and taper of the root canal and the irrigant flow rate (Figure 5.8) [247, 256, 261, 262]. The irrigant cannot reach farther than 1 mm apically to the needle tip in root canals with an apical size less than 30 [263, 264], but penetration is greatly improved in larger canals [256, 261, 262, 264, 265]. An increase in the apical size also reduces the risk of inadvertent irrigant extrusion through the apical foramen [266].

Closed-ended needles can only create a low-intensity jet, which is diverted towards the root canal wall (Figure 5.7) [247]. The irrigant can generally penetrate up to 1 mm apically to the needle tip (Figure 5.8) [247], and this distance

can only be increased very little by increasing the apical size, the taper, or the irrigant flow rate [261, 262, 264, 265, 267]. Thus, closed-ended needles are considered less effective than open-ended ones in terms of apical irrigant penetration and exchange [247, 256, 262, 264, 265, 268]. Another disadvantage is the strongly asymmetric flow that concentrates the mechanical cleaning effect on a small part of the root canal wall facing the vent(s) proximal to the tip [244, 247, 257]; most of the irrigant flows through these vents [245, 247, 262]. Therefore, needle orientation must be taken into account during use. However, closed-ended needles seem to extrude less irrigant through the apical foramen [266, 269].

5.3.1.1.3 Syringe Warmers Various types of syringe warmers have been suggested in order to heat the irrigant prior to delivery into the root canal [270]. Early studies showed that 1% NaOCl at 45 or 60 °C was able to dissolve as much pulp tissue as a 5.25% solution at 20 °C [18]. Yet, more recent work [271], including a clinical study [42], has shown that the temperature of the irrigant inside the root canal is increased only during delivery;

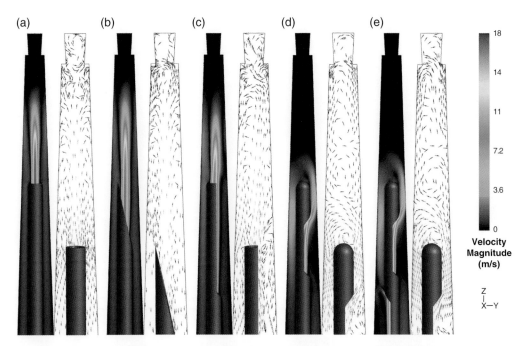

Figure 5.7 Time-averaged contours (left) and vectors (right) of irrigant velocity in the apical part of a size 45/0.06 taper root canal during syringe irrigation by different types of needles, according to computer simulations. Open-ended needles: (a) flat; (b) bevelled; (c) notched. Closed-ended needles: (d) side-vented; (e) double side-vented. All needles are positioned at 3 mm short of working length and are coloured in red. *Source:* Reprinted and modified with permission from Elsevier. Boutsioukis, C., Verhaagen, B., Versluis, M., Kastrinakis, E., Wesselink, P., van der Sluis, L.W.M. Evaluation of irrigant flow in the root canal using different needle types by an unsteady Computational Fluid Dynamics model. *J. Endod.* 2010;36:875–9.

afterwards, it decreases rapidly to 37 °C, which is the physiological core body temperature. Therefore, preheating has only a very short-term effect with limited clinical significance, and there is little justification for the use of such devices. Moreover, the use of rotary NiTi instruments in contact with preheated NaOCl may decrease their resistance to cyclic fatigue considerably [272–274].

5.3.1.1.4 *Technique* In order for the irrigant to penetrate to the apical terminus of the main root canal, needles must be placed close enough to working length without binding and the root canal must be adequately enlarged. Binding of a needle – especially an open-ended one – very close to working length and interruption of the reverse flow towards the root canal orifice could lead to inadvertent irrigant extrusion through the apical foramen,

so this should be carefully avoided at all times [269]. Open-ended needles should be placed at 2–3 mm short of working length, but closed-ended needles must placed even closer (within 1 mm) [247, 256, 261, 262, 264, 265]. A minimum apical size of 30–35 is required for 30G needles to reach these positions. Enlargement of the root canal up to this size is also important for irrigant penetration apically to the needle due to the viscosity of irrigants, which limits their flow in narrow spaces [170]. Root canal taper is less important for irrigant penetration [264, 265].

During irrigant delivery, the needle should be moved in and out along the root canal without exceeding the desired insertion depth. Apart from preventing needle binding, such movement can improve the mechanical cleaning of the canal, not because of agitation, but because the maximum mechanical cleaning is

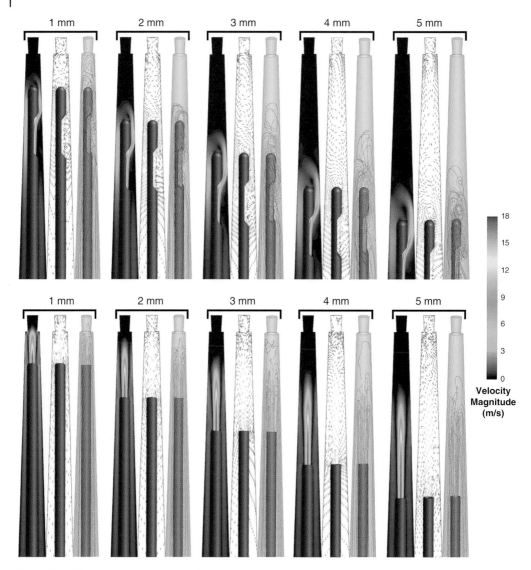

Figure 5.8 Time-averaged irrigant velocity contours (left) and vectors (middle) and stream-lines (right) depicting irrigant flow in a size 45/0.06 taper root canal when a closed-ended (top) or open-ended (bottom) needle is placed at 1–5 mm short of working length, according to computer simulations. Needles are coloured in red. *Source:* Reprinted with permission from Elsevier. Boutsioukis, C., Lambrianidis, T., Verhaagen, B., et al. The effect of needle insertion depth on the irrigant flow in the root canal: evaluation using an unsteady Computational Fluid Dynamics model. *J. Endod.* 2010;36:1664–8.

concentrated on a limited area near the tip of the needle [247, 256, 257, 264, 265]. Finally, the irrigant should be delivered at an adequate flow rate (0.15–0.20 ml/s) – a very low one (<0.05 ml/s) might be unable to drive the irrigant even up to the tip of a closed-ended needle [267].

Syringe irrigation seems to be effective in the main root canal, provided that the requirements concerning root canal size, needle insertion depth, and irrigant flow rate are satisfied. Several *ex vivo* studies and one clinical trial did not find any significant difference between syringe irrigation and a variety of other methods, including negative-pressure irrigation, sonic activation, and ultrasonic activation, regarding the removal of soft-tissue remnants, hard-tissue debris, bacteria, and biofilm from the main root canal or the healing of apical periodontitis [275–283]. Several further studies could not find any difference between syringe irrigation and other methods, although it was unclear whether the aforementioned requirements were met [284–288]. Studies showing inferior cleaning and disinfection of the main root canal by syringe irrigation compared to other methods generally did not enlarge the canals to an adequate size or placed the needles too far from the working length [257, 289–293]. Therefore, syringe irrigation seems to be sufficient for teeth with a single root canal and simple anatomy. Nonetheless, the irrigant appears unable to penetrate anatomic intricacies such as fins and uninstrumented oval extensions [294–302], the isthmus [279, 282, 284, 303–306], and accessory canals [307–310], so other irrigation methods – especially irrigant activation methods – may be necessary in cases with more complex anatomy.

5.3.1.2 Negative-Pressure Irrigation

Negative-pressure delivery techniques are sometimes categorized erroneously as agitation or activation techniques. During negative-pressure irrigation, the irrigant is delivered in the pulp chamber and negative pressure (suction) is applied on the distal end of a cannula placed inside the root canal, so that the irrigant is drawn along the canal from the coronal towards the apical third, where it is evacuated [290, 311]. Negative-pressure irrigation is not a new idea in endodontics [312], but it was reintroduced as an alternative to syringe irrigation in order to remove entrapped air bubbles from the apical third of the root canal (Apical vapor lock) [313] and to minimize the risk of irrigant extrusion through the apical foramen [290, 312] under the assumption that NaOCl accidents are caused by the increased irrigant pressure near the apical foramen. Both of these arguments have since been

questioned [165, 314]. Its popularity appears to be much lower than that of syringe irrigation and other supplementary irrigation techniques [6, 230].

5.3.1.2.1 Cannulas and Systems

A variety of cannulas, both open- and closed-ended, can be used for negative-pressure irrigation, including needles normally used for syringe irrigation (Figure 5.9) [311, 315] as long as there is a suitable adaptor to fit them on the suction hose of the dental unit. Nevertheless, they need to be fine enough to reach the apical third of the root canal, or even full working length, without binding [311]. They are made of stainless steel or plastic and usually have a cylindrical shape, although tapered ones are also available; tapering reduces the resistance to the flow [311]. In order to circumvent the frequent problem of clogging during use, multivented cannulas have been developed, so that if one of the vents is clogged the flow is not completely stopped.

A negative-pressure irrigation system may also include some means of irrigant delivery to the pulp chamber (usually a syringe and needle) and an additional suction hose to evacuate the overflow, together with the necessary tubes and connectors.

5.3.1.2.2 Technique

Placement of cannulas in the apical third of the root canal and effective suction of the irrigant require sufficient enlargement of the root canal. Closed-ended cannulas should be placed at working length without binding, so if a 30G cannula is used, the canal should be enlarged at least to an apical size 35–40/0.04 taper [231, 316]. Open-ended cannulas can be placed slightly farther away, at 2 mm from working length, without compromising irrigant exchange [311], but these are often larger, so the root canal should also be enlarged almost to the same size and taper.

There are no strict protocols for most negative-pressure irrigation systems [311, 315]. However, the manufacturer of the EndoVac system (Kerr, Brea, CA, USA) recommends a specific protocol for its use [317] in order to

(a)   (b)

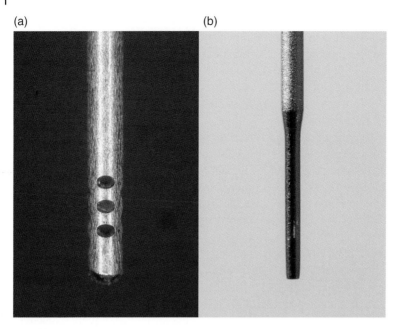

Figure 5.9 Cannulas used for negative pressure irrigation: (a) 30G closed-ended microcannula of the EndoVac system (Kerr, Brea, CA, USA); (b) 28G open-ended iNP cannula (Mikuni Kogyo, Nagano, Japan). Variable magnifications have been used to highlight differences in tip design. *Source:* Christos Boutsioukis. iNP cannula photo courtesy of Dr Carlos Adorno, Asunción, Paraguay.

ensure consistency between clinicians and between the various studies evaluating it. A larger plastic open-ended cannula is initially used to irrigate the pulp chamber and the coronal and middle third of the root canal in order to remove larger particles, before applying a finer cannula apically. This additional step reduces the chances of clogging the finer cannula, but even the larger one may be clogged by debris [316]. The finer cannula is subsequently inserted at working length. In both cases, the irrigant is simultaneously delivered in the pulp chamber by a syringe and the overflow is evacuated by a separate suction hose. All of the steps in this protocol are standardized in terms of time (delivery time and rest time) but not in terms of irrigant volume delivered in the root canal, arguably because it is difficult to determine exactly how much irrigant flows through each part of this complex system during irrigation *in vivo*. Therefore, the protocol relies on a standardized flow rate through each cannula – although in reality this

may fluctuate due to clogging, depletion of the irrigant in the root canal, or changes in the suction pressure used to drive the system.

Dental suction pumps maintain a negative pressure of approximately 20–25 kPa [231, 311], but this is rarely monitored during everyday use. Any decrease in pressure causes a proportional decrease in the irrigant flow rate through the cannulas, which may be difficult to detect. Moreover, the maximum flow rate though a cannula during negative-pressure irrigation is approximately 4–16 times lower than that through a needle of the same type and size used for syringe irrigation [231, 241, 311]. This is mainly attributed to the much lower driving pressure (20–25 kPa); the positive pressure developed inside the syringe reaches up to 540 kPa [241]. As a consequence, the irrigant exchange is much slower during negative-pressure irrigation, and the mechanical cleaning effect is reduced accordingly [261].

Despite claims that negative-pressure irrigation is generally superior to syringe irrigation [290, 316, 318], there seems to be no solid evidence to support this view. Negative-pressure systems have been often compared to suboptimal syringe-irrigation protocols; these comparisons are thus inherently biased [319]. Taking this into account, negative-pressure irrigation doesn't seem to be better than syringe irrigation in terms of cleaning and disinfection of the main root canal, although it may result in improved cleaning of the apical part of the isthmus [319]. A notable advantage of negative-pressure systems is that they extrude much less irrigant through the apical foramen than does syringe irrigation [22]. This difference may not be clinically relevant in most cases, but it could become relevant in cases where a NaOCl accident has already occurred, so that the risk of another one is high [165].

5.3.1.3 Combined Positive- and Negative-Pressure Irrigation

A combination of syringe irrigation and negative-pressure irrigation has been proposed as a way to improve the cleaning of isthmuses *ex vivo* [320]. The two techniques are applied simultaneously in the two root canals associated with the isthmus in order to force the irrigant from one, through the isthmus, and into the other. This combination appears to remove more hard-tissue debris from the isthmus than either technique alone, or than ultrasonic activation [320]. Nonetheless, clinical application of this combined technique may be difficult because the clinician must apply and control irrigant delivery and evacuation in two different root canals using two different techniques at the same time.

5.3.2 Irrigant Activation and Agitation Techniques

5.3.2.1 Ultrasonic Activation

Ultrasonic activation is the most widely used irrigant activation/agitation method [6, 81], so it could also be considered a clinical standard. It relies on the transverse oscillation of an ultrasonic instrument inside an irrigant-filled root canal [321] at a frequency of approximately 25–32 kHz [322]. Instrument oscillation drives the surrounding irrigant and induces a complicated flow inside the root canal [297, 323, 324], which consists of an oscillatory component and a steady component; the latter is also known as '*acoustic streaming*' [325]. This intense flow agitates the irrigant in the main canal, transports it to remote areas of the root canal system, and improves the mechanical cleaning [326]. The rapid instrument motion and the resulting irrigant pressure changes may also give rise to *acoustic cavitation* (formation, behaviour, and collapse of bubbles) [227, 327, 328]. Transient acoustic cavitation may be particularly useful for root canal cleaning because of the shockwaves emitted [327], the high shear stress applied on surfaces, and the local increase of pressure and temperature, which might give rise to sonochemical effects [227, 228, 327–329]. A part of the kinetic energy is inevitably converted to heat and increases the temperature of the irrigant [330–332], which may also accelerate chemical reactions [18, 34]. Thus, ultrasonic activation may augment both the chemical and the mechanical effects of irrigation [5].

5.3.2.1.1 *Ultrasonic Instruments* Various types of ultrasonic files, tips, and wires made of either stainless steel or NiTi have been used for irrigant activation (Figure 5.10). Smooth wires were proposed for this purpose in order to avoid unwanted dentine removal [333], but it appears that they are not immune to this problem [334]. They are made from either a tapered or a nontapered rod with a circular cross-section. Ultrasonic K-files are made by twisting a tapered (2%) blank with a square cross-section, providing sharp edges along the instrument. It should be emphasized that these files were originally designed for dentine cutting rather than irrigant activation. K-files show a gradual decrease in the oscillation amplitude of the antinodes from the free end towards the handpiece, due to their taper [322]. Irrisafe files (Acteon Satelec, Merignac,

(a)   (b)   (c)

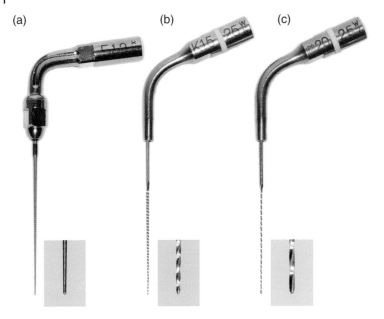

Figure 5.10 Ultrasonic instruments commonly used for irrigant activation: (a) smooth wire (Endo Soft Instrument (ESI), Electro Medical Systems, Nyon, Switzerland); (b) K-file (Acteon Satelec, Merignac, France); (c) Irrisafe file (Acteon Satelec, Merignac, France). *Source:* Christos Boutsioukis.

France) were introduced more recently as an attempt to adapt K-files to the requirements of irrigant activation. They have almost no taper, a larger pitch, rounded edges, and a blunt tip, in an effort to minimize unintentional removal of dentine [335]. Nevertheless, some dentine may still be removed during use [334, 336]. Due to the absence of taper, Irrisafe files have almost equal oscillation amplitude at all antinodes along their length [322, 337]. Ultrasonic K-files and Irrisafe files appear to be almost equally popular, whilst smooth wires are less so [338].

5.3.2.1.2 *Ultrasound Devices* Ultrasonic
instruments can be driven by the standard ultrasound devices typically present in every dental practice, either as standalone devices or built in the main dental units, so long as the power can be adjusted to the required levels (30–50%) and the water spray can be switched off. Continuous ultrasonic activation may also require that the irrigant be delivered through the ultrasonic handpiece, in which case the

device should be connected to an external irrigant tank. Battery-operated handheld ultrasonic handpieces specifically designed for intermittent irrigant activation are also available [339]. Given the fact that most practices are already equipped with the much more powerful and versatile corded units, there seems to be little incentive to obtain and use a separate device just for this purpose.

5.3.2.1.3 *Technique* Ultrasonic activation
can be applied continuously with simultaneous irrigant delivery through the ultrasonic handpiece or by a syringe, or intermittently in combination with irrigant delivery in between activation periods. In the latter case, the irrigant is usually delivered by a syringe and needle [338]. Delivery of the irrigant before, between, and after activation periods is performed according to the same standards described earlier. The aim of ultrasonic activation is not to compensate for suboptimal syringe irrigation but to clean and disinfect areas of the root canal system that syringe

irrigation is unable to reach even when an optimum protocol is followed.

Currently, intermittent ultrasonic activation appears to be more widely used [338], arguably because it allows for delivery of the irrigant in the apical part of the root canal at a precisely known depth instead of the pulp chamber, the volume of irrigant delivered can be monitored, and the repeated start-up of the oscillation increases the cleaning efficacy compared to continuous activation over the same period of time [295, 340, 341]. Moreover, frequent irrigant replenishment in the whole root canal can compensate for the inevitable consumption of the irrigant during activation [29] and the loss of irrigant through splashing out of the pulp chamber [227]. Therefore, it is preferable to apply activation for several shorter periods rather than a single longer one [294, 295]. A popular choice is intermittent activation for 3×20 seconds, although even shorter protocols are used (e.g. 3×10 seconds) [338].

There are no clear guidelines regarding the size of the instrument that should be used in each root canal [322, 338, 342, 343]. Larger instruments may create a more intense flow than smaller ones in the absence of any confinement, but the presence of the root canal wall creates additional obstacles. Since the flow extends only up to 2–3 mm apically to the instrument irrespective of the curvature [344], the instrument should be placed within 2–3 mm of working length and enough space should be available at that level for both the instrument and its 'free' oscillation. The tip oscillation amplitude of small ultrasonic instruments (size 15 or 20) is approximately 50–80 μm [322, 345], so at least 250–360 μm are required at the level of their tip; additional space is required for larger instruments or curved root canals. Therefore, small ultrasonic instruments seem to be the reasonable choice in most cases [326]. In addition, sufficient space for relatively free oscillation is very rarely available until instrumentation is completed, so ultrasonic activation before or during instrumentation makes little sense. Root canals

should be prepared at least to an apical size 30–35 in order to allow effective syringe delivery of the irrigant and relatively unobstructed oscillation of the ultrasonic instruments [326].

Following root canal preparation, the irrigant in the canal should be refreshed and the chosen ultrasonic instrument inserted at the desired depth. Instruments should be pre-bent before use in curved root canals [343, 346]. The power setting of the ultrasound device is a critical parameter; higher power increases the oscillation amplitude, which results in more intense streaming and improved cleaning [345]. However, there are limits to the power settings that can be used clinically, due to instrument fracture [347, 348] and inadvertent dentine removal [334, 336]. Most manufacturers of ultrasound devices and instruments recommend using around 30–35% of the maximum available power for ultrasonic files or wires [335, 349, 350], although some more recent recommendations suggest 40–50% [351]. File-to-wall contact during activation is inevitable, but it should be reduced as much as possible. Any contact results in dampening of the oscillation [352, 353] and reduction of the desired effects. Thus, the instrument should not be pushed intentionally towards the root canal wall; cleaning and disinfection are achieved by the intense flow of the irrigant and not by direct physical contact between the instrument and the wall.

During activation, it should be kept in mind that the streaming created around ultrasonic instruments is more intense along the direction of oscillation (i.e. the direction of the handpiece's longitudinal axis) than in other directions [324], so areas of the root canal in this direction will be cleaned more effectively [354]. Slight rotation of the handpiece around the canal axis may help to direct the streaming to various areas, especially fins and isthmuses, provided that there is sufficient mouth opening and the instrument has not been bent.

Activation may not be beneficial for all irrigants. It seems to augment the removal of pulp-tissue remnants and hard-tissue debris by NaOCl – and in some cases, its antimicrobial effect, too [338]. Other irrigants that are less effective against bacteria (e.g. CHX) may also benefit from activation because their chemical effect is limited and activation is required to boost the mechanical cleaning effect. The same rationale can be applied to inert irrigants such as physiologic saline [326]. Nevertheless, activation may have a negative effect on the calcium binding capacity of EDTA due to the concurrent heating [355].

As already explained, ultrasonic irrigant activation doesn't seem to provide a significant advantage over syringe irrigation in the main root canal [170]. Nevertheless, it may improve the cleaning of uninstrumented oval extensions, fins, isthmuses, and accessory canals (Figure 5.11) [310, 346], although very limited information is available regarding its antimicrobial effect in those areas and no clinical trial has yet shown that it can increase the treatment success rate compared to syringe irrigation alone [326, 338].

5.3.2.2 Sonic Agitation

This technique seems to be the third most popular one following syringe irrigation and ultrasonic activation [6, 230]. It relies again on the transverse oscillation of a tip inside the root canal in order to agitate the irrigant. However, oscillation takes place at much lower frequencies: 160–190 Hz for the EndoActivator (Dentsply Sirona, Charlotte,

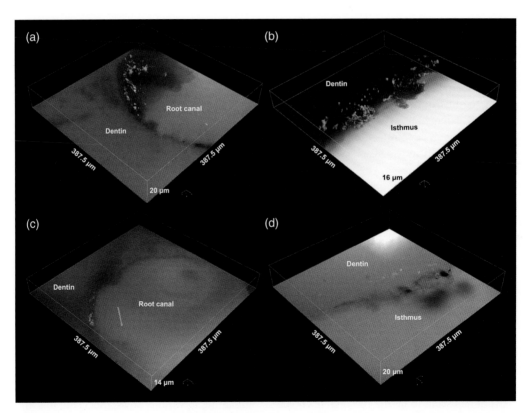

Figure 5.11 Disinfection of the apical third of the main root canal and isthmus by ultrasonic activation of a mixture of NaOCl and HEDP: (a) contaminated root canal wall; (b) contaminated isthmus; (c) root canal wall; and (d) isthmus after treatment with a mixture of NaOCl and HEDP activated ultrasonically for 3 × 20 seconds. Red-coloured bacteria are cells with damaged membranes, green-coloured bacteria are cells with intact membranes viewed under a confocal laser scanning microscope following LIVE/DEAD staining (BacLight; Invitrogen, Eugene, OR, USA). *Source:* Maria Teresa Arias-Moliz.

NC, USA) [297] and up to 6000 Hz for EDDY (VDW, Munich, Germany) [356]. Agitation creates an oscillatory flow in the main root canal, but the frequency is too low and the oscillation amplitude too large to create acoustic streaming and transient acoustic cavitation in this area [297, 324, 328].

5.3.2.2.1 Tips and Devices The currently available tips for sonic irrigant agitation are made of plastic and come in a variety of sizes and tapers. Tips suitable for the EndoActivator, a dedicated battery-operated device, have a size/taper of 15/0.02, 25/0.04, and 35/0.04 (small, medium, and large) [357]. EDDY, a more recently introduced tip that can be driven by a standard air-scaler, has a size 20 [358] and an approximately 0.05 taper (Figure 5.12).

5.3.2.2.2 Technique Sonic agitation is typically applied intermittently but for relatively longer periods compared to ultrasonic activation. Irrigant delivery prior to agitation is accomplished by a syringe and needle. The EndoActivator should be used after root canal preparation. A tip that fits loosely in the root canal within 2 mm of working length is selected in order to reduce dampening of its oscillation. During agitation, it is also recommended to move the tip along the canal in an effort to

reproduce the effect of agitation with a gutta-percha point [357]. There are no specific guidelines regarding the choice of power setting, although the highest setting is normally used for debridement. Agitation should be continued for 30–60 seconds, depending on the irrigant [357].

Regarding EDDY, it should be placed within 1–2 mm of working length [302, 356, 359–361]. According to the manufacturer, the root canal should be prepared to a minimum apical size 25/0.06 taper before applying agitation, but once this size and taper have been reached, EDDY can be used repeatedly after each successive instrument if the canal is further enlarged or as part of a final rinse protocol [362]. Movement of the tip in and out of the root canal during agitation is also recommended [362]. Agitation can be continued for up to 30 seconds at a maximum frequency of 6000 Hz [358].

It is noteworthy that the oscillation amplitude of the EndoActivator tips is around 1200 μm [297], whilst that of EDDY is approximately 350 μm [356, 361], so these tips require at least 2550 and 900 μm of free space, respectively, for unobstructed oscillation. Since it is very unlikely that a root canal will have such a diameter within 1–2 mm of the working length, the tips are expected to make frequent contact

(a)   (b)

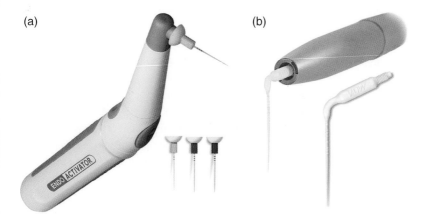

Figure 5.12 (a) EndoActivator (Dentsply Sirona, Charlotte, NC, USA), with its three available plastic tips (small, medium, and large). *Source:* Courtesy Dentsply Sirona, Charlotte, NC, USA. (b) EDDY (VDW, Munich, Germany). *Source:* Courtesy VDW, Munich, Germany.

with the wall of the main root canal in most cases [297]. Such contact is unlikely to result in dentine removal [346], but it probably dampens the oscillation considerably [297]. At the moment, it is unclear whether tip–wall contact enhances the cleaning and disinfection of the root canal system.

A number of studies have failed to detect any advantage of the EndoActivator over conventional syringe irrigation with regards to the cleaning and disinfection of the main root canal [275, 277, 363–365]. Similar findings have been reported regarding isthmuses and uninstrumented fins [277, 365, 366]. Moreover, the EndoActivator seems to be less effective than ultrasonic activation over the same durations [297, 346, 364, 367]. On the other hand, conflicting results have been reported for EDDY. Some studies have shown that it is similar to syringe irrigation in terms of antibacterial efficacy in the main root canal [359] and in terms of hard-tissue debris removal from the isthmus [360], whilst others have concluded that it is more effective than syringe irrigation and possibly equally effective to ultrasonic activation with regards to cleaning of the isthmus and of uninstrumented fins [302, 361].

5.3.2.3 Laser Activation

The term 'laser activation' describes a family of techniques using lasers and irrigants to enhance the cleaning and disinfection of the root canal system. These techniques rely on rapid heating of the irrigant in the vicinity of the laser tip by the light, generating a large vapour bubble (*optic cavitation*), which implodes after the end of the laser pulse [296, 368]. The expansion and, especially, collapse of the bubble force the irrigant inside the root canal to move rapidly. In addition, a shockwave is induced during the collapse, which drives the formation and collapse of smaller bubbles (*secondary cavitation*) in other areas of the root canal system [369]. Nevertheless, the irrigant is pushed towards the apex during the expansion phase, which leads to more irrigant extrusion through the apical foramen compared to techniques relying on lateral oscillation of instruments [370]. Laser activation is one of the least popular irrigation methods (0–1%) [81].

5.3.2.3.1 *Devices and Tips*
Laser activation typically employs Er:YAG or Er,Cr:YSGG lasers (Figure 5.13), which emit light with a wavelength in the infrared range (2940 or 2790 nm); this is absorbed very strongly by water and commonly used root canal irrigants. Nd:YAG and diode lasers with wavelengths in the near-infrared range (760–1400 nm) are much less well absorbed by irrigants, so are not efficient in producing optic cavitation [371]. The laser light is delivered inside the pulp chamber or the root canal by a variety of end- or radial-firing tis with external diameters from 200 up to approximately 600 μm [296, 372–376].

5.3.2.3.2 *Technique*
Traditional laser-activated irrigation (LAI) requires that the laser tip be placed deep inside the irrigant-filled root canal, within a few millimetres of the working length [162, 296, 368, 375–377]. This imposes limitations on the minimum apical size and taper of the root canal, since the laser tips commonly used for this purpose have an external diameter of 300–600 μm. Short high-energy pulses are then delivered repeatedly by the laser tip. The precise settings vary widely between studies, but the energy per pulse is in the order of 10–100 mJ, the pulse duration is approximately 50–100 μs, and the repetition rate is around 15–20 Hz [296, 368, 374–376]. These settings seem to affect the size of the primary bubble created, and hence the cleaning effectiveness of the method [5]. During activation, the irrigant is splashed out of the pulp chamber, so prolonged activation is discouraged; instead, repeated short activation periods (~20–30 seconds) should be alternated with syringe delivery of fresh irrigant [296, 374, 375].

Photon-initiated photoacoustic streaming (PIPS) is another technique that employs a

Figure 5.13 (a) Er:YAG laser (LightWalker ST-E; Fotona, Ljubljana, Slovenia). (b) Laser handpiece used with an Er:YAG laser (H14-N; Fotona). *Source:* Courtesy Fotona, Ljubljana, Slovenia.

(a)   (b)

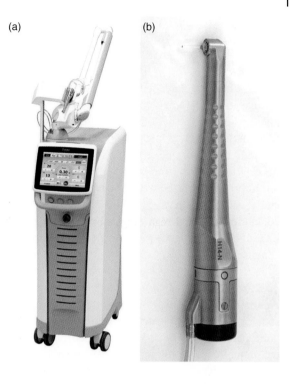

specially modified conical tip allowing lateral emission of the laser light [378]. The tip is placed in the pulp chamber near the root canal orifice, which eliminates the need for root canal enlargement to a specific size [372]. Short low-energy pulses (50 µs, 20 mJ) are delivered at a rate of 15 Hz [372, 373, 379] for approximately 20–30 seconds, and the process is repeated three to four times [373, 375, 380]; slightly different protocols are also used. Continuous irrigant delivery to the pulp chamber by a syringe is necessary in order for the laser tip to remain submerged in the irrigant [372, 378]. Despite the placement of the laser tip in the pulp chamber, this technique is claimed to induce irrigant streaming in the whole root canal through the shockwaves generated. However, placement of the laser tip deep inside the root canal still seems to augment the antimicrobial effect, even if all the other settings remain identical [162].

Shockwave-enhanced emission photoacoustic streaming (SWEEPS) is the most recent addition to the laser activation family.

It is similar to PIPS, but the laser pulses are delivered in pairs, with the second pulse delivered during the initial phase of the collapse of the primary cavitation bubble created by the first (~600 µs delay). This forms a second primary cavitation bubble, whose growth accelerates the collapse of the first bubble. This process is believed to amplify the emitted shockwaves and the accompanying secondary cavitation in other parts of the root canal [381]. The optimum time separation of the two pulses depends on the geometry of the root canal at each level, so the laser device scans through a range of time delays in order to optimize the bubble collapse in the various parts of the root canal system [382]. The rest of the protocol is similar to PIPS.

Regarding the effectiveness of these techniques, LAI appears to be superior to ultrasonic activation, at least for short activation periods (20 seconds), with regards to the removal of hard-tissue debris [296] or biofilm [162]. The two techniques may give similar results if activation is prolonged [375], although other studies reported that LAI is still more effective [361, 376]. Currently, there is no strong evidence that PIPS is superior to LAI [162, 375, 377]. On the contrary, its anti-microbial effect may be similar to that of syringe irrigation when NaOCl is used [379], and the same is true of its cleaning effect in the isthmus in some cases [383]. One study showed that LAI was more effective than PIPS with regards to biofilm removal [162], but others found no difference between the two [375]. A study evaluating the effectiveness of SWEEPS concluded that it was inferior to PIPS [384], although another study came to the opposite conclusion [385].

5.3.2.4 Manual Dynamic Agitation

Another way of agitating the irrigant inside the root canal is to move instruments, brushes, or gutta-percha points in and out of it [386]. This technique relies on the rapid displacement of the irrigant, which is forced both coronally and apically, and also into isthmuses and uninstrumented fins [5]. Thus, well-fitting gutta-percha points are probably the most effective means of bringing about such displacement.

5.3.2.4.1 Gutta-Percha Points Normal gutta-percha points can be used. The only requirement is that they match closely the apical size and taper of the root canal, in order to displace the irrigant as effectively as possible [301].

5.3.2.4.2 Technique Following the end of root canal instrumentation, a gutta-percha point that closely matches its apical size and taper should be selected; a tight fit at working length is very important for the effectiveness of this method [301]. Despite its advantages, manual dynamic agitation (MDA) can extrude significant amounts of irrigant through the apical foramen [387], so it has been recommended that the gutta-percha point be trimmed 1 mm at its tip in order to reduce this untoward effect [386]. Fresh irrigant should subsequently be delivered in the root canal,

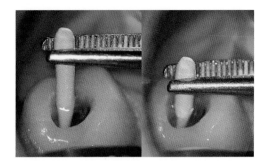

Figure 5.14 Manual dynamic agitation by a well-fitting gutta-percha point. *Source:* Christos Boutsioukis.

usually by a syringe and needle. The gutta-percha point can then be inserted, and push–pull movements applied manually by cotton pliers (Figure 5.14). The technique parameters vary; the displacement ranges between 2 and 5 mm and the frequency between 100 and 180 strokes/min [257, 291, 301, 364, 367, 386]. Agitation is usually continued for 60 seconds per irrigant [364, 386], but shorter times (10 seconds) have also been reported [301]. In some cases, the irrigant is refreshed and agitation is resumed for one or two additional cycles [257, 291].

MDA using well-fitting gutta-percha points may not provide an advantage in the main canal [364], but it can improve the cleaning of uninstrumented fins and oval extensions compared to syringe irrigation [301, 377, 383], and its performance appears similar to that of ultrasonic activation [377, 383]. However, there is no information about its antimicrobial action in these areas, nor its effect on the long-term success of root canal treatment.

5.3.3 Combinations of Techniques

5.3.3.1 Continuous Irrigant Delivery and Ultrasonic Activation

Two of the disadvantages of intermittent ultrasonic activation are that the irrigant is rapidly consumed [29] and the streaming created by the oscillating instruments may be unable to carry bacteria, tissue remnants, and debris out of the root canal system. Therefore, this technique must be supplemented by an irrigant delivery technique in between activation periods. Continuous activation with simultaneous irrigant delivery in the pulp chamber through the handpiece or a syringe is one way of simplifying this process, but irrigant flow to the apical third of the root canal is uncertain. In an effort to circumvent this problem, it has been proposed that specially designed ultrasonic needles be used, which can deliver the irrigant deep inside the root canal and activate it at the same time [284, 305]. This method seems to be less popular than intermittent ultrasonic activation [338].

5.3.3.1.1 Ultrasonic Needles

Ultrasonic needles resemble standard open-ended needles. One commercially available system uses 25G (0.50 mm) needles made of stainless steel (ProUltra PiezoFlow; Dentsply Sirona) (Figure 5.15). These can be connected to a syringe whilst attached to the ultrasonic handpiece. Regular irrigation needles attached to an endodontic file holder suitable for the ultrasonic handpiece can also be used for this purpose [284, 305, 388].

5.3.3.1.2 Technique

According to the manufacturer of the ProUltra PiezoFlow system (Dentsply Sirona), this technique

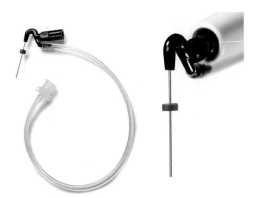

Figure 5.15 ProUltra PiezoFlow ultrasonic needle (Dentsply Sirona, Charlotte, NC, USA). *Source:* Courtesy Dentsply Sirona, Charlotte, NC, USA.

should be applied only in fully-instrumented root canals with a completely formed apex [389]. The open-ended ultrasonic needle is placed 1 mm short of the binding point inside the root canal and no deeper than 75% of the total working length, without any bending [389]. The irrigant is then delivered at a flow rate of 0.25 ml/s by a manually operated syringe or automated pump. A power setting of 30–50% is recommended, depending on the ultrasound device used, and activation is continued for one minute. The needle should be moved along the root canal during this period [389].

It is noteworthy that this technique can be modified so that the irrigant is delivered by negative pressure [388]. In that case, a smaller ultrasonic needle is connected to a high-volume aspiration unit and placed closer to the working length (within 2 mm). The irrigant is delivered into the pulp chamber by a syringe, similar to the technique with negative-pressure irrigation, and activation takes places for repeated 30-second periods [388]. Such a protocol may be preferable to continuous activation for longer periods, because the number of activation start-ups is more important that the total activation time [294, 295]. Movement of the ultrasonic needle along the canal is still advocated [388].

Continuous irrigant delivery and activation by ultrasonic needles seems to be more effective than syringe irrigation with regards to the removal of pulp-tissue remnants and hard-tissue debris, especially from the isthmus [279, 284, 301, 305, 390]. One study reported that the negative-pressure variant of this method performed better than either syringe irrigation or intermittent ultrasonic activation [388]. However, it remains unclear whether biofilm is also removed more effectively.

5.3.3.2 Continuous Irrigant Delivery and Multisonic Activation

Multisonic activation is one of the most recently introduced irrigation techniques. Although it may appear similar to the noninstrumented technique (NIT) proposed in the 1990s [391, 392], its operating principles are quite different. The irrigant is delivered into the pulp chamber by a specially designed handpiece which produces hydrodynamic cavitation in the form of a cloud [393]. The implosion of the bubbles creates acoustic waves with a broad range of frequencies, which travel through the irrigant – hence the term 'multisonic'. Cleaning and disinfection of all the root canals is claimed to be achieved simultaneously by the combined action of the irrigant flow, the acoustic waves, and the chemical effects of the irrigants [393, 394].

5.3.3.2.1 Device

A dedicated standalone device is used with this technique (GentleWave; Sonendo, Laguna Hills, CA, USA). This device includes several components used to deliver and activate multiple irrigants (NaOCl, EDTA, distilled water) and evacuate them from the root canal system.

5.3.3.2.2 Technique

According to the manufacturer, the root canal does not need to be instrumented at all [395], but canals have generally been enlarged to an apical size 15–25 in published studies using this technique [288, 393–396]. Missing tooth structures must be built up in order to create a suitable access cavity for the handpiece to be placed on and to create a coronal seal [394]. The operation of the device is fully automated. Large volumes of sodium hypochlorite 3% (~225 ml), distilled water (~23 ml), 8% EDTA (~90 ml), and further distilled water (~11 ml) are delivered sequentially at high flow rates (~0.75 ml/s) and evacuated [288, 396–398]. The whole cleaning process lasts for approximately five to eight minutes [288, 395, 398]. The precise protocol may differ between cases, and its details have not been disclosed by the manufacturer, which makes standardized comparisons to other methods rather difficult.

Continuous irrigant delivery and multisonic activation by this device appear to clean the isthmus much better than syringe irrigation [288] and to provide a significantly greater reduction of the microbial load compared to ultrasonic activation [395]. High success rates have also been reported 12 months after root canal treatments performed with this technique on both vital pulp cases and cases with apical periodontitis [393, 394], although no control group was included in either case. The main problem is that the manufacturer has been involved in most of the available studies, either through providing funding or as the employer of some of the authors. A recent independent study concluded that this technique is not significantly better than ultrasonic activation with regards to the removal of hard-tissue debris [396].

5.4 Final Remarks

Despite the abundance of *ex vivo* and *in vitro* studies comparing the various irrigating solutions and techniques, it should be underscored that randomized clinical trials, especially those focusing on long-term treatment success, are scarce. Therefore, the use of most solutions and techniques is based only on laboratory studies, which could lead to unnecessarily complicated protocols and unjustified costs. In addition, there are no unanimously accepted protocols for most techniques, so these may vary considerably between studies, and be quite different to those applied in clinical practice. Finally, not all the experimental models and surrogate endpoints used in such studies are equally relevant to the clinical setting [338]. Therefore, the value of each study should be carefully weighed before embracing its conclusions.

One topic closely related to irrigation that has been addressed extensively by clinical studies is whether additional disinfection by a calcium hydroxide dressing is necessary following chemomechanical preparation of infected root canals. The current best available evidence suggests that proper instrumentation and irrigation with NaOCl can reduce the number of bacteria significantly [399, 400], but subsequent medication with calcium hydroxide does not accomplish a further significant reduction [399–401]. In addition, the removal of calcium hydroxide from the root canal presents a number of challenges to irrigation [402–406], and its remnants could potentially affect the root canal filling [407]. Thus, there is little justification for the routine use of calcium hydroxide as an inter-appointment medicament.

References

1 Gulabivala, K., Patel, B., Evans, G., and Ng, Y.L. (2005). Effects of mechanical and chemical procedures on root canal surfaces. *Endod. Topics* 10: 103–122.

2 Zehnder, M. (2006). Root canal irrigants. *J. Endod.* 32: 389–398.

3 Peters, O.A., Schönenberger, K., and Laib, A. (2001). Effects of four Ni-Ti preparation techniques on root canal geometry assessed by micro computed tomography. *Int. Endod. J.* 34: 221–230.

4 Haapasalo, M., Endal, U., Zandi, H., and Coil, J.M. (2005). Eradication of endodontic infection by instrumentation and irrigation solutions. *Endod. Topics* 10: 77–102.

5 van der Sluis, L., Boutsioukis, C., Jiang, L.M. et al. (2015). Root canal irrigation. In: *The Root Canal Biofilm* (eds. L. Chávez de Paz, C.M. Sedgley and A. Kishen), 259–302. New York, NY: Springer.

6 Dutner, J., Mines, P., and Anderson, A. (2012). Irrigation trends among American Association of Endodontists members: a Web-based survey. *J. Endod.* 38: 37–40.

7 Baker, R.W. (1947). Studies on the reaction between sodium hypochlorite and proteins: 1. Physico-chemical study of the course of the reaction. *Biochem. J.* 41: 337–342.

8 Davies, J.M., Horwitz, D.A., and Davies, K.J. (1993). Potential roles of hypochlorous acid and N-chloroamines in collagen breakdown by phagocytic cells in synovitis. *Free Radic. Biol. Med.* 15: 637–643.

9 Jungbluth, H., Marending, M., De-Deus, G. et al. (2011). Stabilizing sodium hypochlorite at high pH: effects on soft tissue and dentin. *J. Endod.* 37: 693–696.

10 Souza, E.M., Calixto, A.M., Lima, C.N. et al. (2014). Similar influence of stabilized alkaline and neutral sodium hypochlorite solutions on the fracture resistance of root canal-treated bovine teeth. *J. Endod.* 40: 1600–1603.

11 Arias-Moliz, M.T., Ferrer-Luque, C.M., Espigares-García, M. et al. (2009). *Enterococcus faecalis* biofilms eradication by root canal irrigants. *J. Endod.* 35: 711–714.

12 Arias-Moliz, M.T., Ordinola-Zapata, R., Baca, P. et al. (2014). Antimicrobial activity of a sodium hypochlorite/etidronic acid irrigant solution. *J. Endod.* 40: 1999–2002.

13 Wong, D.T. and Cheung, G.S. (2014). Extension of bactericidal effect of sodium hypochlorite into dentinal tubules. *J. Endod.* 40: 825–829.

14 Yang, Y., Shen, Y., Wang, Z. et al. (2016). Evaluation of the susceptibility of multispecies biofilms in dentinal tubules to disinfecting solutions. *J. Endod.* 42: 1246–1250.

15 Ruiz-Linares, M., Aguado-Pérez, B., Baca, P. et al. (2017). Efficacy of antimicrobial solutions against polymicrobial root canal biofilm. *Int. Endod. J.* 50: 77–83.

16 Morago, A., Ruiz-Linares, M., Ferrer-Luque, C.M. et al. (2019). Dentine tubule disinfection by different irrigation protocols. *Microsc. Res. Tech.* 82: 558–563.

17 Naenni, N., Thoma, K., and Zehnder, M. (2004). Soft tissue dissolution capacity of currently used and potential endodontic irrigants. *J. Endod.* 30: 785–787.

18 Sirtes, G., Waltimo, T., Schaetzle, M. et al. (2005). The effects of temperature on sodium

hypochlorite short-term stability, pulp dissolution capacity, and antimicrobial efficacy. *J. Endod.* 3: 669–671.

19 Tejada, S., Baca, P., Ferrer-Luque, C.M. et al. (2019). Influence of dentine debris and organic tissue on the properties of sodium hypochlorite solutions. *Int. Endod. J.* 52: 114–122.

20 Hong, S.W., Baik, J.E., Kang, S.S. et al. (2016). Sodium hypochlorite inactivates lipoteichoic acid of *Enterococcus faecalis* by deacylation. *J. Endod.* 42: 1503–1508.

21 Pashley, E.L., Birdsong, N.L., Bowman, K., and Pashley, D.H. (1985). Cytotoxic effects of NaOCl on vital tissue. *J. Endod.* 11: 525–528.

22 Boutsioukis, C., Psimma, Z., and van der Sluis, L.W. (2013). Factors affecting irrigant extrusion during root canal irrigation: a systematic review. *Int. Endod. J.* 46: 599–618.

23 Guivarc'h, M., Ordioni, U., Ahmed, H.M. et al. (2017). Sodium hypochlorite accident: a systematic review. *J. Endod.* 43: 16–24.

24 Slaughter, R.J., Watts, M., Vale, J.A. et al. (2019). The clinical toxicology of sodium hypochlorite. *Clin. Toxicol. (Phila.)* 57: 303–311.

25 Ingram, T.A. (1990). Response of the human eye to accidental exposure to sodium hypochlorite. *J. Endod.* 16: 235–238.

26 Regalado Farreras, D.C., Puente, C.G., and Estrela, C. (2014). Sodium hypochlorite chemical burn in an endodontist's eye during canal treatment using operating microscope. *J. Endod.* 40: 1275–1279.

27 Moorer, W.R. and Wesselink, P.R. (1982). Factors promoting the tissue dissolving capability of sodium hypochlorite. *Int. Endod. J.* 15: 187–196.

28 Macedo, R.G., Wesselink, P.R., Zaccheo, F. et al. (2010). Reaction rate of NaOCl in contact with bovine dentine: effect of activation, exposure time, concentration and pH. *Int. Endod. J.* 43: 1108–1115.

29 Macedo, R.G., Verhaagen, B., Wesselink, P.R. et al. (2014). Influence of refreshment/ activation cycles and temperature rise on the reaction rate of sodium hypochlorite with

bovine dentine during ultrasonic activated irrigation. *Int. Endod. J.* 47: 147–154.

30 Pascon, F.M., Kantovitz, K.R., Sacramento, P.A. et al. (2009). Effect of sodium hypochlorite on dentine mechanical properties. A review. *J. Dent.* 37: 903–908.

31 Zehnder, M., Schmidlin, P., Sener, B. et al. (2005). Chelation in root canal therapy reconsidered. *J. Endod.* 31: 817–820.

32 Prado, M., Santos Júnior, H.M., Rezende, C.M. et al. (2013). Interactions between irrigants commonly used in endodontic practice: a chemical analysis. *J. Endod.* 39: 505–510.

33 Ragnarsson, K.T., Rechenberg, D.K., Attin, T., and Zehnder, M. (2015). Available chlorine consumption from NaOCl solutions passively placed in instrumented human root canals. *Int. Endod. J.* 48: 435–440.

34 Stojicic, S., Zivkovic, S., Qian, W. et al. (2010). Tissue dissolution by sodium hypochlorite: effect of concentration, temperature, agitation, and surfactant. *J. Endod.* 36: 1558–1562.

35 Gernhardt, C.R., Eppendorf, K., Kozlowski, A. et al. (2004). Toxicity of concentrated sodium hypochlorite used as an endodontic irrigant. *Int. Endod. J.* 37: 272–280.

36 de Sermeño, R.F., da Silva, L.A., Herrera, H. et al. (2009). Tissue damage after sodium hypochlorite extrusion during root canal treatment. *Oral Surg. Oral Med. Oral Pathol. Oral Radiol. Endod.* 108: e46–e49.

37 Siqueira, J.F. Jr., Rôças, I.N., Favieri, A. et al. (2000). Chemomechanical reduction of the bacterial population in the root canal after instrumentation and irrigation with 1%, 2.5%, and 5.25% sodium hypochlorite. *J. Endod.* 26: 331–334.

38 Hülsmann, M. and Hahn, W. (2000). Complications during root canal irrigation – literature review and case reports. *Int. Endod. J.* 33: 186–193.

39 Cunningham, W.T. and Joseph, S.W. (1980). Effect of temperature on the bactericidal action of sodium hypochlorite endodontic irrigant. *Oral Surg. Oral Med. Oral Pathol.* 50: 569–571.

40 Dumitriu, D. and Dobre, T. (2015). Effects of temperature and hypochlorite concentration on the rate of collagen dissolution. *J. Endod.* 41: 903–906.

41 Berutti, E. and Marini, R. (1996). A scanning electron microscopic evaluation of the debridement capability of sodium hypochlorite at different temperatures. *J. Endod.* 22: 467–470.

42 de Hemptinne, F., Slaus, G., Vandendael, M. et al. (2015). *In vivo* intracanal temperature evolution during endodontic treatment after the injection of room temperature or preheated sodium hypochlorite. *J. Endod.* 41: 1112–1115.

43 Bartolo, A., Koyess, E., Camilleri, J., and Micallef, C. (2016). Model assessing thermal changes during high temperature root canal irrigation. *Healthc. Technol. Lett.* 3: 247–251.

44 Leonardi, D.P., Grande, N.M., Tomazinho, F.S.F. et al. (2019). Influence of activation mode and preheating on intracanal irrigant temperature. *Aust. Endod. J.* 45: 373–377.

45 van der Waal, S.V., van Dusseldorp, N.E., and de Soet, J.J. (2014). An evaluation of the accuracy of labeling of percent sodium hypochlorite on various commercial and professional sources: is sodium hypochlorite from these sources equally suitable for endodontic irrigation? *J. Endod.* 40: 2049–2052.

46 Nicoletti, M.A., Siqueira, E.L., Bombana, A.C. et al. (2009). Shelf-life of a 2.5% sodium hypochlorite solution as determined by Arrhenius equation. *Braz. Dent. J.* 20: 27–31.

47 Johnson, B.R. and Remeikis, N.A. (1993). Effective shelf-life of prepared sodium hypochlorite solution. *J. Endod.* 1: 40–43.

48 Frais, S., Ng, Y.L., and Gulabivala, K. (2001). Some factors affecting the concentration of available chlorine in commercial sources of sodium hypochlorite. *Int. Endod. J.* 34: 206–215.

49 Vianna, M.E., Gomes, B.P., Berber, V.B. et al. (2004). *In vitro* evaluation of the antimicrobial activity of chlorhexidine and sodium hypochlorite. *Oral Surg. Oral Med. Oral Pathol. Oral Radiol. Endod.* 97: 79–84.

50 Ferraz, C.C., Gomes, B.P., Zaia, A.A. et al. (2007). Comparative study of the antimicrobial efficacy of chlorhexidine gel, chlorhexidine solution and sodium hypochlorite as endodontic irrigants. *Braz. Dent. J.* 18: 294–298.

51 Greenstein, G., Berman, C., and Jaffin, R. (1986). Chlorhexidine. An adjunct to periodontal therapy. *J. Periodontol.* 57: 370–377.

52 Fardal, O. and Turnbull, R.S. (1986). A review of the literature on use of chlorhexidine in dentistry. *J. Am. Dent. Assoc.* 112: 863–869.

53 Gomes, B.P., Vianna, M.E., Zaia, A.A. et al. (2013). Chlorhexidine in endodontics. *Braz. Dent. J.* 24: 89–102.

54 Ringel, A.M., Patterson, S.S., Newton, C.W. et al. (1982). *In vivo* evaluation of chlorhexidine gluconate solution and sodium hypochlorite solution as root canal irrigants. *J. Endod.* 8: 200–204.

55 Ferraz, C.C., Gomes, B.P., Zaia, A.A. et al. (2001). *In vitro* assessment of the antimicrobial action and the mechanical ability of chlorhexidine gel as an endodontic irrigant. *J. Endod.* 27: 452–455.

56 Bonez, P., Dos Santos Alves, C.F., Dalmolin, T.V. et al. (2013). Chlorhexidine activity against bacterial biofilms. *Am. J. Infect. Control* 41: e119–e122.

57 Busanello, F.H., Petridis, X., So, M.V.R. et al. (2019). Chemical biofilm removal capacity of endodontic irrigants as a function of biofilm structure: optical coherence tomography, confocal microscopy and viscoelasticity determination as integrated assessment tools. *Int. Endod. J.* 52: 461–474.

58 Du, T., Shi, Q., Shen, Y. et al. (2013). Effect of modified nonequilibrium plasma with chlorhexidine digluconate against endodontic biofilms *in vitro*. *J. Endod.* 39: 1438–1443.

59 Arias-Moliz, M.T., Ordinola-Zapata, R., Baca, P. et al. (2015). Antimicrobial activity of chlorhexidine, peracetic acid and sodium hypochlorite/etidronate irrigant solutions

against *Enterococcus faecalis* biofilms. *Int. Endod. J.* 48: 1188–1193.

60 Gonçalves, L.S., Rodrigues, R.C., Andrade Junior, C.V. et al. (2016). The effect of sodium hypochlorite and chlorhexidine as irrigant solutions for root canal disinfection: a systematic review of clinical trials. *J. Endod.* 42: 527–532.

61 Marinho, A.C., Martinho, F.C., Leite, F.R. et al. (2015). Proinflammatory activity of primarily infected endodontic content against macrophages after different phases of the root canal therapy. *J. Endod.* 41: 817–823.

62 Okino, L.A., Siqueira, E.L., Santos, M. et al. (2004). Dissolution of pulp tissue by aqueous solution of chlorhexidine digluconate and chlorhexidine digluconate gel. *Int. Endod. J.* 37: 38–41.

63 Dandakis, C., Lambrianidis, T., and Boura, P. (2000). Immunologic evaluation of dental patient with history of hypersensitivity reaction to sodium hypochlorite. *Endod. Dent. Traumatol.* 16: 184–187.

64 Rosenthal, S., Spangberg, L., and Safavi, K. (2004). Chlorhexidine substantivity in root canal dentin. *Oral Surg. Oral Med. Oral Pathol. Oral Radiol. Endod.* 98: 488–492.

65 Khademi, A.A., Mohammadi, Z., and Havaee, A. (2006). Evaluation of the antibacterial substantivity of several intra-canal agents. *Aust. Endod. J.* 32: 112–115.

66 Mohammadi, Z. and Abbott, P.V. (2009). Antimicrobial substantivity of root canal irrigants and medicaments: a review. *Aust. Endod. J.* 35: 131–139.

67 Carrilho, M.R., Carvalho, R.M., Sousa, E.N. et al. (2010). Substantivity of chlorhexidine to human dentin. *Dent. Mater.* 26: 779–785.

68 Baca, P., Junco, P., Arias-Moliz, M.T. et al. (2012). Antimicrobial substantivity over time of chlorhexidine and cetrimide. *J. Endod.* 38: 927–930.

69 Barrios, R., Ferrer-Luque, C.M., Arias-Moliz, M.T. et al. (2013). Antimicrobial substantivity of alexidine and chlorhexidine in dentin. *J. Endod.* 39: 1413–1415.

70 Mohammadi, Z. and Abbott, P.V. (2008). The properties and applications of chlorhexidine in endodontics. *Int. Endod. J.* 42: 288–302.

71 Souza, M., Cecchin, D., Farina, A.P. et al. (2012). Evaluation of chlorhexidine substantivity on human dentin: a chemical analysis. *J. Endod.* 38: 1249–1252.

72 Moreira, D.M., Almeida, J.F., Ferraz, C.C. et al. (2009). Structural analysis of bovine root dentin after use of different endodontics auxiliary chemical substances. *J. Endod.* 35: 1023–1027.

73 Gendron, R., Grenier, D., Sorsa, T. et al. (1999). Inhibition of the activities of matrix metalloproteinases 2, 8, and 9 by chlorhexidine. *Clin. Diagn. Lab. Immunol.* 6: 437–439.

74 Wang, Y. and Spencer, P. (2003). Hybridization efficiency of the adhesive/dentin interface in wet bonding. *J. Dent. Res.* 82: 141–145.

75 Vouzara, T., Koulaouzidou, E., Ziouti, F. et al. (2016). Combined and independent cytotoxicity of sodium hypochlorite, ethylenediaminetetraacetic acid and chlorhexidine. *Int. Endod. J.* 49: 764–773.

76 Scott, M.B., Zilinski, G.S., Kirkpatrick, T.C. et al. (2018). The effects of irrigants on the survival of human stem cells of the apical papilla, including endocyn. *J. Endod.* 44: 263–268.

77 Trevino, E.G., Patwardhan, A.N., Henry, M.A. et al. (2011). Effect of irrigants on the survival of human stem cells of the apical papilla in a platelet-rich plasma scaffold in human root tips. *J. Endod.* 37: 1109–1115.

78 Basrani, B.R., Manek, S., Sodhi, R.N. et al. (2007). Interaction between sodium hypochlorite and chlorhexidine gluconate. *J. Endod.* 33: 966–969.

79 Lanigan, R.S. and Yamarik, T.A. (2002). Final report on the safety assessment of EDTA, calcium disodium EDTA, diammonium EDTA, dipotassium EDTA, disodium EDTA, TEA-EDTA, tetrasodium EDTA, tripotassium EDTA, trisodium EDTA, HEDTA, and trisodium HEDTA. *Int. J. Toxicol.* 21: 95–142.

80 Hart, J.R. (2012). Ethylenediaminetetraacetic acid and related chelating agents. In: *Ullmann's Encyclopedia of Industrial Chemistry* (ed. B. Elvers), 573–578. Weinheim: Wiley-VCH.

81 Willershausen, I., Wolf, T.G., Schmidtmann, I. et al. (2015). Survey of root canal irrigating solutions used in dental practices within Germany. *Int. Endod. J.* 48: 654–660.

82 Calt, S. and Serper, A. (2002). Time-dependent effects of EDTA on dentin structures. *J. Endod.* 28: 17–19.

83 Hülsmann, M., Heckendorff, M., and Lennon, A. (2003). Chelating agents in root canal treatment: mode of action and indications for their use. *Int. Endod. J.* 36: 810–830.

84 De-Deus, G., Zehnder, M., Reis, C. et al. (2008). Longitudinal co-site optical microscopy study on the chelating ability of etidronate and EDTA using a comparative single-tooth model. *J. Endod.* 34: 71–75.

85 Tartari, T., Souza, P.A.R.S., Almeida, B.V.N. et al. (2013). A new weak chelator in endodontics: effects of different irrigation regimens with etidronate on root dentin microhardness. *Int. J. Dent.* 2013: ID743018.

86 Taneja, S., Kumari, M., and Anand, S. (2014). Effect of QMix, peracetic acid and ethylenediaminetetraacetic acid on calcium loss and microhardness of root dentine. *J. Conserv. Dent.* 17: 155–158.

87 Goldman, M., Goldman, L.B., Cavaleri, R. et al. (1982). The efficacy of several endodontic irrigating solutions: part 2. *J. Endod.* 8: 487–492.

88 Haapasalo, M., Qian, W., and Shen, Y. (2012). Irrigation: beyond the smear layer. *Endod. Topics* 27: 35–53.

89 Baldasso, F.E.R., Roleto, L., Silva, V.D.D. et al. (2017). Effect of final irrigation protocols on microhardness reduction and erosion of root canal dentin. *Braz. Oral Res.* 31: e40.

90 Schwartz, R.S. (2006). Adhesive dentistry and endodontics. Part 2: bonding in the root canal system-the promise and the problems: a review. *J. Endod.* 32: 1125–1134.

91 De-Deus, G., Namen, F., Galan, J. Jr. et al. (2008). Soft chelating irrigation protocol optimizes bonding quality of Resilon/ Epiphany root fillings. *J. Endod.* 34: 703–705.

92 Grawehr, M., Sener, B., Waltimo, T. et al. (2003). Interactions of ethylenediaminetetraacetic acid with sodium hypochlorite in aqueous solutions. *Int. Endod. J.* 36: 411–415.

93 Yamada, R.S., Armas, A., Goldman, M. et al. (1983). A scanning electron microscopic comparison of a high volume final flush with several irrigating solutions: part 3. *J. Endod.* 9: 137–142.

94 Peters, O.A., Boessler, C., and Zehnder, M. (2005). Effect of liquid and paste-type lubricants on torque values during simulated rotary root canal instrumentation. *Int. Endod. J.* 38: 223–229.

95 Boessler, C., Peters, O.A., and Zehnder, M. (2007). Impact of lubricant parameters on rotary instrument torque and force. *J. Endod.* 33: 280–283.

96 Boutsioukis, C. and Lambrianidis, T. (2018). Factors affecting intracanal instrument fracture. In: *Management of Separated Instruments: A Clinical Guide* (ed. T. Lambrianidis), 31–60. New York, NY: Springer.

97 Arias-Moliz, M.T., Ferrer-Luque, C.M., Espigares-Rodríguez, E. et al. (2008). Bactericidal activity of phosphoric acid, citric acid, and EDTA solutions against *Enterococcus faecalis. Oral Surg. Oral Med. Oral Pathol. Oral Radiol. Endod.* 106: e84–e89.

98 Ordinola-Zapata, R., Bramante, C.M., Cavenago, B. et al. (2012). Antimicrobial effect of endodontic solutions used as final irrigants on a dentine biofilm model. *Int. Endod. J.* 45: 162–168.

99 Leive, L. (1965). Release of lipopolysaccharide by EDTA treatment of *E. coli. Biochem. Biophys. Res. Commun.* 21: 290–296.

100 de Almeida, J., Hoogenkamp, M., Felippe, W.T. et al. (2016). Effectiveness of EDTA

and modified salt solution to detach and kill cells from *Enterococcus faecalis* biofilm. *J. Endod.* 42: 320–323.

101 Kim, H.J., Park, S.J., Park, S.H. et al. (2013). Efficacy of flowable gel-type EDTA at removing the smear layer and inorganic debris under manual dynamic activation. *J. Endod.* 39: 910–914.

102 Sen, B.H., Akdeniz, B.G., and Denizci, A.A. (2000). The effect of ethylenediamine-tetraacetic acid on *Candida albicans*. *Oral Surg. Oral Med. Oral Pathol. Oral Radiol. Endod.* 90: 651–655.

103 Ates, M., Akdeniz, B.G., and Sen, B.H. (2005). The effect of calcium chelating or binding agents on *Candida albicans*. *Oral Surg. Oral Med. Oral Pathol. Oral Radiol. Endod.* 100: 626–630.

104 Tartari, T., Guimarães, B.M., Amoras, L.S. et al. (2015). Etidronate causes minimal changes in the ability of sodium hypochlorite to dissolve organic matter. *Int. Endod. J.* 48: 399–404.

105 Tartari, T., Oda, D.F., Zancan, R.F. et al. (2017). Mixture of alkaline tetrasodium EDTA with sodium hypochlorite promotes *in vitro* smear layer removal and organic matter dissolution during biomechanical preparation. *Int. Endod. J.* 50: 106–114.

106 Marins, J.S., Sassone, L.M., Fidel, S.R. et al. (2012). *In vitro* genotoxicity and cytotoxicity in murine fibroblasts exposed to EDTA, NaOCl, MTAD and citric acid. *Braz. Dent. J.* 23: 527–533.

107 Segura, J.J., Calvo, J.R., Guerrero, J.M. et al. (1997). EDTA inhibits *in vitro* substrate adherence capacity of macrophages: endodontic implications. *J. Endod.* 23: 205–208.

108 Dioguardi, M., Di Gioia, G., Illuzzi, G. et al. (2018). Endodontic irrigants: different methods to improve efficacy and related problems. *Eur. J. Dent.* 12: 459–466.

109 O'Connell, M.S., Morgan, L.A., Beeler, W.J. et al. (2000). A comparative study of smear layer removal using different salts of EDTA. *J. Endod.* 26: 739–743.

110 Solana, C., Ruiz-Linares, M., Baca, P. et al. (2017). Antibiofilm activity of sodium hypochlorite and alkaline tetrasodium EDTA solutions. *J. Endod.* 43: 2093–2096.

111 Biel, P., Mohn, D., Attin, T. et al. (2017). Interactions between the tetrasodium salts of EDTA and 1-hydroxyethane 1,1-diphosphonic acid with sodium hypochlorite irrigants. *J. Endod.* 43: 657–661.

112 Wright, P.P., Kahler, B., and Walsh, L.J. (2019). The effect of heating to intracanal temperature on the stability of sodium hypochlorite admixed with etidronate or EDTA for continuous chelation. *J. Endod.* 45: 57–61.

113 Wayman, B.E., Kopp, W.M., Pinero, G.J. et al. (1979). Citric acid and lactic acids as root canal irrigants *in vitro*. *J. Endod.* 5: 258–265.

114 Pérez-Heredia, M., Ferrer-Luque, C.M., and González-Rodríguez, M.P. (2006). The effectiveness of different acid irrigating solutions in root canal cleaning after hand and rotary instrumentation. *J. Endod.* 32: 993–997.

115 Prado, M., Gusman, H., Gomes, B.P. et al. (2011). Scanning electron microscopic investigation of the effectiveness of phosphoric acid in smear layer removal when compared with EDTA and citric acid. *J. Endod.* 37: 255–258.

116 Haznedaroğlu, F. (2003). Efficacy of various concentrations of citric acid at different pH values for smear layer removal. *Oral Surg. Oral Med. Oral Pathol. Oral Radiol. Endod.* 96: 340–344.

117 Malheiros, C.F., Marques, M.M., and Gavini, G. (2005). *In vitro* evaluation of the cytotoxic effects of acid solutions used as canal irrigants. *J. Endod.* 31: 746–748.

118 Amaral, K.F., Rogero, M.M., Fock, R.A. et al. (2007). Cytotoxicity analysis of EDTA and citric acid applied on murine resident macrophages culture. *Int. Endod. J.* 40: 338–343.

119 Qian, W., Shen, Y., and Haapasalo, M. (2011). Quantitative analysis of the effect of irrigant solution sequences on dentin erosion. *J. Endod.* 37: 1437–1441.

120 Eswaranandam, S., Hettiarchchy, N.S., and Johnson, M.G. (2004). Antimicrobial activity of citric, lactic, malic, or tartaric acids and nisin-incorporated soy protein film against *Listeria monocytogenes, Escherichia coli* O157:H7, and *Salmonella graminara. J. Food Sci.* 69: 79–84.

121 Zeng, B., Li, M.D., Zhu, Z.P. et al. (2013). Application of 1-hydroxyethylidene-1, 1-diphosphonic acid in boiler water for industrial boilers. *Water Sci. Technol.* 67: 1544–1550.

122 Russell, R.G. and Rogers, M.J. (1999). Bisphosphonates: from the laboratory to the clinic and back again. *Bone* 25: 97–106.

123 Ganguli, A., Henderson, C., Grant, M.H. et al. (2002). The interactions of bisphosphonates in solution and as coatings on hydroxyapatite with osteoblasts. *J. Mater. Sci. Mater. Med.* 13: 923–931.

124 Lottanti, S., Gautschi, H., Sener, B. et al. (2009). Effects of ethylenediaminetetraacetic, etidronic and peracetic acid irrigation on human root dentine and the smear layer. *Int. Endod. J.* 42: 335–343.

125 Paqué, F., Rechenberg, D.K., and Zehnder, M. (2012). Reduction of hard-tissue debris accumulation during rotary root canal instrumentation by etidronic acid in a sodium hypochlorite irrigant. *J. Endod.* 38: 692–695.

126 Ulusoy, Ö.I., Savur, I.G., Alaçam, T. et al. (2018). The effectiveness of various irrigation protocols on organic tissue removal from simulated internal resorption defects. *Int. Endod. J.* 51: 1030–1036.

127 Arias-Moliz, M.T., Morago, A., Ordinola-Zapata, R. et al. (2016). Effects of dentin debris on the antimicrobial properties of sodium hypochlorite and etidronic acid. *J. Endod.* 42: 771–775.

128 Morago, A., Ordinola-Zapata, R., Ferrer-Luque, C.M. et al. (2016). Influence of

smear layer on the antimicrobial activity of a sodium hypochlorite/etidronic acid irrigating solution in infected dentin. *J. Endod.* 42: 1647–1650.

129 Zollinger, A., Mohn, D., Zeltner, M. et al. (2018). Short-term storage stability of NaOCl solutions when combined with dual rinse HEDP. *Int. Endod. J.* 51: 691–696.

130 Ballal, N.V., Das, S., Rao, B.S.S. et al. (2019). Chemical, cytotoxic and genotoxic analysis of etidronate in sodium hypochlorite solution. *Int. Endod. J.* 52: 1228–1234.

131 Ballal, N.V., Gandhi, P., Shenoy, P.A. et al. (2019). Safety assessment of an etidronate in a sodium hypochlorite solution: randomized double-blind trial. *Int. Endod. J.* 52: 1274–1282.

132 Wright, P.P., Cooper, C., Kahler, B., and Walsh, L.J. (2020). From an assessment of multiple chelators, clodronate has potential for use in continuous chelation. *Int. Endod. J.* 53: 122–134.

133 Wright, P.P., Scott, S., Kahler, B., and Walsh, L.J. (2020). Organic tissue dissolution in clodronate and etidronate mixtures with sodium hypochlorite. *J. Endod.* 46: 289–294.

134 Ballal, N.V., Kandian, S., Mala, K. et al. (2009). Comparison of the efficacy of maleic acid and ethylenediaminetetraacetic acid in smear layer removal from instrumented human root canal: a scanning electron microscopic study. *J. Endod.* 35: 1573–1576.

135 Ulusoy, Ö.İ. and Görgül, G. (2013). Effects of different irrigation solutions on root dentine microhardness, smear layer removal and erosion. *Aust. Endod. J.* 39: 66–72.

136 Ballal, N.V., Jain, I., and Tay, F.R. (2016). Evaluation of the smear layer removal and decalcification effect of QMix, maleic acid and EDTA on root canal dentine. *J. Dent.* 51: 62–68.

137 Jaiswal, S., Patil, V., Satish Kumar, K.S. et al. (2018). Comparative analysis of smear layer removal by conventional endodontic

irrigants with a newly experimented irrigant-fumaric acid: a scanning electron microscopic study. *J. Conserv. Dent.* 21: 419–423.

138 Ballal, N.V., Kundabala, M., Bhat, S. et al. (2009). A comparative *in vitro* evaluation of cytotoxic effects of EDTA and maleic acid: root canal irrigants. *Oral Surg. Oral Med. Oral Pathol. Oral Radiol. Endod.* 108: 633–638.

139 Ballal, N.V., Rao, B.N., Mala, K. et al. (2013). Assessment of genotoxic effect of maleic acid and EDTA: a comparative *in vitro* experimental study. *Clin. Oral Investig.* 17: 1319–1327.

140 Gadang, V.P., Hettiarachchy, N.S., Johnson, M.G. et al. (2008). Evaluation of antibacterial activity of whey protein isolate coating incorporated with nisin, grape seed extract, malic acid, and EDTA on a Turkey frankfurter system. *J. Food Sci.* 73: M389–M394.

141 Ferrer-Luque, C.M., Arias-Moliz, M.T., González-Rodríguez, M.P. et al. (2010). Antimicrobial activity of maleic acid and combinations of cetrimide with chelating agents against *Enterococcus faecalis biofilm*. *J. Endod.* 36: 1673–1675.

142 Prabhu, S.G., Rahim, N., Bhat, K.S. et al. (2003). Comparison of removal of endodontic smear layer using NaOCl, EDTA, and different concentrations of maleic acid – an SEM study. *Endodontology* 15: 20–25.

143 Huth, K.C., Quirling, M., Maier, S. et al. (2009). Effectiveness of ozone against endodontopathogenic microorganisms in a root canal biofilm model. *Int. Endod. J.* 42: 3–13.

144 Oizumi, M., Suzuki, T., Uchida, M. et al. (1998). *In vitro* testing of a denture cleaning method using ozone. *J. Med. Dent. Sci.* 45: 135–139.

145 Zanacic, E., Stavrinides, J., and McMartin, D.W. (2016). Field-analysis of potable water quality and ozone efficiency in ozone-assisted biological filtration systems for surface water treatment. *Water Res.* 104: 397–407.

146 Brodowska, A.J., Nowak, A., and Śmigielski, K. (2018). Ozone in the food industry: principles of ozone treatment, mechanisms of action, and applications: an overview. *Crit. Rev. Food Sci. Nutr.* 58: 2176–2201.

147 Bocci, V., Zanardia, I., Valacchi, G. et al. (2015). Validity of oxygen–ozone therapy as integrated medication form in chronic inflammatory diseases. *Cardiovasc. Hematol. Disord. Drug Targets* 15: 127–138.

148 Braidy, N., Izadi, M., Sureda, A. et al. (2018). Therapeutic relevance of ozone therapy in degenerative diseases: focus on diabetes and spinal pain. *J. Cell. Physiol.* 233: 2705–2714.

149 Nagayoshi, M., Kitamura, C., Fukuizumi, T. et al. (2004). Antimicrobial effect of ozonated water on bacteria invading dentinal tubules. *J. Endod.* 30: 778–781.

150 Hems, R.S., Gulabivala, K., Ng, Y.L. et al. (2005). An *in vitro* evaluation of the ability of ozone to kill a strain of *Enterococcus faecalis*. *Int. Endod. J.* 38: 22–29.

151 Case, P.D., Bird, P.S., Kahler, W.A. et al. (2012). Treatment of root canal biofilms of *Enterococcus faecalis* with ozone gas and passive ultrasound activation. *J. Endod.* 38: 523–526.

152 Cardoso, M.G., de Oliveira, L.D., Koga-Ito, C.Y. et al. (2008). Effectiveness of ozonated water on *Candida albicans*, *Enterococcus faecalis*, and endotoxins in root canals. *Oral Surg. Oral Med. Oral Pathol. Oral Radiol. Endod.* 105: e85–e91.

153 Silva, E.J.N.L., Prado, M.C., Soares, D.N. et al. (2020). The effect of ozone therapy in root canal disinfection: a systematic review. *Int. Endod. J.* 53: 317–332.

154 Gulabivala, K., Stock, C.J., Lewsey, J.D. et al. (2004). Effectiveness of electrochemically activated water as an irrigant in an infected tooth model. *Int. Endod. J.* 37: 624–631.

155 Solovyeva, A.M. and Dummer, P.M. (2000). Cleaning effectiveness of root canal irrigation with electrochemically activated anolyte and catholyte solutions: a pilot study. *Int. Endod. J.* 33: 494–504.

156 Rossi-Fedele, G., Guastalli, A.R., Doğramacı, E.J. et al. (2011). Influence of pH changes on chlorine-containing endodontic irrigating solutions. *Int. Endod. J.* 44: 792–799.

157 Selkon, J.B., Babb, J.R., and Morris, R. (1999). Evaluation of the antimicrobial activity of a new super-oxidized water, Sterilox, for the disinfection of endoscopes. *J. Hosp. Infect.* 41: 59–70.

158 Cheng, X., Tian, Y., Zhao, C. et al. (2016). Bactericidal effect of strong acid electrolyzed water against flow *Enterococcus faecalis* biofilms. *J. Endod.* 42: 1120–1125.

159 Marais, J.T. and Williams, W.P. (2001). Antimicrobial effectiveness of electro-chemically activated water as an endodontic irrigation solution. *Int. Endod. J.* 34: 237–243.

160 Rossi-Fedele, G., Figueiredo, J.A., Steier, L. et al. (2010). Evaluation of the antimicrobial effect of super-oxidized water (Sterilox®) and sodium hypochlorite against *Enterococcus faecalis* in a bovine root canal model. *J. Appl. Oral Sci.* 18: 498–502.

161 Rossi-Fedele, G., Steier, L., Dogramaci, E.J. et al. (2013). Bovine pulp tissue dissolution ability of HealOzone®, Aquatine Alpha Electrolyte® and sodium hypochlorite. *Aust. Endod. J.* 39: 57–61.

162 De Meyer, S., Meire, M.A., Coenye, T., and De Moor, R.J. (2017). Effect of laser-activated irrigation on biofilms in artificial root canals. *Int. Endod. J.* 50: 472–479.

163 Robinson, J.P., Macedo, R.G., Verhaagen, B. et al. (2018). Cleaning lateral morphological features of the root canal: the role of streaming and cavitation. *Int. Endod. J.* 51 (Suppl. 1): e55–e64.

164 Krishnamurthy, S. and Sudhakaran, S. (2010). Evaluation and prevention of the precipitate formed on interaction between sodium hypochlorite and chlorhexidine. *J. Endod.* 36: 1154–1157.

165 Psimma, Z. and Boutsioukis, C. (2019). A critical view on sodium hypochlorite accidents. *ENDO* 13: 165–175.

166 Abou-Rass, M. and Patonai, F.J. Jr. (1982). The effects of decreasing surface tension on the flow of irrigating solutions in narrow root canals. *Oral Surg. Oral Med. Oral Pathol.* 53: 524–526.

167 Taşman, F., Cehreli, Z.C., Oğan, C., and Etikan, I. (2000). Surface tension of root canal irrigants. *J. Endod.* 26: 586–587.

168 Giardino, L., Ambu, E., Becce, C. et al. (2006). Surface tension comparison of four common root canal irrigants and two new irrigants containing antibiotic. *J. Endod.* 32: 1091–1093.

169 Palazzi, F., Morra, M., Mohammadi, Z. et al. (2012). Comparison of the surface tension of 5.25% sodium hypochlorite solution with three new sodium hypochlorite-based endodontic irrigants. *Int. Endod. J.* 45: 129–135.

170 Boutsioukis, C. (2019). Syringe irrigation revisited. *ENDO* 13: 101–113.

171 Simões, M., Pereira, M.O., and Vieira, M.J. (2005). Effect of mechanical stress on biofilms challenged by different chemicals. *Water Res.* 39: 5142–5152.

172 Wang, Z., Shen, Y., Ma, J. et al. (2012). The effect of detergents on the antibacterial activity of disinfecting solutions in dentin. *J. Endod.* 38: 948–953.

173 Arias-Moliz, M.T., Ferrer-Luque, C.M., González-Rodríguez, M.P. et al. (2010). Eradication of *Enterococcus faecalis* biofilms by cetrimide and chlorhexidine. *J. Endod.* 36: 87–90.

174 Ferrer-Luque, C.M., Conde-Ortiz, A., Arias-Moliz, M.T. et al. (2012). Residual activity of chelating agents and their combinations with cetrimide on root canals infected with *Enterococcus faecalis*. *J. Endod.* 38: 826–828.

175 Ferrer-Luque, C.M., González-Castillo, S., Ruiz-Linares, M. et al. (2015). Antimicrobial residual effects of irrigation regimens with maleic acid in infected root canals. *J. Biol. Res.* 22: 1.

176 Bukiet, F., Couderc, G., Camps, J. et al. (2012). Wetting properties and critical micellar concentration of benzalkonium chloride mixed in sodium hypochlorite. *J. Endod.* 38: 1525–1529.

177 Baron, A., Lindsey, K., Sidow, S.J. et al. (2016). Effect of a benzalkonium chloride surfactant-sodium hypochlorite combination on elimination of *Enterococcus faecalis*. *J. Endod.* 42: 145–149.

178 Clarkson, R.M., Kidd, B., Evans, G.E., and Moule, A.J. (2012). The effect of surfactant on the dissolution of porcine pulpal tissue by sodium hypochlorite solutions. *J. Endod.* 38: 1257–1260.

179 Jungbluth, H., Peters, C., Peters, O. et al. (2012). Physicochemical and pulp tissue dissolution properties of some household bleach brands compared with a dental sodium hypochlorite solution. *J. Endod.* 38: 372–375.

180 De-Deus, G., de Berredo Pinho, M.A., Reis, C. et al. (2013). Sodium hypochlorite with reduced surface tension does not improve *in situ* pulp tissue dissolution. *J. Endod.* 39: 1039–1043.

181 Guastalli, A.R., Clarkson, R.M., and Rossi-Fedele, G. (2015). The effect of surfactants on the stability of sodium hypochlorite preparations. *J. Endod.* 41: 1344–1348.

182 Shen, Y., Stojicic, S., and Haapasalo, M. (2011). Antimicrobial efficacy of chlorhexidine against bacteria in biofilms at different stages of development. *J. Endod.* 37: 657–661.

183 Zehnder, M., Schicht, O., Sener, B., and Schmidlin, P. (2005). Reducing surface tension in endodontic chelator solutions has no effect on their ability to remove calcium from instrumented root canals. *J. Endod.* 31: 590–592.

184 De-Deus, G., Reis, C., Fidel, S. et al. (2008). Dentine demineralization when subjected to EDTA with or without various wetting agents: a co-site digital optical microscopy study. *Int. Endod. J.* 41: 279–287.

185 da Silva, L.A., Sanguino, A.C., Rocha, C.T. et al. (2008). Scanning electron microscopic preliminary study of the efficacy of SmearClear and EDTA for smear layer removal after root canal instrumentation in permanent teeth. *J. Endod.* 34: 1541–1544.

186 Torabinejad, M., Khademi, A.A., Babagoli, J. et al. (2003). A new solution for the removal of the smear layer. *J. Endod.* 29: 170–175.

187 Torabinejad, M., Cho, Y., Khademi, A.A. et al. (2003). The effect of various concentrations of sodium hypochlorite on the ability of MTAD to remove the smear layer. *J. Endod.* 29: 233–239.

188 Newberry, B.M., Shabahang, S., Johnson, N. et al. (2007). The antimicrobial effect of biopure MTAD on eight strains of *Enterococcus faecalis*: an *in vitro* investigation. *J. Endod.* 33: 1352–1354.

189 Haznedaroğlu, F. and Ersev, H. (2001). Tetracycline HCl solution as a root canal irrigant. *J. Endod.* 27: 738–740.

190 Mozayeni, M.A., Javaheri, G.H., Poorroosta, P. et al. (2009). Effect of 17% EDTA and MTAD on intracanal smear layer removal: a scanning electron microscopic study. *Aust. Endod. J.* 35: 13–17.

191 Tay, F.R., Pashley, D.H., Loushine, R.J. et al. (2006). Ultrastructure of smear layer covered intraradicular dentin after irrigation with BioPure MTAD. *J. Endod.* 32: 218–221.

192 Baker, P., Evans, R., and Coburn, R. (1983). Tetracycline and its derivatives strongly bind to and are released from the tooth surface in active form. *J. Periodontol.* 54: 580–585.

193 Mohammadi, Z. and Shahriari, S. (2008). Residual antibacterial activity of chlorhexidine and MTAD in human root dentin *in vitro*. *J. Oral Sci.* 50: 63–67.

194 Shabahang, S., Pouresmail, M., and Torabinejad, M. (2003). *In vitro* antimicrobial efficacy of MTAD and sodium hypochlorite. *J. Endod.* 29: 450–452.

195 Shabahang, S. and Torabinejad, M. (2003). Effect of MTAD on *Enterococcus faecalis*-contaminated root canals of extracted human teeth. *J. Endod.* 29: 576–579.

196 Torabinejad, M., Shabahang, S., Aprecio, R.M. et al. (2003). The antimicrobial effect of MTAD: an *in vitro* investigation. *J. Endod.* 29: 400–403.

197 Prabhakar, J., Senthilkumar, M., Priya, M.S. et al. (2010). Evaluation of antimicrobial efficacy of herbal alternatives (Triphala and green tea polyphenols), MTAD, and 5% sodium hypochlorite against *Enterococcus faecalis* biofilm formed on tooth substrate: an *in vitro* study. *J. Endod.* 36: 83–86.

198 Clegg, M.S., Vertucci, F.J., Walker, C. et al. (2006). The effect of exposure to irrigant solutions on apical dentin biofilms *in vitro*. *J. Endod.* 32: 434–437.

199 Dunavant, T.R., Regan, J.D., Glickman, G.N. et al. (2006). Comparative evaluation of endodontic irrigants against *Enterococcus faecalis* biofilms. *J. Endod.* 32: 527–531.

200 Kho, P. and Baumgartner, J.C. (2006). A comparison of the antimicrobial efficacy of NaOCl/biopure MTAD versus NaOCl/EDTA against *Enterococcus faecalis*. *J. Endod.* 32: 652–655.

201 Tay, F.R., Hiraishi, N., Schuster, G.S. et al. (2006). Reduction in antimicrobial substantivity of MTAD after initial sodium hypochlorite irrigation. *J. Endod.* 32: 970–975.

202 Johal, S., Baumgartner, J.C., and Marshall, J.G. (2007). Comparison of the antimicrobial efficacy of 1.3% NaOCl/BioPure MTAD to 5.25% NaOCl/15% EDTA for root canal irrigation. *J. Endod.* 33: 48–51.

203 Giardino, L., Andrade, F.B., and Beltrami, R. (2016). Antimicrobial effect and surface tension of some chelating solutions with added surfactants. *Braz. Dent. J.* 27: 584–588.

204 Malkhassian, G., Manzur, A.J., Legner, M. et al. (2009). Antibacterial efficacy of MTAD final rinse and two percent chlorhexidine gel medication in teeth with apical periodontitis: a randomized double-blinded clinical trial. *J. Endod.* 35: 1483–1490.

205 Stojicic, S., Shen, Y., Qian, W. et al. (2012). Antibacterial and smear layer removal ability of a novel irrigant, QMiX. *Int. Endod. J.* 45: 363–371.

206 Zhang, W., Torabinejad, M., and Li, Y. (2003). Evaluation of cytotoxicity of MTAD using the MTT-tetrazolium method. *J. Endod.* 29: 654–657.

207 Tay, F.R. and Mazzoni, A. (2006). Potential iatrogenic tetracycline staining of endodontically treated teeth with NaOCl/MTAD irrigation. A preliminary report. *J. Endod.* 32: 354–358.

208 Singla, M.G., Garg, A., and Gupta, S. (2011). MTAD in endodontics: an update review. *Oral Surg. Oral Med. Oral Pathol. Oral Radiol. Endod.* 112: e70–e76.

209 Giardino, L., Ambu, E., Savoldi, E. et al. (2007). Comparative evaluation of antimicrobial efficacy of sodium hypochlorite, MTAD, and Tetraclean against *Enterococcus faecalis* biofilm. *J. Endod.* 33: 852–855.

210 Pappen, F.G., Shen, Y., Qian, W. et al. (2010). *In vitro* antibacterial action of Tetraclean, MTAD, and five experimental irrigation solutions. *Int. Endod. J.* 43: 528–535.

211 Poggio, C., Dagna, A., Colombo, M. et al. (2012). Decalcifying effect of different ethylenediaminetetraacetic acid irrigating solutions and tetraclean on root canal dentin. *J. Endod.* 38: 1239–1243.

212 Mohammadi, Z., Mombeinipour, A., Giardino, L. et al. (2011). Residual antibacterial activity of a new modified sodium hypochlorite-based endodontic irrigation solution. *Med. Oral Patol. Oral Cir. Bucal* 16: e588–e592.

213 Mohammadi, Z., Giardino, L., and Mombeinipour, A. (2012). Antibacterial substantivity of a new antibiotic-based endodontic irrigation solution. *Aust. Endod. J.* 38: 26–30.

214 Mohammadi, Z., Giardino, L., Palazzi, F. et al. (2013). Effect of initial irrigation with sodium hypochlorite on residual antibacterial activity of tetraclean. *N. Y. State Dent. J.* 79: 32–36.

215 Dai, L., Khechen, K., Khan, S. et al. (2011). The effect of QMix, an experimental antibacterial root canal irrigant, on removal of canal wall smear layer and debris. *J. Endod.* 37: 80–84.

216 Wang, Z., Shen, Y., and Haapasalo, M. (2012). Effectiveness of endodontic disinfecting solutions against young and old *Enterococcus faecalis* biofilms in dentin canals. *J. Endod.* 38: 1376–1379.

217 Ordinola-Zapata, R., Bramante, C.M., Garcia, R.B. et al. (2013). The antimicrobial effect of new and conventional endodontic irrigants on intra-orally infected dentin. *Acta Odontol. Scand.* 71: 424–431.

218 Balić, M., Lucić, R., Mehadžić, K. et al. (2016). The efficacy of photon-initiated photoacoustic streaming and sonic-activated irrigation combined with QMiX solution or sodium hypochlorite against intracanal *E. faecalis* biofilm. *Lasers Med. Sci.* 31: 335–342.

219 Ye, W.H., Fan, B., Purcell, W. et al. (2018). Anti-biofilm efficacy of root canal irrigants against *in-situ Enterococcus faecalis* biofilms in root canals, isthmuses and dentinal tubules. *J. Dent.* 79: 68–76.

220 Souza, M.A., Montagner, A., Lana, D.L. et al. (2017). Comparative evaluation of the retaining of QMix and chlorhexidine formulations on human dentin: a chemical analysis. *Clin. Oral Investig.* 21: 873–878.

221 Gomes-Filho, J.E., Aurélio, K.G., Costa, M.M. et al. (2008). Comparison of the biocompatibility of different root canal irrigants. *J. Appl. Oral Sci.* 16: 137–144.

222 Chandrasekhar, V., Amulya, V., Rani, V.S. et al. (2013). Evaluation of biocompatibility of a new root canal irrigant Q Mix™ 2 in 1 – an *in vivo* study. *J. Conserv. Dent.* 16: 36–40.

223 Tay, F.R., Hosoya, Y., Loushine, R.J. et al. (2006). Ultrastructure of intraradicular dentin after irrigation with BioPure MTAD. II. The consequence of obturation with an epoxy resin-based sealer. *J. Endod.* 32: 473–477.

224 Vilanova, W.V., Carvalho-Junior, J.R., Alfredo, E. et al. (2012). Effect of intracanal irrigants on the bond strength of epoxy resin-based and methacrylate resin-based sealers to root canal walls. *Int. Endod. J.* 45: 42–48.

225 Stelzer, R., Schaller, H.G., and Gernhardt, C.R. (2014). Push-out bond strength of RealSeal SE and AH plus after using different irrigation solutions. *J. Endod.* 40: 1654–1657.

226 Collares, F.M., Portella, F.F., Rodrigues, S.B. et al. (2016). The influence of methodological variables on the push-out resistance to dislodgement of root filling materials: a meta-regression analysis. *Int. Endod. J.* 49: 836–849.

227 Macedo, R.G., Verhaagen, B., Fernandez Rivas, D. et al. (2014). Sonochemical and high-speed optical characterization of cavitation generated by an ultrasonically oscillating dental file in root canal models. *Ultrason. Sonochem.* 21: 324–335.

228 Tiong, T.J. and Price, G.J. (2012). Ultrasound promoted reaction of Rhodamine B with sodium hypochlorite using sonochemical and dental ultrasonic instruments. *Ultrason. Sonochem.* 19: 358–364.

229 Savani, G.M., Sabbah, W., Sedgley, C.M., and Whitten, B. (2014). Current trends in endodontic treatment by general dental practitioners: report of a United States national survey. *J. Endod.* 40: 618–624.

230 de Gregorio, C., Arias, A., Navarrete, N. et al. (2015). Differences in disinfection protocols for root canal treatments between general dentists and endodontists: a web-based survey. *J. Am. Dent. Assoc.* 146: 536–543.

231 Brunson, M., Heilborn, C., Johnson, J.D., and Cohenca, N. (2010). Effect of apical preparation size and preparation taper on irrigant volume delivered by using negative pressure irrigation system. *J. Endod.* 36: 721–724.

232 Boutsioukis, C. and van der Sluis, L.W.M. (2015). Syringe irrigation: blending Endodontics and Fluid Dynamics. In: *Endodontic Irrigation: Chemical Disinfection of the Root Canal System* (ed. B. Basrani), 45–64. New York, NY: Springer.

233 Senia, E.S., Marshall, J.F., and Rosen, S. (1971). The solvent action of sodium hypochlorite on pulp tissue of extracted teeth. *Oral Surg. Oral Med. Oral Pathol.* 31: 96–103.

234 Abou-Rass, M. and Piccinino, M.V. (1982). The effectiveness of four clinical irrigation methods on the removal of root canal debris. *Oral Surg. Oral Med. Oral Pathol.* 54: 323–328.

235 Moser, J.B. and Heuer, M.A. (1982). Forces and efficacy in endodontic irrigation systems. *Oral Surg. Oral Med. Oral Pathol.* 53: 425–428.

236 Chow, T.W. (1983). Mechanical effectiveness of root canal irrigation. *J. Endod.* 9: 475–479.

237 Kahn, F.H., Rosenberg, P.A., and Gliksberg, J. (1995). An *in vitro* evaluation of the irrigating characteristics of ultrasonic and subsonic handpieces and irrigating needles and probes. *J. Endod.* 21: 277–280.

238 Sabins, R.A., Johnson, J.D., and Hellstein, J.W. (2003). A comparison of the cleaning efficacy of short term sonic and ultrasonic passive irrigation after hand instrumentation in molar root canals. *J. Endod.* 29: 674–678.

239 Sedgley, C.M., Nagel, A.C., Hall, D., and Applegate, B. (2005). Influence of irrigant needle depth in removing bacteria inoculated into instrumented root canals using real-time imaging *in vitro*. *Int. Endod. J.* 38: 97–104.

240 Haapasalo, M., Shen, Y., Qian, W., and Gao, Y. (2010). Irrigation in endodontics. *Dent. Clin. N. Am.* 54: 291–312.

241 Boutsioukis, C., Lambrianidis, T., Kastrinakis, E., and Bekiaroglou, P. (2007). Measurement of pressure and flow rates during irrigation of a root canal *ex vivo* with three endodontic needles. *Int. Endod. J.* 40: 504–513.

242 Goldman, M., Kronman, J.H., Goldman, L.B. et al. (1976). New method of irrigation during endodontic treatment. *J. Endod.* 2: 257–260.

243 Goldman, L.B., Goldman, M., Kronman, J.H., and Lin, P.S. (1979). Scanning electron microscope study of a new irrigation method in endodontic treatment. *Oral Surg. Oral Med. Oral Pathol.* 48: 79–83.

244 Yamamoto, A., Otogoto, J., Kuroiwa, A. et al. (2006). The effect of irrigation using trial-manufactured washing needle. *Jpn. J. Conserv. Dent.* 49: 64–70.

245 Vinothkumar, T.S., Kavitha, S., Lakshminarayanan, L. et al. (2007). Influence of irrigating needle-tip designs in removing bacteria inoculated into instrumented root canals measured using single-tube luminometer. *J. Endod.* 33: 746–748.

246 Hülsmann, M., Rödig, T., and Nordmeyer, S. (2009). Complications during root canal irrigation. *Endod. Topics* 16: 27–63.

247 Boutsioukis, C., Verhaagen, B., Versluis, M. et al. (2010). Evaluation of irrigant flow in the root canal using different needle types by an unsteady Computational Fluid Dynamics model. *J. Endod.* 36: 875–879.

248 Boutsioukis, C., Lambrianidis, T., and Vasiliadis, L. (2007). Clinical relevance of standardization of endodontic irrigation needle dimensions according to the ISO 9626:1991 & 9626:1991/Amd 1:2001 specification. *Int. Endod. J.* 40: 700–706.

249 ISO 9626 (2001). Stainless steel needle tubing for manufacture of medical devices. Amendment 1, 1–5. Geneva: International Organization for Standardization.

250 Brown, J.I. and Doran, J.E. (1975). An *in vitro* evaluation of the particle flotation capability of various irrigating solutions. *J. Calif. Dent. Assoc.* 3: 60–63.

251 Ram, Z. (1977). Effectiveness of root canal irrigation. *Oral Surg. Oral Med. Oral Pathol.* 44: 306–312.

252 Salzgeber, R.M. and Brilliant, J.D. (1977). An *in vivo* evaluation of the penetration of an irrigating solution in root canals. *J. Endod.* 3: 394–398.

253 Teplitsky, P.E., Chenail, B.L., Mack, B., and Machnee, C.H. (1987). Endodontic irrigation--a comparison of endosonic and syringe delivery systems. *Int. Endod. J.* 20: 233–241.

254 Druttman, A.C.S. and Stock, C.J.R. (1989). An *in vitro* comparison of ultrasonic and conventional methods of irrigant replacement. *Int. Endod. J.* 22: 174–178.

255 Bronnec, F., Bouillaguet, S., and Machtou, P. (2010). *Ex vivo* assessment of irrigant penetration and renewal during the final irrigation regimen. *Int. Endod. J.* 43: 663–672.

256 Boutsioukis, C., Lambrianidis, T., Verhaagen, B. et al. (2010). The effect of needle insertion depth on the irrigant flow in the root canal: evaluation using an unsteady Computational Fluid Dynamics model. *J. Endod.* 36: 1664–1668.

257 Huang, T.Y., Gulabivala, K., and Ng, Y.L. (2008). A bio-molecular film *ex-vivo* model to evaluate the influence of canal dimensions and irrigation variables on the efficacy of irrigation. *Int. Endod. J.* 41: 60–71.

258 Sedgley, C., Applegate, B., Nagel, A., and Hall, D. (2004). Real-time imaging and quantification of bioluminescent bacteria in root canals *in vitro*. *J. Endod.* 30: 893–898.

259 Nguy, D. and Sedgley, C. (2006). The influence of canal curvature in the mechanical efficacy of root canal irrigation *in vitro* using real-time imaging of bioluminescent bacteria. *J. Endod.* 32: 1077–1080.

260 Gluskin, A.H., Peters, C.I., and Peters, O.A. (2014). Minimally invasive endodontics: challenging prevailing paradigms. *Br. Dent. J.* 216: 347–353.

261 Chen, J.E., Nurbakhsh, B., Layton, G. et al. (2014). Irrigation dynamics associated with positive pressure, apical negative pressure and passive ultrasonic irrigations: a Computational Fluid Dynamics analysis. *Aust. Endod. J.* 40: 54–60.

262 Verhaagen, B., Boutsioukis, C., Heijnen, G.L. et al. (2012). Role of the confinement of a root canal on jet impingement during endodontic irrigation. *Exp. Fluids* 53: 1841–1853.

263 Hsieh, Y.D., Gau, C.H., Kung Wu, S.F. et al. (2007). Dynamic recording of irrigating fluid distribution in root canals using thermal image analysis. *Int. Endod. J.* 40: 11–17.

264 Boutsioukis, C., Gogos, C., Verhaagen, B. et al. (2010). The effect of apical preparation size on irrigant flow in root canals evaluated using an unsteady Computational Fluid Dynamics model. *Int. Endod. J.* 43: 874–881.

265 Boutsioukis, C., Gogos, C., Verhaagen, B. et al. (2010). The effect of root canal taper on the irrigant flow: evaluation using an unsteady Computational Fluid Dynamics model. *Int. Endod. J.* 43: 909–916.

266 Psimma, Z., Boutsioukis, C., Vasiliadis, L., and Kastrinakis, E. (2013). A new method for real-time quantification of irrigant extrusion during root canal irrigation *ex vivo*. *Int. Endod. J.* 46: 619–631.

267 Boutsioukis, C., Lambrianidis, T., and Kastrinakis, E. (2009). Irrigant flow within a prepared root canal using different flow rates: a Computational Fluid Dynamics study. *Int. Endod. J.* 42: 144–155.

268 Šnjarić, D., Carija, Z., Braut, A. et al. (2012). Irrigation of human prepared root canal – *ex vivo* based Computational Fluid Dynamics analysis. *Croat. Med. J.* 53: 470–479.

269 Psimma, Z., Boutsioukis, C., Kastrinakis, E., and Vasiliadis, L. (2013). Effect of needle insertion depth and root canal curvature on irrigant extrusion *ex vivo*. *J. Endod.* 39: 521–524.

270 Rossi-Fedele, G. and De Figueiredo, J.A. (2008). Use of a bottle warmer to increase 4% sodium hypochlorite tissue dissolution ability on bovine pulp. *Aust. Endod. J.* 34: 39–42.

271 Macedo, R.G., Verhaagen, B., Versluis, M. et al. (2017). Temperature evolution of preheated irrigant injected into a root canal *ex vivo*. *Clin. Oral Investig.* 21: 2841–2850.

272 de Vasconcelos, R.A., Murphy, S., Carvalho, C.A. et al. (2016). Evidence for reduced fatigue resistance of contemporary rotary instruments exposed to body temperature. *J. Endod.* 42: 782–787.

273 Plotino, G., Grande, N.M., Mercadé Bellido, M. et al. (2017). Influence of temperature on cyclic fatigue resistance of Protaper Gold and Protaper Universal rotary files. *J. Endod.* 43: 200–202.

274 Huang, X., Shen, Y., Wei, X., and Haapasalo, M. (2017). Fatigue resistance of nickel-titanium instruments exposed to high-concentration hypochlorite. *J. Endod.* 43: 1847–1851.

275 Brito, P.R., Souza, L.C., Machado de Oliveira, J.C. et al. (2009). Comparison of the effectiveness of three irrigation techniques in reducing intracanal *Enterococcus faecalis* populations: an *in vitro* study. *J. Endod.* 35: 1422–1427.

276 Bhuva, B., Patel, S., Wilson, R. et al. (2010). The effectiveness of passive ultrasonic irrigation on intraradicular *Enterococcus faecalis* biofilms in extracted single-rooted human teeth. *Int. Endod. J.* 43: 241–250.

277 Klyn, S.L., Kirkpatrick, T.C., and Rutledge, R.E. (2010). *In vitro* comparisons of debris removal of the EndoActivator system, the F file, ultrasonic irrigation, and NaOCl irrigation alone after hand-rotary instrumentation in human mandibular molars. *J. Endod.* 36: 1367–1371.

278 Howard, R.K., Kirkpatrick, T.C., Rutledge, R.E., and Yaccino, J.M. (2011). Comparison of debris removal with three different irrigation techniques. *J. Endod.* 37: 1301–1305.

279 Adcock, J.M., Sidow, S.J., Looney, S.W. et al. (2011). Histologic evaluation of canal and isthmus debridement efficacies of two different irrigant delivery techniques in a closed system. *J. Endod.* 37: 544–548.

280 Johnson, M., Sidow, S.J., Looney, S.W. et al. (2012). Canal and isthmus debridement efficacy using a sonic irrigation technique in a closed-canal system. *J. Endod.* 38: 1265–1268.

281 Sarno, M.U., Sidow, S.J., Looney, S.W. et al. (2012). Canal and isthmus debridement efficacy of the VPro EndoSafe negative-pressure irrigation technique. *J. Endod.* 38: 1631–1634.

282 Versiani, M.A., Alves, F.R., Andrade-Junior, C.V. et al. (2016). Micro-CT evaluation of the efficacy of hard tissue removal from the root canal and isthmus area by positive and negative pressure irrigation systems. *Int. Endod. J.* 49: 1079–1087.

283 Liang, Y.H., Jiang, L.M., Jiang, L. et al. (2013). Radiographic healing after a root canal treatment performed in single-rooted teeth with and without ultrasonic activation of the irrigant: a randomized controlled trial. *J. Endod.* 39: 1218–1225.

284 Burleson, A., Nusstein, J., Reader, A., and Beck, M. (2007). The *in vivo* evaluation of hand/rotary/ultrasound instrumentation in necrotic, human mandibular molars. *J. Endod.* 33: 782–787.

285 Miller, T.A. and Baumgartner, J.C. (2010). Comparison of the antimicrobial efficacy of irrigation using the EndoVac to endodontic needle delivery. *J. Endod.* 36: 509–511.

286 Miranda, R.G., Santos, E.B., Souto, R.M. et al. (2013). *Ex vivo* antimicrobial efficacy of the EndoVac system plus photodynamic therapy associated with calcium hydroxide against intracanal *Enterococcus faecalis*. *Int. Endod. J.* 46: 499–505.

287 Paiva, S.S., Siqueira, J.F. Jr., Rôças, I.N. et al. (2013). Molecular microbiological evaluation of passive ultrasonic activation as a supplementary disinfecting step: a clinical study. *J. Endod.* 39: 190–194.

288 Molina, B., Glickman, G., Vandrangi, P., and Khakpour, M. (2015). Evaluation of root canal debridement of human molars using the Gentlewave system. *J. Endod.* 41: 1701–1705.

289 Hockett, J.L., Dommisch, J.K., Johnson, J.D., and Cohenca, N. (2008). Antimicrobial efficacy of two irrigation techniques in tapered and nontapered canal preparations: an *in vitro* study. *J. Endod.* 34: 1374–1377.

290 Nielsen, B.A. and Baumgartner, J.C. (2007). Comparison of the EndoVac system to needle irrigation of root canals. *J. Endod.* 33: 611–615.

291 McGill, S., Gulabivala, K., Mordan, N., and Ng, Y.L. (2008). The efficacy of dynamic irrigation using a commercially available system (RinsEndo) determined by removal of a collagen 'bio-molecular film' from an *ex vivo* model. *Int. Endod. J.* 41: 602–608.

292 Azim, A.A., Aksel, H., Zhuang, T. et al. (2016). Efficacy of 4 irrigation protocols in killing bacteria colonized in dentinal tubules examined by a novel confocal laser scanning microscope analysis. *J. Endod.* 42: 928–934.

293 Kishen, A., Shrestha, A., and Del Carpio-Perochena, A. (2018). Validation of biofilm assays to assess antibiofilm efficacy in instrumented root canals after syringe irrigation and sonic agitation. *J. Endod.* 44: 292–298.

294 van der Sluis, L., Wu, M.K., and Wesselink, P. (2009). Comparison of 2 flushing methods used during passive ultrasonic irrigation of the root canal. *Quintessence Int.* 40: 875–879.

295 van der Sluis, L.W.M., Voogels, M.P.J.M., Verhaagen, B. et al. (2010). Study on the influence of refreshment/activation cycles and irrigants on mechanical cleaning efficiency during ultrasonic activation of the irrigant. *J. Endod.* 36: 737–740.

296 de Groot, S.D., Verhaagen, B., Versluis, M. et al. (2009). Laser-activated irrigation within root canals: cleaning efficacy and flow visualization. *Int. Endod. J.* 42: 1077–1083.

297 Jiang, L.M., Verhaagen, B., Versluis, M., and van der Sluis, L.W.M. (2010). Evaluation of a sonic device designed to activate irrigant in the root canal. *J. Endod.* 36: 143–146.

298 Rödig, T., Bozkurt, M., Konietschke, F., and Hülsmann, M. (2010). Comparison of the Vibringe system with syringe and passive ultrasonic irrigation in removing debris from simulated root canal irregularities. *J. Endod.* 36: 1410–1413.

299 Rödig, T., Sedghi, M., Konietschke, F. et al. (2010). Efficacy of syringe irrigation, RinsEndo and passive ultrasonic irrigation in removing debris from irregularities in root canals with different apical sizes. *Int. Endod. J.* 43: 581–589.

300 Amato, M., Vanoni-Heineken, I., Hecker, H., and Weiger, R. (2011). Curved versus straight root canals: the benefit of activated irrigation techniques on dentin debris removal. *Oral Surg. Oral Med. Oral Pathol. Oral Radiol. Endod.* 111: 529–534.

301 Jiang, L.M., Lak, B., Eijsvogels, L.M. et al. (2012). Comparison of the cleaning efficacy of different final irrigation techniques. *J. Endod.* 38: 838–841.

302 Conde, A.J., Estevez, R., Loroño, G. et al. (2017). Effect of sonic and ultrasonic activation on organic tissue dissolution from simulated grooves in root canals using sodium hypochlorite and EDTA. *Int. Endod. J.* 50: 976–982.

303 Paqué, F., Boessler, C., and Zehnder, M. (2011). Accumulated hard tissue debris levels in mesial roots of mandibular molars after sequential irrigation steps. *Int. Endod. J.* 44: 148–153.

304 Leoni, G.B., Versiani, M.A., Silva-Sousa, Y.T. et al. (2017). *Ex vivo* evaluation of four final irrigation protocols on the removal of hard-tissue debris from the mesial root canal system of mandibular first molars. *Int. Endod. J.* 50: 398–406.

305 Gutarts, R., Nusstein, J., Reader, A., and Beck, M. (2005). *In vivo* debridement efficacy of ultrasonic irrigation following hand-rotary instrumentation in human mandibular molars. *J. Endod.* 31: 166–170.

306 Al-Ali, M., Sathorn, C., and Parashos, P. (2012). Root canal debridement efficacy of different final irrigation protocols. *Int. Endod. J.* 45: 898–906.

307 Al-Jadaa, A., Paqué, F., Attin, T., and Zehnder, M. (2009). Necrotic pulp tissue dissolution by passive ultrasonic irrigation in simulated accessory canals: impact of canal location and angulation. *Int. Endod. J.* 42: 59–65.

308 de Gregorio, C., Estevez, R., Cisneros, R. et al. (2010). Efficacy of different irrigation and activation systems on the penetration of sodium hypochlorite into simulated lateral canals and up to working length: an *in vitro* study. *J. Endod.* 36: 1216–1221.

309 de Gregorio, C., Paranjpe, A., Garcia, A. et al. (2012). Efficacy of irrigation systems on penetration of sodium hypochlorite to working length and to simulated uninstrumented areas in oval shaped root canals. *Int. Endod. J.* 45: 475–481.

310 Malentacca, A., Uccioli, U., Zangari, D. et al. (2012). Efficacy and safety of various active irrigation devices when used with either positive or negative pressure: an *in vitro* study. *J. Endod.* 38: 1622–1626.

311 Adorno, C.G., Fretes, V.R., Ortiz, C.P. et al. (2016). Comparison of two negative pressure systems and syringe irrigation for root canal irrigation: an *ex vivo* study. *Int. Endod. J.* 49: 174–183.

312 Gutmann, J.L., Zehnder, M., and Levermann, V.M. (2014). Historical perspectives on the roots of the apical negative pressure irrigation technique in endodontics. *J. Hist. Dent.* 62: 32–40.

313 Tay, F.R., Gu, L.S., Schoeffel, G.J. et al. (2010). Effect of vapor lock on root canal debridement by using a side-vented needle for positive-pressure irrigant delivery. *J. Endod.* 36: 745–750.

314 Boutsioukis, C., Kastrinakis, E., Lambrianidis, T. et al. (2014). Formation and removal of apical vapor lock during syringe irrigation: a combined experimental and Computational Fluid Dynamics approach. *Int. Endod. J.* 47: 191–201.

315 Fukumoto, Y., Kikuchi, I., Yoshioka, T. et al. (2006). An *ex vivo* evaluation of a new root canal irrigation technique with intracanal aspiration. *Int. Endod. J.* 39: 93–99.

316 Glassman, G. and Charara, K. (2015). Apical negative pressure: safety, efficacy and efficiency. In: *Endodontic Irrigation: Chemical Disinfection of the Root Canal System* (ed. B. Basrani), 157–171. New York, NY: Springer.

317 Kerr Endodontics. (2018). EndoVac™ apical negative pressure irrigation system. Instructions for use. 8–10.

318 Schoeffel, G.J. (2008). The EndoVac method of endodontic irrigation, part 2 – efficacy. *Dent. Today* 27: 82, 84, 86–87.

319 Konstantinidi, E., Psimma, Z., Chávez de Paz, L.E., and Boutsioukis, C. (2017). Apical negative pressure irrigation versus syringe irrigation: a systematic review of cleaning and disinfection of the root canal system. *Int. Endod. J.* 50: 1034–1054.

320 Thomas, A.R., Velmurugan, N., Smita, S., and Jothilatha, S. (2014). Comparative evaluation of canal isthmus debridement efficacy of modified EndoVac technique with different irrigation systems. *J. Endod.* 40: 1676–1680.

321 van der Sluis, L.W., Versluis, M., Wu, M.K., and Wesselink, P.R. (2007). Passive ultrasonic irrigation of the root canal: a review of the literature. *Int. Endod. J.* 40: 415–426.

322 Verhaagen, B., Lea, S.C., de Bruin, G.J. et al. (2012). Oscillation characteristics of endodontic files: numerical model and its validation. *IEEE Trans. Ultrason. Ferroelectr. Freq. Control* 59: 2448–2459.

323 Duck, P.W. and Smith, F.T. (1979). Steady streaming induced between oscillating cylinders. *J. Fluid Mech.* 91: 93–110.

324 Verhaagen, B., Boutsioukis, C., van der Sluis, L.W., and Versluis, M. (2014). Acoustic streaming induced by an ultrasonically oscillating endodontic file. *J. Acoust. Soc. Am.* 135: 1717–1730.

325 Yasui, K. (2018). *Acoustic Cavitation and Bubble Dynamics*, 37–97. New York, NY: Springer.

326 Retsas, A. and Boutsioukis, C. (2019). An update on ultrasonic irrigant activation. *ENDO* 13: 115–129.

327 Brennen, C.E. (1995). *Cavitation and Bubble Dynamics*, 1e, 1–290. New York, NY: Oxford University Press.

328 Macedo, R., Verhaagen, B., Rivas, D.F. et al. (2014). Cavitation measurement during sonic and ultrasonic activated irrigation. *J. Endod.* 40: 580–583.

329 Suslick, K.S. (1990). Sonochemistry. *Science* 247: 1439–1445.

330 Cunningham, W.T., Martin, H., and Forrest, W.R. (1982). Evaluation of root canal debridement by the endosonic ultrasonic synergistic system. *Oral Surg. Oral Med. Oral Pathol.* 53: 401–404.

331 Cameron, J.A. (1988). The effect of ultrasonic endodontics on the temperature of the root canal wall. *J. Endod.* 14: 554–559.

332 Zeltner, M., Peters, O.A., and Paqué, F. (2009). Temperature changes during ultrasonic irrigation with different inserts and modes of activation. *J. Endod.* 35: 573–577.

333 Weller, R.N., Brady, J.M., and Bernier, W.E. (1980). Efficacy of ultrasonic cleaning. *J. Endod.* 6: 740–743.

334 Retsas, A., Koursoumis, A., Tzimpoulas, N., and Boutsioukis, C. (2016). Uncontrolled removal of dentin during *in vitro* ultrasonic irrigant activation in curved root canals. *J. Endod.* 42: 1545–1549.

335 Acteon-Satelec (2015). Tip book. Available from http://www.satelecsupport.com/Documentation/TIPS/TIPBOOK.pdf (accessed 10 August 2020).

336 Boutsioukis, C. and Tzimpoulas, N. (2016). Uncontrolled removal of dentin during *in vitro* ultrasonic irrigant activation. *J. Endod.* 42: 289–293.

337 Lea, S.C., Walmsley, A.D., and Lumley, P.J. (2010). Analyzing endosonic root canal file oscillations: an *in vitro* evaluation. *J. Endod.* 36: 880–883.

338 Căpuță, P.E., Retsas, A., Kuijk, L. et al. (2019). Ultrasonic Irrigant activation during root canal treatment: a systematic review. *J. Endod.* 45: 31–44.

339 Pedullà, E., Genovese, C., Messina, R. et al. (2019). Antimicrobial efficacy of cordless sonic or ultrasonic devices on *Enterococcus faecalis*-infected root canals. *J. Investig. Clin. Dent.* 00: e12434.

340 van der Sluis, L.W.M., Gambarini, G., Wu, M.K., and Wesselink, P.R. (2006). The influence of volume, type of irrigant and flushing method on removing artificially placed dentine debris from the apical root canal during passive ultrasonic irrigation. *Int. Endod. J.* 39: 472–476.

341 Jiang, L.M., Verhaagen, B., Versluis, M. et al. (2010). An evaluation of the effect of pulsed ultrasound on the cleaning efficacy of passive ultrasonic irrigation. *J. Endod.* 36: 1887–1891.

342 Ahmad, M., Roy, R.A., and Kamarudin, A.G. (1992). Observations of acoustic streaming fields around an oscillating ultrasonic file. *Endod. Dent. Traumatol.* 8: 189–194.

343 Lumley, P.J. and Walmsley, A.D. (1992). Effect of precurving on the performance of endosonic K files. *J. Endod.* 18: 232–236.

344 Malki, M., Verhaagen, B., Jiang, L.M. et al. (2012). Irrigant flow beyond the insertion depth of an ultrasonically oscillating file in straight and curved root canals: visualization and cleaning efficacy. *J. Endod.* 38: 657–661.

345 Jiang, L.M., Verhaagen, B., Versluis, M. et al. (2011). The influence of the ultrasonic intensity on the cleaning efficacy of passive ultrasonic irrigation. *J. Endod.* 37: 688–692.

346 Al-Jadaa, A., Paque, F., Attin, T., and Zehnder, M. (2009). Acoustic hypochlorite activation in simulated curved canals. *J. Endod.* 35: 1408–1411.

347 Ahmad, M. and Roy, R.A. (1994). Some observations on the breakage of ultrasonic files driven piezoelectrically. *Endod. Dent. Traumatol.* 10: 71–76.

348 Verhaagen, B. (2012). Root canal cleaning through cavitation and microstreaming. PhD thesis, 94–98. Enschede: Physics of Fluids Group, University of Twente.

349 Electro Medical Systems (EMS) Piezon® Systems (2012). Operation instructions. Available from https://www.ems-dental.com/sites/default/files/2019-11/FB-439_3_ed_2012-06_Piezon_instruments.compressed_1.pdf (accessed 10 August 2020).

350 NSK (2017). Tip guide. Available from https://www.nsk-dental.com/admin/wp-content/uploads/oral_hygiene_tip_guide.pdf (accessed 10 August 2020).

351 Acteon-Satelec (2018). User manual. Available from https://www.acteongroup.com/en/uploads/media/default/0001/01/a264bc99fb3e386a7d8e6269957ffc225bc2efb3.pdf (accessed 10 August 2020).

352 Walmsley, A.D. and Williams, A.R. (1989). Effect of constraint on the oscillatory pattern of endosonic files. *J. Endod.* 15: 189–184.

353 Boutsioukis, C., Verhaagen, B., Walmsley, A.D. et al. (2013). Measurement and visualization of file-to-wall contact during ultrasonically activated irrigation in simulated canals. *Int. Endod. J.* 46: 1046–1055.

354 Jiang, L.M., Verhaagen, B., Versluis, M., and van der Sluis, L.W. (2010). Influence of the oscillation direction of an ultrasonic file on the cleaning efficacy of passive ultrasonic irrigation. *J. Endod.* 36: 1372–1376.

355 Zehnder, M. and Paqué, F. (2011). Disinfection of the root canal system during root canal re-treatment. *Endod. Topics* 19: 58–73.

356 Neuhaus, K.W., Liebi, M., Stauffacher, S. et al. (2016). Antibacterial efficacy of a new sonic irrigation device for root canal disinfection. *J. Endod.* 42: 1799–1803.

357 Ruddle, C.J. (2007). Hydrodynamic disinfection: tsunami endodontics. *Dent. Today* 26: 114–117.

358 VDW (2017). EDDY Innovative sonic power irrigation. Available from https://www.vdw-dental.com/fileadmin/Dokumente/Sortiment/Spuelung/Eddy/VDW-Dental-EDDY-Product-Brochure-EN.pdf (accessed 10 August 2020).

359 Zeng, C., Willison, J., Meghil, M.M. et al. (2018). Antibacterial efficacy of an endodontic sonic-powered irrigation system: an *in vitro* study. *J. Dent.* 75: 105–112.

360 Rödig, T., Koberg, C., Baxter, S. et al. (2019). Micro-CT evaluation of sonically and ultrasonically activated irrigation on the removal of hard-tissue debris from isthmus-containing mesial root canal systems of mandibular molars. *Int. Endod. J.* 52: 1173–1181.

361 Swimberghe, R.C.D., De Clercq, A., De Moor, R.J.G., and Meire, M.A. (2019). Efficacy of sonically, ultrasonically and laser-activated irrigation in removing a biofilm-mimicking hydrogel from an isthmus model. *Int. Endod. J.* 52: 515–523.

362 VDW (2017). EDDY Innovative sonic power irrigation: step by step card. Available from https://www.vdw-dental.com/fileadmin/Dokumente/Sortiment/Spuelung/Eddy/VDW-Dental-EDDY-Step-by-Step-Card-EN.pdf (accessed 10 August 2020).

363 Rödig, T., Zimmermann, F., Konietschke, F. et al. (2018). Comparison of the

antibacterial efficacy of sonic- and two ultrasonic-activated irrigation techniques in reducing intracanal *Enterococcus faecalis* populations. *Quintessence Int.* 49: 689–697.

364 Varela, P., Souza, E., de Deus, G. et al. (2019). Effectiveness of complementary irrigation routines in debriding pulp tissue from root canals instrumented with a single reciprocating file. *Int. Endod. J.* 52: 475–483.

365 Duque, J.A., Duarte, M.A., Canali, L.C. et al. (2017). Comparative effectiveness of new mechanical irrigant agitating devices for debris removal from the canal and isthmus of mesial roots of mandibular molars. *J. Endod.* 43: 326–331.

366 Arslan, H., Capar, I.D., Saygili, G. et al. (2014). Effect of photon-initiated photoacoustic streaming on removal of apically placed dentinal debris. *Int. Endod. J.* 47: 1072–1077.

367 Mohmmed, S.A., Vianna, M.E., Penny, M.R. et al. (2016). A novel experimental approach to investigate the effect of different agitation methods using sodium hypochlorite as an irrigant on the rate of bacterial biofilm removal from the wall of a simulated root canal model. *Dent. Mater.* 32: 1289–1300.

368 Matsumoto, H., Yoshimine, Y., and Akamine, A. (2011). Visualization of irrigant flow and cavitation induced by Er:YAG laser within a root canal model. *J. Endod.* 37: 839–843.

369 van der Sluis, L.W.M., Verhaagen, B., Macedo, R., and Versluis, M. (2016). The role of irrigation in endodontics. In: *Lasers in Endodontics: Scientific Background and Clinical Applications* (eds. G. Olivi, R. De Moor and E. DiVito), 45–69. New York, NY: Springer.

370 Yost, R.A., Bergeron, B.E., Kirkpatrick, T.C. et al. (2015). Evaluation of 4 different irrigating systems for apical extrusion of sodium hypochlorite. *J. Endod.* 41: 1530–1534.

371 Meire, M.A., Poelman, D., and De Moor, R.J. (2014). Optical properties of root canal irrigants in the 300–3000-nm wavelength region. *Lasers Med. Sci.* 29: 1557–1562.

372 DiVito, E., Peters, O.A., and Olivi, G. (2012). Effectiveness of the Erbium:YAG laser and new design radial and stripped tips in removing the smear layer after root canal instrumentation. *Lasers Med. Sci.* 27: 273–280.

373 Guneser, M.B., Arslan, D., and Usumez, A. (2015). Tissue dissolution ability of sodium hypochlorite activated by photon-initiated photoacoustic streaming technique. *J. Endod.* 41: 729–732.

374 Meire, M.A., Havelaerts, S., and De Moor, R.J. (2016). Influence of lasing parameters on the cleaning efficacy of laser-activated irrigation with pulsed erbium lasers. *Lasers Med. Sci.* 31: 653–658.

375 Verstraeten, J., Jacquet, W., De Moor, R.J.G., and Meire, M.A. (2017). Hard tissue debris removal from the mesial root canal system of mandibular molars with ultrasonically and laser-activated irrigation: a micro-computed tomography study. *Lasers Med. Sci.* 32: 1965–1970.

376 De Moor, R.J., Meire, M., Goharkhay, K. et al. (2010). Efficacy of ultrasonic versus laser-activated irrigation to remove artificially placed dentin debris plugs. *J. Endod.* 36: 1580–1583.

377 Deleu, E., Meire, M.A., and De Moor, R.J. (2015). Efficacy of laser-based irrigant activation methods in removing debris from simulated root canal irregularities. *Lasers Med. Sci.* 30: 831–835.

378 Peters, O.A., Bardsley, S., Fong, J. et al. (2011). Disinfection of root canals with photon-initiated photoacoustic streaming. *J. Endod.* 37: 1008–1012.

379 Pedullà, E., Genovese, C., Campagna, E. et al. (2012). Decontamination efficacy of photon-initiated photoacoustic streaming (PIPS) of irrigants using low-energy laser settings: an *ex vivo* study. *Int. Endod. J.* 45: 865–870.

380 Ordinola-Zapata, R., Bramante, C.M., Aprecio, R.M. et al. (2014). Biofilm removal by 6% sodium hypochlorite activated by different irrigation techniques. *Int. Endod. J.* 47: 659–666.

381 Lukač, N. and Jezeršek, M. (2018). Amplification of pressure waves in laser-assisted endodontics with synchronized delivery of Er:YAG laser pulses. *Lasers Med. Sci.* 33: 823–833.

382 Lukac, N., Tasic Muc, B., Jezersek, M., and Lukac, M. (2017). Photoacoustic endodontics using the novel SWEEPS Er:YAG laser modality. *J. Laser Health Acad.* 1: 1–7.

383 Passalidou, S., Calberson, F., De Bruyne, M. et al. (2018). Debris removal from the mesial root canal system of mandibular molars with laser-activated irrigation. *J. Endod.* 44: 1697–1701.

384 Galler, K.M., Grubmüller, V., Schlichting, R. et al. (2019). Penetration depth of irrigants into root dentine after sonic, ultrasonic and photoacoustic activation. *Int. Endod. J.* 52: 1210–1217.

385 Yang, Q., Liu, M.W., Zhu, L.X., and Peng, B. (2020). Micro-CT study on the removal of accumulated hard-tissue debris from the root canal system of mandibular molars when using a novel laser-activated irrigation approach. *Int. Endod. J.* 53: 529–538.

386 Machtou, P. (2015). Manual dynamic activation (MDA). In: *Endodontic Irrigation: Chemical Disinfection of the Root Canal System* (ed. B. Basrani), 149–155. New York, NY: Springer.

387 Boutsioukis, C., Psimma, Z., and Kastrinakis, E. (2014). The effect of flow rate and agitation technique on irrigant extrusion *ex vivo*. *Int. Endod. J.* 47: 487–496.

388 Malentacca, A., Uccioli, U., Mannocci, F. et al. (2018). The comparative effectiveness and safety of three activated irrigation techniques in the isthmus area using a transparent tooth model. *Int. Endod. J.* 51 (Suppl. 1): e35–e41.

389 Dentsply Tulsa Dental Specialties (2019). ProUltra PiezoFlow ultrasonic irrigation needle – directions for use. Available from: https://www.dentsplysirona.com/content/dam/dentsply/pim/manufacturer/Endodontics/Irrigation__Activation/Ultrasonics/ProUltra_PiezoFlow_Ultrasonic_Irrigation_Needle/Proultra-PiezoFlow-Irrigation-Needle-fpamuc7-en-1402 (accessed 10 August 2020).

390 Curtis, T.O. and Sedgley, C.M. (2012). Comparison of a continuous ultrasonic irrigation device and conventional needle irrigation in the removal of root canal debris. *J. Endod.* 38: 1261–1264.

391 Lussi, A., Nussbächer, U., and Grosrey, J. (1993). A novel noninstrumented technique for cleansing the root canal system. *J. Endod.* 19: 549–553.

392 Lussi, A., Portmann, P., Nussbächer, U. et al. (1999). Comparison of two devices for root canal cleansing by the noninstrumentation technology. *J. Endod.* 25: 9–13.

393 Sigurdsson, A., Garland, R.W., Le, K.T., and Rassoulian, S.A. (2018). Healing of periapical lesions after endodontic treatment with the GentleWave procedure: a prospective multicenter clinical study. *J. Endod.* 44: 510–517.

394 Sigurdsson, A., Garland, R.W., Le, K.T., and Woo, S.M. (2016). 12-month healing rates after endodontic therapy using the novel GentleWave system: a prospective multicenter clinical study. *J. Endod.* 42: 1040–1048.

395 Zhang, D., Shen, Y., de la Fuente-Núñez, C., and Haapasalo, M. (2019). *In vitro* evaluation by quantitative real-time PCR and culturing of the effectiveness of disinfection of multispecies biofilms in root canals by two irrigation systems. *Clin. Oral Investig.* 23: 913–920.

396 Chan, R., Versiani, M.A., Friedman, S. et al. (2019). Efficacy of 3 supplementary irrigation protocols in the removal of hard tissue debris from the mesial root canal system of mandibular molars. *J. Endod.* 45: 923–929.

397 Haapasalo, M., Wang, Z., Shen, Y. et al. (2014). Tissue dissolution by a novel multisonic ultracleaning system and sodium hypochlorite. *J. Endod.* 40: 1178–1181.

398 Ma, J., Shen, Y., Yang, Y. et al. (2015). *In vitro* study of calcium hydroxide removal from mandibular molar root canals. *J. Endod.* 41: 553–558.

399 Peters, L.B., van Winkelhoff, A.J., Buijs, J.F., and Wesselink, P.R. (2002). Effects of instrumentation, irrigation and dressing with calcium hydroxide on infection in pulpless teeth with periapical bone lesions. *Int. Endod. J.* 35: 13–21.

400 Waltimo, T., Trope, M., Haapasalo, M., and Ørstavik, D. (2005). Clinical efficacy of treatment procedures in endodontic infection control and one year follow-up of periapical healing. *J. Endod.* 31: 863–866.

401 Sathorn, C., Parashos, P., and Messer, H. (2007). Antibacterial efficacy of calcium hydroxide intracanal dressing: a systematic review and meta-analysis. *Int. Endod. J.* 40: 2–10.

402 Lambrianidis, T., Margelos, J., and Beltes, P. (1999). Removal efficiency of calcium

hydroxide dressing from the root canal. *J. Endod.* 25: 85–88.

403 Lambrianidis, T., Kosti, E., Boutsioukis, C., and Mazinis, M. (2006). Removal efficacy of various calcium hydroxide/chlorhexidine medicaments from the root canal. *Int. Endod. J.* 39: 55–61.

404 van der Sluis, L.W., Wu, M.K., and Wesselink, P.R. (2007). The evaluation of removal of calcium hydroxide paste from an artificial standardized groove in the apical root canal using different irrigation methodologies. *Int. Endod. J.* 40: 52–57.

405 Rödig, T., Vogel, S., Zapf, A., and Hülsmann, M. (2010). Efficacy of different irrigants in the removal of calcium hydroxide from root canals. *Int. Endod. J.* 43: 519–527.

406 Yaylali, I.E., Kececi, A.D., and Ureyen, K.B. (2015). Ultrasonically activated irrigation to remove calcium hydroxide from apical third of human root canal system: a systematic review of *in vitro* studies. *J. Endod.* 41: 1589–1599.

407 Margelos, J., Eliades, G., Verdelis, C., and Palaghias, G. (1997). Interaction of calcium hydroxide with zinc oxide-eugenol type sealers: a potential clinical problem. *J. Endod.* 23: 43–48.

6

Root Canal Filling Materials and Techniques

Bun San Chong[1] and Nicholas Chandler[2]

[1] *Institute of Dentistry, Barts and The London School of Medicine and Dentistry, Queen Mary University of London, London, UK*
[2] *Sir John Walsh Research Institute, University of Otago, Dunedin, New Zealand*

TABLE OF CONTENTS

Endodontic Materials in Clinical Practice, First Edition. Edited by Josette Camilleri.

6.1 Introduction

According to the American Association of Endodontists (AAE), 'The ultimate goal of endodontic treatment is the long-term retention in function of teeth with pulpal or periapical pathosis' [1]. Following chemomechanical cleaning and shaping of the root canal system, a root canal filling is meant to provide a permanent, biocompatible, microbial-, and fluid-tight seal.

Root fillings consisting of gutta-percha cones as a core material combined with a root canal sealer have been standard practice for many years. However, variations in obturation materials include [1]:

- A sealer (cement/paste/resin) only.
- A sealer and a single cone of a rigid or semi-rigid core material.
- A sealer coating combined with cold compaction of core materials.
- A sealer coating combined with warm compaction of core materials.
- A sealer coating combined with carrier-based core materials.

Newer materials focus on the deficiencies of the key groups of sealers and of gutta-percha, whilst improved placement techniques have provided time and cost savings. Some improvements are aimed at replacing gutta-percha, often accompanied by newer sealers. Newer cores are produced from materials designed to match the size and taper of the canal preparation instruments, such that single-cone obturation is now considered acceptable.

Following its success in the treatment of the 'open' apices of immature teeth, mineral trioxide aggregate (MTA) may now be used as a root filling material on its own in selected cases. In addition, MTA and related hydraulic calcium silicate cements (HCSCs) have an increasing role as root canal sealers. Despite these developments, some root canal shapes – especially oval ones – remain challenging to fill.

Root canal obturation aims to:

1) Seal the pulp chamber and canal system from coronal microleakage.
2) Prevent remaining microorganisms from proliferating.
3) Stop microorganisms entering the pulp space through the apical foramen and other pathways (lateral/furcation canals opening into the gingival sulcus, exposed and open dentinal tubules around the tooth).

Both a quality canal obturation and a well-sealing coronal restoration are critical to long-term success [2, 3]. Although canals can be filled immediately following preparation, in cases of infection the use of intracanal medicaments reduces the microbial population and the presence of endotoxins and may provide an improved prognosis [4]. Regardless, it is a requirement that canals be dried appropriately prior to obturation.

The smear layer influences sealer adaptation, tubular penetration, and leakage; the greatest potential for leakage is at the interface between the sealer and canal wall [5]. Removal of the smear layer and irrigation protocols is discussed in Chapter 5. Although the sealing ability and methods used to measure leakage are now considered outdated [6], they will be covered in this chapter as they have been employed for a number of years specifically in order to evaluate sealer performance and compare obturation methods.

6.2 Root Canal Obturation Materials

6.2.1 Sealers

Sealers play a critical role in sealing the root canal system by filling areas that are not occupied by the core filling material and through the entombment of remaining microorganisms after chemomechanical preparation [7]. They also act as lubricants and antimicrobial agents [8]. A dense appearance of obturated canals on radiographs is desirable, but some voids are likely with all root fillings [9]. Currently, no sealer is available that completely prevents leakage [10]. In general, conventional root canal sealers tend to shrink on setting, and many are hydrophobic; therefore, moisture in the apical region of the root canal system can prevent the formation of an effective seal. All sealers are soluble to an extent, and all differ in their setting times and their release of leachates [11]. These leachates can migrate through dentinal tubules and the apical foramina, creating porosities within the materials. Most conventional root canal sealers do not possess any biological activity, and some have been found to be cytotoxic to the periapical tissues when freshly mixed, causing cellular degeneration and delayed wound healing [12].

Sealer flow may be affected by root canal morphology, the core root filling material, dentine tubules, and the smear layer [13]. Increasing the rate of sealer insertion may increase volumetric flow and reduce the viscosity of the sealer. However, with a reduced internal canal width, there is reduced volumetric flow and increased viscosity. In addition, increasing the rate of insertion does not necessarily improve sealer flow; this depends on the sealer used and the width of a root canal. Similarly, reducing the powder–liquid ratio of a sealer may not improve flow, as it has been shown that flow may be reduced at a higher rate of insertion [13]. Furthermore, the flow of root canal sealers is temperature- and shear-dependent, and varies between sealers [14].

No sealer is ideal, but many work well in clinical practice. Some are initially toxic and many may be absorbed to some degree after setting, so that their volume is decreased; a low solubility and a film thickness <50 μm are requirements [15]. Sealers penetrate into dentinal tubules (Figure 6.1), which can be facilitated by methods such as ultrasonic obturation. This also improves the incidence of filled accessory channels [16]. However, all sealers must be regarded as implantable materials, and so caution is necessary during the

development of novel sealer types and delivery methods.

Whilst their characteristics differ, there is only limited evidence that different types of sealers influence treatment outcome [4]. Nonetheless, the choice is important when considering the obturation technique employed [17]. Commonly used sealers can be divided into six groups based on their constituents:

1) Zinc oxide-eugenol (ZOE) sealers: e.g. Tubli-Seal and Pulp Canal Sealer (Kerr Endodontics, Brea, CA, USA) and Roth's Sealer (Roth International, Chicago, IL, USA).
2) Calcium hydroxide sealers: e.g. Sealapex (Kerr Endodontics) and Apexit and Apexit Plus (Ivoclar Vivadent, Liechtenstein, Germany).
3) Glass ionomer sealers: e.g. Ketac Endo (3M ESPE, Seefeld, Germany).
4) Resin sealers: e.g. AH 26, AH Plus (Dentsply De Trey GmbH, Konstanz, Germany), SimpliSeal (Kerr Endodontics), 2Seal (VDW GmbH, Munich, Germany), and Obturys (Itena, Paris, France).
5) Silicone-based sealers: e.g. Roekoseal (Coltène/Whaledent, Langenau, Germany).
6) HCSC sealers: e.g. BioRoot RCS (Septodont, Saint-Maur-des Fosses, France), EndoSequence BC Sealer (Brasseler, Savannah, GA, USA), and Totalfill BC sealer (FKG Dentaire, La Chaux-de-Fonds, Switzerland).

6.2.1.1 Zinc Oxide-Eugenol Sealers

ZOE sealers have a long history of use in endodontics, and have commonly been considered the standard sealer for many decades. The original formulation took the form of a powder/liquid with silver particles to provide radiopacity [18]. Unfortunately, the presence of these particles caused this sealer to stain the teeth.

Rickert's formula is commercially marketed as Pulp Canal Sealer, in both a standard and an

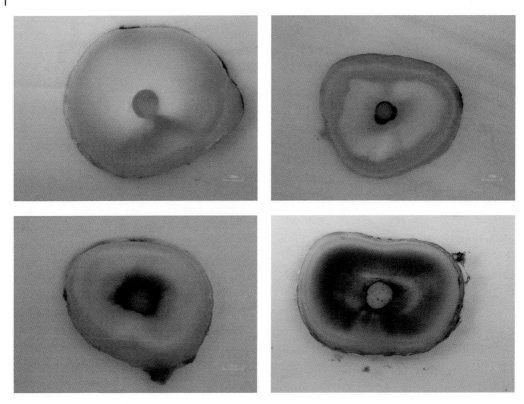

Figure 6.1 Penetration of a sealer, dyed with Sudan Black B, at different levels of filled roots: absent (top left), inner third (top right), middle third (lower left), and outer third (lower right). *Source:* Humza Ahmed.

extended working time (EWT) version. According to the manufacturer, it is a non-irritating, radiopaque sealer. The EWT version has a setting time in excess of 6 hours, compared to 20–40 minutes for the basic formulation. Grossman modified Rickert's formula, introducing a nonstaining ZOE sealer in 1958. This formulation is marketed as Roth's Sealer and Tubli-Seal; the latter is a catalyst/base sealer, which means that it has a faster setting time when compared to the earlier powder/liquid versions. These sealers also exhibit antimicrobial activity [19]. Proco-Sol (Star Dental, Lancaster, PA, USA) is a nonstaining modification of Rickert's original sealer with the silver particles removed. Another ZOE sealer, Wach's Paste, has Canada balsam added, which makes it more viscous.

As a group, ZOE sealers require water in their setting process, are cytotoxic to the periapical tissues, shrink on setting, are soluble, and can stain tooth structures [20]. Since gutta-percha soaked in eugenol shows an increase in volumetric expansion, and eugenol may exist in fresh mixes where it is not crystallized fully as zinc eugenolate, this combination of root filling materials may counteract the shrinkage sustained by any sealer [21].

6.2.1.2 Calcium Hydroxide Sealers

Calcium hydroxide sealers were initially developed to take advantage of the antimicrobial properties of calcium hydroxide, with the idea that they would display bioactive potential [22]. However, they have not shown bioactivity [20]. Sealapex, Apexit, and Apexit Plus are popular commercially available versions.

Calcium hydroxide sealers have been reported to be both soluble and cytotoxic [23]. The seal achieved is similar to that produced by ZOE sealers [24]. Dentalis (Neo Dental, Federal Way, WA, USA) is a calcium hydroxide sealer with iodoform, which gained US Food and Drug Administration (FDA) approval in 1997; this material exhibits excellent radiopacity but must be avoided in patients with an allergy to iodine.

6.2.1.3 Glass Ionomer Sealers

Glass ionomer cement (GIC) sealers were developed as restorative materials in the early 1970s [25]. They offered the potential to bond to dentine, suggesting a leak-free root filling might be achievable. Initial research [26] on their endodontic use showed greater dye leakage compared to AH 26. The first GIC sealer set too rapidly to allow the use of the lateral condensation filling technique. For endodontic application, radiopacifiers were required, and modifications had to be made to the powder to increase its setting time. Prototype materials had similar leakage to Pulp Canal Sealer [26].

A commercial GIC sealer, Ketac Endo, was formulated in the early 1990s. The manufacturer's data of the time stated particle sizes from less than 1 μm to a maximum of 25 μm and a working time of 40 minutes. It was claimed that the adhesion to dentine would cause treated teeth to be strengthened. Initial research reported a snap set, leaving a working time of just 60 seconds. Considering the time needed to transport the sealer to the root canal system, this resulted in radiographically detectable voids in the resultant root filling [27].

A single-cone gutta-percha technique is necessary with GIC sealers in order to allow retreatment; this way, space can be created to reinstrument the canal following gutta-percha removal. Later work investigated Vitrebond (3M ESPE), a resin-modified GIC, as a sealer; it was found that the bond to gutta-percha was not better than that with a ZOE sealer, but there was good adaptation to the root canal wall and it penetrated into dentinal tubules [28]. Vitrebond has a mean particle size of 25 μm and a range 8–40 μm; its fluoride release may have a caries inhibitory effect.

The seal of Ketac Endo sealer was compared with AH 26 [29] and showed a higher leakage, which was attributed to its fast setting, higher volumetric shrinkage, and adhesive failure during setting. Support for the clinical use of Ketac Endo is derived from a 1995 study of 486 teeth treated by three operators [30]; the authors observed that any extruded material was not absorbed by the tissues in their 6–18-month observation period.

Bond strengths of GIC sealers to root canal walls were investigated [31], and it was found that phosphoric and citric acid were preferable for smear layer removal to ethylene diamine tetracetic acid (EDTA) when using Ketac Endo. Bonding without prior removal of the smear layer could not be measured. The bond strength of Ketac Endo and AH Plus to gutta-percha was better than that to tooth structures [32]. It was speculated that the GIC would chelate with zinc components in the gutta-percha cones. This work draws attention to apical leakage at different interfaces. The disadvantages of GIC as a sealer include its poor antibacterial activity [19] and the difficulties it presents during retreatment, as there is no known solvent.

GICs exhibit some antimicrobial properties due to fluoride release, low pH values when setting, and the presence of cations such as strontium and zinc [33]. An experimental GIC-based root canal sealer, ZUT, was developed at the University of Toronto, with an emphasis on enhancing antimicrobial properties. This consisted of a GIC base combined with antimicrobial zeolites: porous ceramic (aluminosilicate) structures that can enclose a core material, which may be either an alkali earth metal ion or an organic molecule (e.g. pharmaceutical). The proportion of the zeolite in the GIC powder can vary depending on the desired physical properties of the material and the antimicrobial dose required. A study was conducted to compare the antimicrobial effects of ZUT with Ketac Endo, using *Enterococcus faecalis* as the test organism [34]. Ketac Endo suppressed *E. faecalis* effectively 24 hours after preparation, but failed to do so one week later. ZUT formulations showed a strong antimicrobial effect that was sustained for long periods. They had better or similar cytotoxicity to Ketac Endo and two AH 26 formulations (with and without silver) [35].

6.2.1.4 Resin Sealers

There are two main categories of resin sealers: epoxy resin sealers and methacrylate resin sealers. Epoxy resin sealers have repeatedly demonstrated excellent physicochemical properties and are considered the gold standard in many experiments. AH Plus, for example, has been widely used for over two decades [36]. It superseded the original AH 26, which became unpopular due to its release of formaldehyde, which reacted with the bismuth oxide in the preparation, leading to tooth and material discolouration [37]. AH Plus contains zirconium oxide and calcium tungstate instead of bismuth oxide. It is less cytotoxic than AH 26, can be used in a thinner film (Figure 6.2), has a lower solubility, and releases only a minimal amount of formaldehyde. It is now one of the most commonly used sealers as it forms a strong bond with dentine and has a low

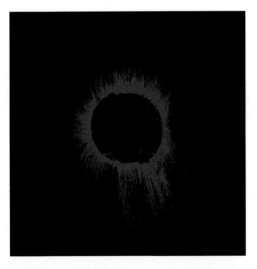

Figure 6.2 Confocal microscope image (×10) of penetration of AH Plus (Dentsply De Trey GmbH) into dentinal tubules. *Source:* Assil Russell.

solubility and satisfactory dimensional stability [38–41]. Its disadvantage is that it does not display any bioactivity or osteogenic potential [42, 43]; however, this means that it is more stable. An excellent literature review is available [44].

Complex canal systems require considerable time to obturate and thus need sealers with extended working times. Furthermore, if heat is used during obturation then sealer setting time will become even more extended. When AH Plus is used with warm gutta-percha techniques, the chemical changes involved will adversely affect its physical properties [45, 46]; its setting time will be reduced and its film thickness increased [17]. The choice of irrigant should be carefully considered when selecting resin-based sealers, as the final rinse can have a positive influence on adhesion to dentine. The use of EDTA and sodium hypochlorite increases the bond strength of AH Plus to dentine; neither solution affects the bond strength of resin-based root canal sealers, whilst both have a negative effect on HCSC sealers [47].

Methacrylate resin root canal sealers first appeared in the 1970s. As existing root canal filling materials did not bond to root canal dentine, methacrylate resin sealers were promoted as being adaptable and bondable, creating a 'monoblock' system. Many generations of these sealers have since been developed. A fourth-generation one is marketed as Epiphany/RealSeal (SybronEndo, Kerr Endodontics); the manufacturer claims that it bonds to the Resilon (Pentron, Wallingford, CT, USA) core (see later) and attaches to the etched root surface, resulting in a gap-free, solid mass in the root canal. It has been concluded, however, that methacrylate resin sealers do not create a monoblock root filling and fail to prevent leakage [48].

An experimental resin sealer composed of 70 wt% vinylidene fluoride/hexafluoropropylene copolymer, methyl methacrylate, zirconia, and tributylborane catalyst has been developed, called Endoresin [49]. Its dentine bonding and sealing ability were evaluated, and good adhesion to both dentine and gutta-percha was demonstrated in comparison to controls (Pulp Canal Sealer EWT and Sealapex). Endoresin-2, a modified version, was subsequently developed to overcome the problem of supply of the fluoropolymer, which was a key component of the initial formulation. This fluoropolymer is substituted with polymethylmethacrylate. The new material has been found to have good sealing ability, high adhesiveness to dentine, and easy removability [50].

6.2.1.5 Silicone Sealers

RoekoSeal is a polydimethylsiloxane-based sealer which expands slightly on setting (0.2%) and is very radiopaque; the claimed advantages include good sealing ability [51], excellent biocompatibility [52], and very low cytotoxicity [53].

GuttaFlow (Coltène/Whaledent) is a modified version containing particles of gutta-percha <30 µm in size. It expands similarly on curing and is considered almost insoluble. It is used with a single master gutta-percha cone, without mechanical compaction, although lateral or vertical condensation is acceptable. Its flow into lateral grooves and depressions in the apical regions of root canals is significantly better than the lateral condensation or warm compaction of gutta-percha combined with AH 26 sealer [54]. It is also effective in filling oval-shaped canals [55]. Its sealing qualities are similar to obturations obtained by lateral compaction or the System B technique with AH 26 [56]. All traces of irrigants must be thoroughly removed by rinsing the canal with water or isopropyl alcohol prior to its introduction. GuttaFlow has a working time of 15 minutes and a setting time of about 30 minutes, whilst GuttaFlow FAST has a working time of 5 minutes and a setting time of 10 minutes. A potential concern is extrusion of material beyond the apex [54], although its cytotoxicity is lower than that of some other sealers.

GuttaFlow and GuttaFlow2 (Coltène/Whaledent) consist of a small amount of gutta-percha in RoekoSeal in a capsulated form. The material is injected into a canal, and then a single gutta-percha master cone is then placed.

6.2.1.6 HCSC Sealers

HCSC sealers feature a hydration setting reaction and have a hydraulic nature, representing a major shift in the chemistry of sealer types. They are mostly based on tricalcium or dicalcium silicate, and their main characteristic is the formation of calcium hydroxide when setting in contact with water [57, 58]. Unlike other sealer types, HCSC sealers interact with the clinical environment, leading their chemistry to change accordingly; this characteristic has been termed 'bioactivity'. They do not conform to the ISO 6876;2012 standard for sealer ideal properties [15], which was developed for materials that are stable and whose chemistry does not change in use [59].

Based on the classification proposed in Chapter 1, there are five types of HCSCs. Most are composed of a cement and a radiopacifer, and are either mixed with water or delivered in a nonaqueous vehicle. They set when in contact with the surrounding tissues. Endo CPM Sealer (Egeo, Buenos Aires, Argentina) is composed of Portland cement and a radiopacifer and is mixed with water and an accelerator [60]. It is a good example of a Type 2 HCSC, since it is a Portland cement type with additives and mixed with water. MTA Fillapex (Angelus, Londrina, Brazil) has a salicylate-resin matrix and thus can be classed with the calcium hydroxide sealers. However, Type 3 HCSCs are Portland cement-based with additives and a nonaqueous carrier, so it could fit in this category as well. Furthermore, MTA Fillapex only sets in a moist environment [59], another typical property of the Type 3 HCSCs. Endoseal (Maruchi, Wonju, Korea) is another premixed Type 3 HCSC. Type 4 HCSCs include those that are tricalcium silicate-based with additives and mixed with water, such as BioRoot RCS. Type 5 HCSCs are all premixed sealers based on tricalcium silicate, such as the Totalfill BC sealer.

Endodontic hydraulic sealers are hydrophilic, setting by reaction with water. They are dimensionally sound, expand on setting, and have excellent properties for root canal sealing [61, 62]. However, their dimensional stability is dependent on the environment, as drying out will lead to shrinkage [63]. The pH of unset hydraulic sealers is above 12, due to the formation of calcium hydroxide and subsequent dissociation into calcium and hydroxyl ions [64, 65]. When mixed with water, a matrix of calcium silicate hydrates and calcium hydroxide is formed, which hardens with time. The calcium hydroxide is then released, which has been linked to bioactivity [66]. It has been shown *in vitro* that it reacts with phosphate ions in physiologic fluid, resulting in the precipitation of hydroxyapatite [67, 68]. This is a similar interaction to that of bioactive glass [69]. It is enhanced by the availability of phosphates in the canal, such as with a final phosphate-rich irrigating solution [70]. This has been shown for a number of sealers when in contact with dentine [71]. The hydroxyapatite coprecipitates with the calcium silicate hydrate, reinforcing the set material. These properties improve the tissue attachment of bioactive materials [72]. HCSC sealers demonstrate radiopacity, which is enhanced with a radiopacifier, and they flow in accordance with ISO 6876/2012 [15], with a minimum radiopacity equivalent to 3 mm of aluminium [73].

6.2.1.6.1 Type 2 HCSC Sealers

Endo CPM Sealer is based on MTA but has additives to improve its performance. These include silicon dioxide, calcium carbonate, propyleneglycol alginate, sodium citrate, and calcium chloride [60]. It also contains bismuth trioxide and barium sulphate, which give it a radiopacity equivalent to 6 mm of aluminium [60]. The material sets within an hour [74]. Endo CPM Sealer has been found to be dimensionally stable, but it exhibits significantly more leakage when compared with MTA Fillapex

and a conventional calcium hydroxide-based sealer [75, 76]. It has been found to have a significantly higher bond strength to root dentine compared to MTA Fillapex and AH Plus [77]. It displays antibacterial activity against *Staphylococcus aureus* and *Streptococcus mutans* when freshly mixed, although less than that displayed by AH Plus [78]. It also displays biocompatibility [74, 79].

ProRoot Endo Sealer (Dentsply Tulsa Dental Specialties, Tulsa, OK, USA) was developed from ProRoot MTA root repair material (Dentsply Tulsa Dental Specialties) and introduced in 2016. The major powder components are tricalcium silicate and dicalcium silicate, with calcium sulphate included as the setting retardant, bismuth oxide as a radiopacifier, and a small amount of tricalcium aluminate; these are the same components found in ProRoot MTA, but ProRoot Endo Sealer is claimed to be enhanced, and it has thus been grouped with the Type 2 HCSCs. It is available as a predosed powder and liquid, and is designed for use with all obturation techniques. It has been indicated for use as a sealer in both cold and warm root canal filling techniques with a working time of 65 minutes and a setting time of 12 hours. It demonstrates superior sealing to a conventional ZOE sealer and exhibits bioactivity when in contact with physiological fluids [80, 81].

MTA Obtura (Angelus), from the same manufacturer as MTA Fillapex, is similar to grey MTA (Angelus) in composition. It exhibits a flow rate similar to AH Plus [82]. When used as a root canal sealing material, it has been found to demonstrate higher leakage than AH Plus [83].

6.2.1.6.2 Type 3 HCSC Sealers

MTA Fillapex (Angelus) sealer is an HCSC-based, salicylate resin root canal sealer. It was created in an attempt to combine the biocompatibility and bioactive potential of MTA with a synthetic resin, which demonstrates sound physical properties. It consists of a yellow-coloured base paste and white catalyst paste. It is indicated for use in cold and warm root canal filling techniques [84]. It has a high pH and therefore displays antimicrobial activity. It was found to produce a greater zone of inhibition against *E. faecalis* in an agar diffusion test when compared to Endo CPM Sealer; however, neither sealer material was able to sustain this antibacterial effect seven days after mixing [85].

MTA Fillapex is more radiopaque than BioRoot RCS, a tricalcium silicate root canal sealer, but less so than the conventional sealers, such as AH Plus and Pulp Canal Sealer [86]. It has a radiopacity equivalent to 7 mm of aluminium, due to the presence of bismuth trioxide [87]. Other researchers report a lower radiopacity value [84]. According to the manufacturer, its composition after mixing is essentially MTA, salicylate resin, natural resin, bismuth, and silica, and it has a setting time of less than 240 minutes. It has a high flow rate (Figure 6.3) and can fill lateral and accessory canals. It has been reported to have higher solubility, dimensional and volumetric change, and porosity compared to AH Plus [88], as well as significantly less leakage [89]. When compared to a ZOE sealer, depending on whether there is bismuth oxide in its formulation,

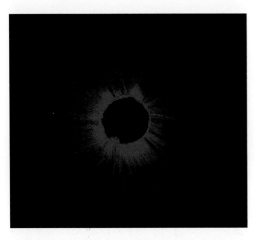

Figure 6.3 Confocal microscope image (×10) of penetration of MTA Fillapex (Angelus) sealer into dentinal tubules. *Source:* Assil Russell.

discolouration is minimal on placement in the pulp chambers of molar teeth [90]. Recent studies have demonstrated contradictory results regarding cytotoxicity and genotoxicity, with MTA Fillapex displaying no biocompatibility or bone tissue repair and instead inducing an irritating effect on tissues [91–96]. Other recent studies have concluded that it is cytotoxic [97, 98]. Therefore, despite the presence of MTA, this formulation may not have the intended biological advantages.

Other sealers based on Portland cement and using nonaqueous vehicles have been introduced. One is Bio-C Sealer (Angelus, Londrina, Brazil), which is based on Portland cement, a radiopacifier, and additives and is delivered in a propylene glycol nonaqueous matrix [99–101].

6.2.1.6.3 *Type 4 and Type 5 HCSC Sealers*

The tricalcium silicate-based sealers were developed to avoid the trace element contamination of Portland cement. The water-based ones include BioRoot RCS, a powder/liquid hydraulic tricalcium silicate-based cement which has been on the market since early 2015. This Type 4 HCSC is recommended for single-cone or cold lateral condensation techniques. Heating results in evaporation of the water component, a reduction in setting time and flow, and an increase in film thickness [17]. The manufacturer claims it has a minimum working time of over 10 minutes and a maximum setting time of 4 hours [102], although studies have found the actual final setting time to be 300 ± 5 min [86]. The powder contains tricalcium silicate, povidone, and zirconium oxide, whilst the liquid component is an aqueous solution of calcium chloride and polycarboxylate. BioRoot RCS is formulated so that it does not stain teeth and has great flowability, and retreatment is simple to carry out [86, 102]. Obturations have shown higher void volumes compared with AH Plus [103]. Although the material is radiopaque, this property is significantly less than that of conventional sealers such as AH Plus and Pulp

Canal Sealer [86]. A recent *in vitro* study reported that BioRoot RCS was bioactive and biocompatible [104]. Unfortunately, it has also exhibited some degree of cytotoxicity, although lower than that of conventional root canal sealers [105, 106]. It shows exceptional antimicrobial properties [107] regardless of the irrigation protocol used [108].

EndoSequence BC Sealer, also known as iRoot SP (Innovative Bioceramix Inc., Vancouver, BC, Canada) or TotalFill BC Sealer depending on the region where it is sold, is a calcium silicate-based, premixed, ready-to-use, injectable white hydraulic cement paste; the term 'bioceramic' was coined for this sealer type [109, 110]. It is composed of tricalcium silicate, dicalcium silicate, calcium phosphate monobasic, calcium hydroxide, and a thickening agent. The working time of the material is 30 minutes, and in normal conditions it sets within 4 hours [10]; if the dentine is very dry, it can take up to 10 hours. It has a radiopacity equivalent to 3.83 mm of aluminium, just above the minimum reference standard – although one study reports an equivalent of 6.09 mm of aluminium [111]. It has been found to increase the force to fracture of root-filled premolar teeth [112]. Specifically developed for warm obturation techniques, EndoSequence BC Sealer HiFlow (Brasseler) and TotalFill BC Sealer HiFlow (FKG) exhibit a lower viscosity when heated and are more radiopaque [113]. Neither show any chemical changes when subjected to high temperatures [113, 114], with their nonaqueous vehicle preventing desiccation.

iRoot SP sealer has an initial antibacterial effect against *E. faecalis in vitro*, but this has been found to dramatically decrease just seven days after setting [64]. The manufacturer claims that there is no shrinkage on setting. *In vitro* studies have shown that it demonstrates some degree of cytotoxicity, although less than that of AH Plus [62, 115, 116]. A recent study found that it displayed a higher cytocompatibility when compared to MTA Fillapex and AH Plus [96]. It has antibacterial properties due to its high alkalinity during setting [64]. It also

shows promising *in vitro* results in providing increased resistance to root fracture [117]. It has higher dentinal tubule penetration following various irrigation protocols when compared to AH Plus, GuttaFlow, and MTA Fillapex [118], and it produces a higher resistance to dislodgement from root dentine compared to AH Plus, Epiphany, and MTA Fillapex [119].

6.2.1.7 Other Sealer Types

Use of chloroform-based sealers such as Rosin-chloroform, Chloropercha (Tanrac Ltd, Gavle, Sweden), and Kloropercha has declined due to concerns about their toxicity. Formaldehyde-containing sealers are no longer recommended because they contain substantial amounts of paraformaldehyde and are considered unsafe.

Calcium phosphate-based sealers such as Capseal I and II and Sankin Apatite Root Canal Sealer (Sankin Kogyo, Tokyo, Japan) are available. The presence of iodoform and polyacrylic acids in these formulations is said to cause cytotoxicity [120], and questionable results have been found with regard to their biocompatibility [121].

Almost all endodontic materials can discolour teeth, so it is unlikely that any sealer will guarantee colour stability in a root-filled tooth [122]. This emphasizes the need to terminate the root filling well clear of the clinical crown, protect it with an orifice barrier, and carefully clean the access cavity before placement of the final coronal restoration.

6.2.2 Core Materials

6.2.2.1 Silver Points

Due to the limitations of early root canal preparation instruments, curved root canals were difficult to enlarge adequately to accept semi-rigid materials such as gutta-percha cones. Rigid core materials such as silver points, first used in 1931 [123], which could be forced down narrow canals, offered easier placement to the correct depth. Since placement was easier, the silver point technique could sometimes lead to less care being taken during root canal preparation, with infected dentine and debris being left in the canals, resulting in treatment failure (Figure 6.4). Silver points could also corrode when exposed to tissue fluids or saliva [124], and their round cross-section led to obturations with excessive sealer. Being made of 99.9% silver, they were initially thought to offer valuable antimicrobial properties, but in fact the corrosion products were toxic and could reach the periapical tissues and compound the problems caused by sealer dissolution [125]. Silver points

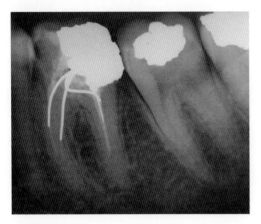

Figure 6.4 Mandibular left first molar root filled with silver points. *Source:* Bun San Chong, Nicholas Chandler.

are thus no longer recommended as a core root filling material.

6.2.2.2 Acrylic Points

'PD' Acrylic Points (Produits Dentaires SA, Vevey, Switzerland) are colour-coded and radiopaque. They are made of a methyl methacrylate polymer, bismuth oxide, zinc oxide, and a cadmium-free colouring agent. As a rigid core material, they are meant to offer all of the advantages and none of the disadvantages of silver points, and they are promoted as being removable with burs, solvents, or essential oils if retreatment is necessary.

6.2.2.3 Gutta-Percha

Over 2000 plant species produce natural rubber latex (NRL), the main constituent of which is poly(*cis*-1,4 isoprene). The main constituent of endodontic gutta-percha, on the other hand, is 19–22% poly(*trans*-1,4 isoprene); other constituents added to it for endodontic use include zinc oxide (59–75%) and various waxes, colouring agents, antioxidants, and metal salts as radiopacifiers. The proportions vary from brand to brand, so there are considerable variations in stiffness, brittleness, and tensile strength. To facilitate fit, gutta-percha cones are available in different sizes and tapers (Figure 6.5).

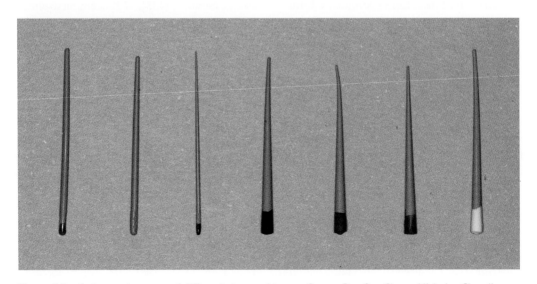

Figure 6.5 Gutta-percha cones of different sizes and tapers. *Source:* Bun San Chong, Nicholas Chandler.

Gutta-percha has two crystalline forms. In its unheated β-phase, the material is solid and compactable. When heated, it changes to the α-phase, becoming more pliable and capable of being made to flow under pressure. The α-phase shrinks as it cools and sets, which is a disadvantage clinically. The thermomechanical properties of gutta-percha have been well reported [126–130]. Most of the changes in phase occur from room temperature to around 60 °C.

Gutta-percha has many advantages, being:

1) inert;
2) dimensionally stable after treatment;
3) nonallergenic;
4) antibacterial;
5) nonstaining to dentine;
6) radiopaque;
7) compactable;
8) softenable by heat;
9) softenable by organic solvents; and
10) easily removable from the canal, when necessary.

It also has some disadvantages (Figure 6.6), being:

1) nonrigid;
2) nonadherent to dentine; and
3) capable of being stretched.

As early as 1961, Ingle commented that 'There has been no serious attempt to replace the time-honored plastic gutta-percha with a modern plastic . . . with a strong possibility it will be replaced by a newer plastic' [131]. Gutta-percha may be disinfected prior to use at the chairside in solutions of sodium hypochlorite for one minute [132]. Its biggest drawback is that it does not adhere to dentine. This can lead to penetration of bacteria along the space between the gutta-percha and the canal walls in the absence of an adequate coronal seal [133], resulting in treatment failure. Microbial degradation of rubber is a relatively new area of research; fortunately, there is currently no evidence of the poly(*trans*-1,4 isoprene) in gutta-percha

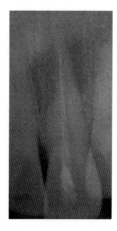

Figure 6.6 Suboptimal, poorly condensed gutta-percha root filling in a maxillary left central incisor. *Source:* Bun San Chong, Nicholas Chandler.

being associated with biodegradation by microbial enzymes [134].

6.2.2.3.1 Coated Cones

To enhance the bonding of GIC sealer to gutta-percha, one product consists of gutta-percha coated with 2 μm of GIC particles on its surface (ActiV GP Precision Obturation System, Brasseler, Savannah, GA, USA). This was compared with AH Plus and gutta-percha in a bacterial leakage model and no significant difference was found [135]. Bioceramic-coated/impregnated gutta-percha cones are also available (TotalFill gutta-percha cone, FKG); the gutta-percha is impregnated and coated with calcium silicate nanoparticles and used as a single cone. When combined with TotalFill BC sealer (FKG), no difference was found in fracture load compared with teeth filled with gutta-percha and AH Plus [136]; the bioceramic combination, however, demonstrated higher bond strength and greater sealer penetration at all root levels.

6.2.2.3.2 Chlorhexidine-Impregnated Gutta-Percha Points

Some studies have shown that *E. faecalis* is relatively resistant to calcium hydroxide [137, 138]. In order to take advantage of the antibacterial properties of chlorhexidine, especially to *E. faecalis*, a chlorhexidine-impregnated gutta-percha point, Activ point (Roeko), has been marketed. According to the manufacturer, it contains a gutta-percha matrix embedded with 5% chlorhexidine diacetate. Studies have been undertaken to investigate the antimicrobial activity of Activ points, concluding that they do not possess an inhibitory activity strong enough to completely eliminate a moderately large number of *E. faecalis* organisms from infected human dentinal tubules [139, 140]. An *in vitro* study testing the cellular toxicity of medicated and nonmedicated gutta-percha points found that chlorhexidine-impregnated gutta-percha points were more cytotoxic than either calcium hydroxide-impregnated or nonmedicated gutta-percha points [141].

6.2.2.3.3 *Gutta-Percha Points Impregnated with Metronidazole*

According to the abstract of a study conducted at Shandong University in China [142], controlled-release delivery gutta-percha points (CDGMCs) containing metronidazole compounds were made and placed in prepared extracted teeth. A non-drug CDGMC was used as the control. The absorbency of the drugs in normal saline (37 °C, pH 7.4) was determined, and the percentage of release and cumulated release of the drugs were calculated according to the concentrations in medium. The authors concluded that CDGMCs could continuously release effective drug concentrations for more than 10 days [142].

The introduction of antimicrobials into gutta-percha points and their disinfection prior to clinical use has recently been reviewed [132].

6.2.2.3.4 *Gutta-Percha Allergy*

Cases of allergy to gutta-percha arise but are unusual. There has been speculation regarding potential cross-reactivity between NRL and gutta-percha allergens in latex-allergic patients, as they are related materials from the same family of trees. In case reports [143, 144], lip and gingival swelling, throbbing sensation, diffuse urticaria, and tachycardia have been noticed following the placement of gutta-percha root fillings; these symptoms resolved completely after removal of the fillings. In contrast, investigations of cross-reactivity between different latex materials using the radioallergosorbent test (RAST) inhibition assay concluded that there was an absence of cross-reactivity between raw or manufactured gutta-percha and NRL antibodies. However, gutta-balata (if added to gutta-percha products) may cross-react with latex-specific immunoglobulin E (IgE) antibodies [145]. Similarly, a study using the enzyme-linked immunosorbent assay (ELISA) reported no cross-reactivity between gutta-percha and NRL protein allergens; the authors speculated that additives in gutta-percha cone manufacture, such as zinc oxide, barium sulphate, waxes, formaldehyde, and paraformaldehyde, might be responsible for eliciting allergic reactions in patients [146]. For these rare cases, consideration should be given to providing root fillings of MTA, as an example.

6.3 Root Filling Techniques

Since gutta-percha remains the most commonly used core root filling material, the main focus of this section will be on techniques utilizing gutta-percha.

During obturation, sealer may be extruded beyond the apex (Figure 6.7) or out of a lateral/accessory canal (Figure 6.8). A radiographic study of 92 overextension cases involving ZOE sealers (Procosol and Roth's 801) in well-obturated canals found that 96% showed evidence of periapical repair at recall and that the extruded material remained unchanged in only three cases (1.6%). Extruded materials disappeared over time and did not prevent healing [147].

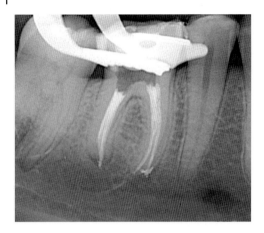

Figure 6.7 Extrusion of sealer from the mesiolingual canal of a mandibular right first molar. *Source:* David Yong.

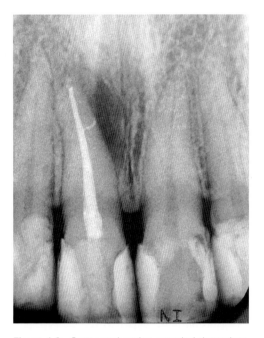

Figure 6.8 Root canal sealer extruded through to reveal a lateral canal in a maxillary right central incisor, explaining the adjacent bone loss. *Source:* Finn Gilroy.

6.3.1 Cold Gutta-Percha Condensation Techniques

6.3.1.1 Lateral Condensation

Gutta-percha may be used cold or softened by heat or solvents. Lateral condensation is the most popular cold obturation method (Figure 6.9). Today's preparation techniques produce a flared canal which cannot be filled with just one 0.02 taper gutta-percha cone, so standardized sizes with larger tapers (e.g. 0.04 or 0.06) are available. A laboratory study of curved canals found a single tapered cone method comparable to lateral condensation in terms of the quantity of gutta-percha in the root canal space; the technique was also faster than lateral condensation [148].

It has been said that lateral condensation is 'single cone filling with a conscience', as the space that must be created can lead to over-preparation, weakening the tooth and leading to the risk of root fracture, given the forces involved [149]. Nevertheless, lateral condensation is taught and practised throughout the world and is the technique of choice of many clinicians. It offers excellent length control and can be employed with a wide variety of sealers.

The master gutta-percha cone selected should ideally present some resistance to withdrawal (tug-back), and its size will often correspond to the master apical file used to prepare the apical termination. The positioned cone will be marked, and spreaders can be pre-curved for treatment of curved canals. For greater flexibility, spreaders made of nickel–titanium (NiTi) should be considered. Finger-rather than handheld spreaders may also be used; these reduce the forces applied inside the tooth and reduces the risk of root fractures.

The sealer should be mixed and smeared on to the canal wall either using a hand file rotated anticlockwise, on a paper point or by coating the master cone. The cone should then be 'buttered' lightly with sealer and inserted. Apical pressure can be applied with a spreader for about 20 seconds to compact the gutta-percha. The first accessory cone should be inserted into the space created and the spreader reinserted without delay. A second accessory cone can then be inserted, and the sequence continued until the canal is adequately filled. Following this, excess gutta-percha should be removed to well below the gingival level in

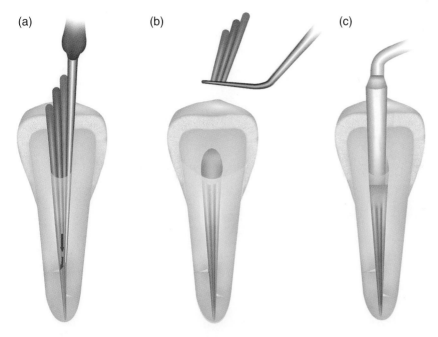

(a) (b) (c)

Figure 6.9 Cold lateral condensation. (a) Spreader inserted and force used to compress gutta-percha laterally and vertically. (b) Heated instrument used to remove excess gutta-percha coronally. (c) Condensor used to compact gutta-percha vertically. *Source:* Humza Ahmed.

order to maintain the colour of the crown and prevent the possibility of staining by sealers. Covering the gutta-percha by placing a protective orifice barrier of suitable material (often a GIC) reduces the risk of microleakage.

If a post-retained coronal restoration is to be provided, condensation of gutta-percha can cease when the apical 5–6 mm has been filled, with any excess removed immediately without disturbing the apical filling [150]. This has the advantages that the clinician will be aware of the canal length and anatomy and the dental dam will already be in place. Lateral condensation remains the most commonly taught obturation technique in dental schools, but over the past decade many dentists worldwide have changed to single-cone obturation, warm vertical condensation, or a carrier-based system.

6.3.1.2 Single-Cone Obturation

The single-cone obturation technique uses a gutta-percha cone which matches the final preparation size, so that there is no need for any accessory gutta-percha cones, heat, or sequential compaction (Figure 6.10). It has gained much popularity since the advent of HCSC sealers as it is comparatively quick and easy to use [151].

A study compared single-cone obturation and warm vertical condensation techniques using two sealers, iRoot SP and AH Plus [152]; the results showed no significant difference in filling quality or sealer penetration regardless of obturation technique or sealer type. Hence, there is some evidence to suggest that single-cone obturation can be an effective root canal obturation technique, especially if the canal is round and uniform in shape [153]. Since it is heavily reliant on the sealer to fill any deficiencies, there is an increased likelihood of voids in the resultant root filling [151, 153–155]. Therefore, root fillings produced using single-cone obturation may be at greater risk of long-term failure. However, there is also a suggestion that the volume of voids is greater in the

(a) (b)

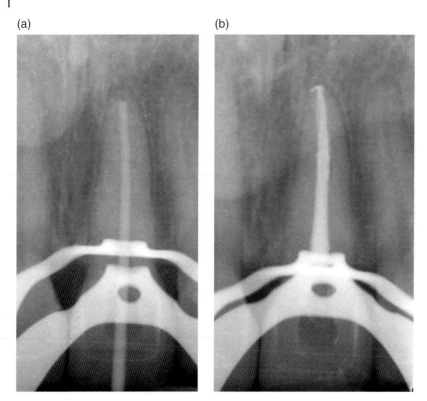

Figure 6.10 Maxillary left central incisor obturated using the single-cone technique. (a) Cone fit radiograph, ensuring the master gutta-percha cone is well-fitting, with very little space left for the sealer. (b) Master gutta-percha cone and sealer placement following checking. *Source:* Bun San Chong, Nicholas Chandler.

coronal rather than the apical portion of the root canal with this technique [156]. The application of ultrasonic activation directly to the master cone may help produce a better-quality root filling with fewer voids [157]. The single-cone obturation technique relies on the anti-microbial properties of the HCSC sealers, aiming at a biological seal.

A clinical study of 307 patients treated by endodontists in private practice using single-cone obturation with a hydraulic sealer (EndoSequence BC Sealer) reported a success-ful outcome of 90.9%, based on clinical and radiographic findings with a minimum follow-up of one year [158]. Although single-cone obturation with an HCSC sealer is a viable technique, there is still a need for further high-quality clinical research.

6.3.2 Heat-Softened Gutta-Percha Techniques

Thermoplastic gutta-percha can fill canal irregularities better than solid gutta-percha cones, with a better gutta-percha to sealer ratio and hence, theoretically, a better seal [159]. Gutta-percha shows two phase changes with a changing temperature, going from a β- to an α-phase as it rises and then from amorphous to a β-phase as it cools again. The maximum tem-perature required to reach the amorphous phase is 60 °C [128]. Cold gutta-percha may be placed in the canal and warmed, or else gutta-percha heated outside the canal may be deliv-ered to it.

Thermoplasticized gutta-percha can pene-trate patent dentinal tubules with or without the presence of sealer, particularly in the middle third of root canals [160]. The movement of sealer assists the flow of gutta-percha apically. It is important that the highest percentage of sealer/dentine interface is sealer-covered, that the sealer film thickness is minimal, and that tubule penetration is as high as possible. In a confocal microscopy evaluation of the penetration of three root canal sealers during lateral condensation [161], Sealapex showed the greatest penetration at the two levels assessed; its mean penetration at the 3 mm level was 360 μm. Sealer 26 (Dentsply Maillefer), an epoxy resin-based material, was not significantly different from GuttaFlow, and the percentage adaptation to the canals walls was the same for all three materials [161].

6.3.2.1 Intracanal Heating Techniques

Schilder's [162] warm vertical condensation method remains popular, with several newer techniques available. It involves filling the canal with heat-softened gutta-percha packed to flow into the entire system, including accessory and lateral canals. A flared canal preparation matches the pluggers used to condense the gutta-percha. The traditional technique uses condensing instruments heated in an open flame, but vertical condensation has been simplified by the introduction of electrically heated spreaders and pluggers such as the Touch 'n Heat, System B Heat Source, and Elements Free units (SybronEndo, Kerr Endodontics). It produces homogeneous, compact fillings, with gutta-percha present in all irregularities, but no substantial improvement in apical or coronal seal has been demonstrated compared to cold lateral condensation [163]. Intracanal heating of gutta-percha using ultrasound has also been described and is reported to save time [164].

The continuous-wave-of-condensation technique (Figure 6.11) uses a System B-type heat source and involves two stages: down-packing and back-packing [165]. Heat is carried along the length of a master gutta-percha cone, starting coronally and ending in apical 'corkage' in a wave of condensation. Although it requires time to master, this is simpler and more rapid than other techniques, as down-packing is completed in a single continuous vertical movement. A tapering canal shape is required, and the taper of the plugger matches this, but without contacting the canal walls. The System B unit is set to a power level of 10 and a temperature of 200 °C, although the actual peak

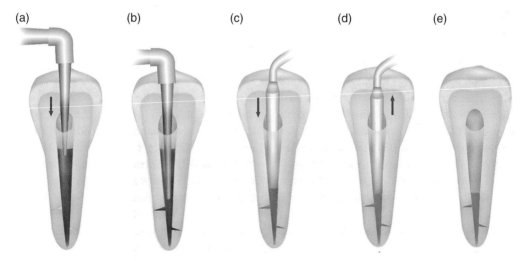

(a)   (b)   (c)   (d)   (e)

Figure 6.11 Continuous wave of condensation. (a) Down-pack, heat, and vertical force. (b) Separation and withdrawal. (c, d) Vertical compaction of gutta-percha. (e) Dense apical plug of gutta-percha. *Source:* Humza Ahmed.

temperature of the plugger tips is lower than this and is affected by the taper of the chosen plugger [166]. Following sealer application and cone placement, the plugger is positioned and activated and is pushed through the gutta-percha to the level of the binding point, indicated by a silicone stop. After one second, the activating button is released and further vertical pressure is applied on the cooling plugger for another 10 seconds, counteracting shrinkage. Finally, the heat source is activated for a further one second whilst apical pressure is maintained, before the plugger is withdrawn. Backpacking of the remainder of the canal may be carried out with a warm gutta-percha injection system. A study of the percentage of sealer and the distance between the gutta-percha and canal wall has shown that there is no benefit in a second application of AH Plus sealer during the down-pack stage of this process [167].

Choice of sealer is important when considering heated gutta-percha techniques. The setting time of the sealer will depend on its constituents and particle size, the ambient temperature, and the relative humidity. The continuous-wave technique produces a higher temperature within a sealer than the warm backfill technique, whilst temperature rises using carrier-based gutta-percha (Thermafil; Dentsply Tulsa Dental) are negligible [168]. The chemistry of AH Plus and its physical properties alter on heating, its setting time decreasing and its film thickness increasing [17]. As for ZOE sealers, increasing temperatures increases their setting time [169] and provokes irreversible chemical changes [114]. EndoSequence BC Sealer HiFlow and TotalFill BC Sealer HiFlow have been specifically developed for warm gutta-percha techniques, as their viscosities decrease on heating, improving sealer flow [113].

6.3.2.2 Extracanal Heating Techniques

6.3.2.2.1 Carrier-Based Systems

A method using a metal carrier to introduce heat-softened gutta-percha into canals was introduced commercially in 1989, and plastic carriers are now in use today (Thermafil) [170]. A verifier device can be used to check the diameter of the preparation and to assist in obturator size selection. Obturators are now made to match the tapers of canal preparation systems.

Logically, carrier-based obturation systems should stop 1 mm short of the canal length to prevent overfills. The amount of sealer is important: if it is adequate, fears of the gutta-percha stripping from the carrier in a curved canal are probably unfounded. A study found that Thermafil, System B, and single-point cold gutta-percha obturations featured similar percentages of filling material and void distribution [171]. New research using the technique in simulated canals shows it to be very effective for obturating C-shaped canals [172].

These carrier-based obturation systems require a dedicated oven which heats the material in less than one minute. A disadvantage of some of these devices, particularly when a post-retained restoration is planned, is that the shaft of the carrier remains in the canal; this is also a concern if retreatment is necessary. Current Thermafil obturators feature a V-shaped groove in the shaft of the carrier to facilitate removal, and research shows that they may be removed from moderately curved canals using rotary NiTi files [173].

GuttaCore (Dentsply Tulsa Dental) is a recently introduced obturator system intended to replace Thermafil. Initial production used a grey-coloured cross-linked gutta-percha core, but a newer version with a pink-coloured core is said to be slightly more rigid. Canals should be prepared to a minimum size of 20 and a 0.06 taper. The device aims to provide the same quality of obturation as Thermafil, but its removal with files is easier and faster if retreatment or post-space preparation is necessary [174]. Using GuttaCore, it is easier to sever the obturator's handle off at orifice level and to make a space for a post. This and related techniques may save time, especially when treating molars. Using micro-CT and scanning electron microscopy data, oval canals obturated with this system had a lower incidence of interfacial gaps and voids than those filled with lateral condensation or warm vertical methods [175]; it was thus suggested as a valuable alternative for the root filling of these challenging canal types. Guttafusion (VDW) is a similar system designed to match the same manufacturer's Reciproc NiTi reciprocating instrumentation system.

6.3.2.2.2 Thermoplastic Delivery Systems

These devices inject molten gutta-percha into a canal. Vertical condensation is then applied to adapt the material to the canal walls. In the earliest commercial delivery system (Obtura, Obtura Spartan Endodontics, Algonquin, IL, USA), the gutta-percha was heated to 160 °C and delivered at approximately 60 °C. Examples of newer devices are the Elements Free unit (Figure 6.12) and the Beefill (VDW). The Elements Free unit contains a gutta-percha extruder and a System B heated-tip device; it heats to 200 °C in 0.5 seconds and can be set to a temperature range of 100–400 °C. The extruder works similarly to previous motorized and manual devices. These high-temperature machines have been shown to produce

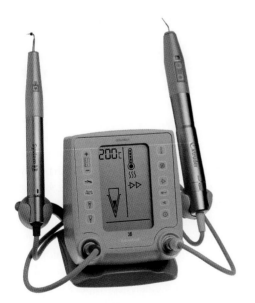

Figure 6.12 Elements Free obturation unit (Kerr Endodontics). *Source:* Bun San Chong, Nicholas Chandler.

clinically acceptable results and as good an apical seal as lateral condensation, with the warm gutta-percha penetrating patent dentinal tubules to some degree [160]. They are also popular for back-filling of the middle and coronal portions of a canal following vertical or lateral condensation. Nevertheless, some canals – especially those with oval shapes – remain challenging to obturate adequately [176, 177].

6.3.3 Thermomechanical Compaction

6.3.3.1 Vibration and Heat

A combination of heat and vibration may be used to condense gutta-percha using the DownPak Obturation Device (Hu-Friedy Co., Chicago, IL, USA). This cordless instrument provides low-frequency (100 Hz) pulses and heats to 350 °C. It can be used for lateral and warm vertical condensation techniques with any core material. A master cone is heated in vibration mode and accessory cones are then placed. Heated plugger tips, available in NiTi or soft stainless steel, allow great flexibility in curved canals. This can provide improved condensation and homogeneity in tortuous root canal systems, which would otherwise need more canal enlargement to accommodate conventional warm obturation techniques [178].

6.3.3.2 Rotating Condenser

An engine-driven rotating compactor capable of softening and condensing gutta-percha vertically and laterally was described by McSpadden [179]. The specially designed stainless-steel instrument could be rotated within the root canal to generate frictional heat in order to plasticize a cold gutta-percha cone and drive the thermomechanically plasticized gutta-percha apically. The original instruments have been discontinued, but the Gutta-Condensor (Dentsply Maillefer; Figure 6.13), which operates at 8000 rpm in a high-torque handpiece, and Thermal Lateral Condensor (Brasseler) are both available.

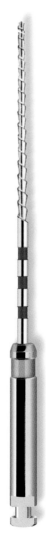

Figure 6.13 Gutta-Condensor (Dentsply Maillefer). *Source:* Bun San Chong, Nicholas Chandler.

The original technique involved the condenser being activated in the canal, alongside the master gutta-percha cone, at approximately 12 000 rpm, without apical pressure. The friction created softened the gutta-percha very rapidly and the plasticized material is driven apically on advancement of the condenser to about 2 mm from the termination of the preparation. As the apical region filled, the condenser backed out of the canal and is slowly withdrawn, whilst still rotating at the optimum speed. In large canals, the procedure is repeated with additional gutta-percha cones to fill any coronal deficiencies.

The method was later modified to meet certain concerns, particularly over apical extrusion of material and instrument fracture [180]. The hybrid technique combines the predictability of lateral condensation near the apex with the speed and efficacy of the condenser in the remainder of the canal. A master cone is cemented and lateral condensation of accessory points is carried out in the apical 3–4 mm before using the compactor in the rest of the canal. In addition to stainless steel, modern condensers are also manufactured from NiTi.

6.3.4 Other Obturation Techniques

6.3.4.1 Pastes

Paste fillers were introduced in order to speed up root canal treatment. They are related to the historic use of pulp mummification agents [181]. These materials should not be confused with sealers for use with solid or semi-solid root canal filling materials. They may contain strong disinfectants (e.g. paraformaldehyde) and anti-inflammatory agents (e.g. corticosteroids), and were first used to circumvent conventional root canal preparation, disinfection, and filling; advocates argued that thorough cleaning and shaping were not necessary, and that the anti-inflammatory agents would reduce the host response. Some patients suffered injury as a result of these toxic materials being extruded into the periapical tissues and beyond. Most pastes (Endomethasone, Septodont; N2, Indrag-Agsa, Bologna, Italy; SPAD, Quetigny, France) contain paraformaldehyde. If deposited in the periapical tissues, this may give rise to severe inflammatory reactions and long-lasting or permanent injury, particularly to adjacent nerves. The corticosteroid in paste fillers severely affects the defence responses by suppressing phagocytosis, and their use may cause unwanted systemic side-effects. Paraformaldehyde applied to vital tissue will

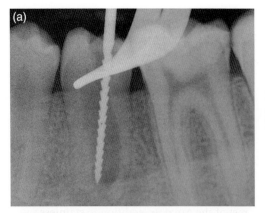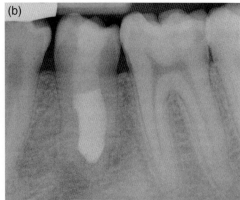

Figure 6.14 Malformed mandibular left second premolar. (a) Root canal treatment. (b) Root filled with MTA (ProRoot MTA, Dentsply). *Source:* Shreya Aggarwala.

also result in traces of the material or its components being spread throughout the body. Some patients may show a hypersensitivity response, and the material may have both mutagenic and carcinogenic potentials. A more recent development is Endomethasone N (Septodont), which does not contain paraformaldehyde and claims improved biocompatibility. In one study, it was no longer cytotoxic after one week [53].

6.3.4.2 HCSCs

MTA has been shown to have excellent sealing ability, biocompatibilty, and promotion of tissue regeneration. Its use as an apical plug for teeth with immature, open apices has proved very successful [182, 183]. This technique is discussed in Chapter 3 for the management of nonvital immature teeth. The material creates a hard barrier and the remainder of the canal is then filled with MTA or gutta-percha, or else the root is reinforced by appropriate materials [184]. The MTA apical-plug technique avoids the long-term use of calcium hydroxide dressings to bring about apical closure, which may weaken the already thin dentine walls [185]. Apart from MTA, other HCSC-based material may be used as apical plugs for teeth with immature, open apices.

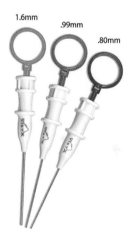

Figure 6.15 Disposable MTA carriers with different tip sizes. *Source:* Courtesy of Vista-Dental.

MTA can be used for obturation without a filling core (Figure 6.14). Canals may be obturated incrementally with pluggers, using a series of K-files (the Lawaty technique) or tapered rotary NiTi files used in reverse as augers [186]; MTA carriers may also be used to deliver the MTA into the root canal (Figure 6.15). Manual condensation using pluggers will produce a dense fill [187]. Ultrasound, applied indirectly, has been suggested as an aid to MTA condensation, but there is some controversy regarding its effectiveness [188]. It may be that ultrasound of certain durations creates a shock effect which separates cement particles and creates voids.

There is evidence that obturation with MTA may strengthen roots [189]. However, it has also been reported that MTA affects the flexural properties of dentine [190]. Root fillings of MTA should be considered for patients concerned about the use of gutta-percha root fillings. They may be valuable in problematic teeth where apicectomy is likely to be necessary in the future. In these cases, during surgery, the root resection can be made through the set material, so that root-end cavity preparation and root-end fillings are not required [191]. Another clinical consideration is expansion of MTA during setting. Teeth requiring retreatment may have preexisting undetected radicular infractions from heavy occlusal loads or extensive coronal restorations and posts. MTA obturation must be considered a permanent procedure in teeth with curved roots. It may be removed using ultrasonics in straight canals, but in curved canals its removal is extremely challenging [192].

The recent discovery of crystal growth in dentinal tubules adjacent to MTA may be significant, as it might enhance bacterial entombment, reduce the need for retreatment, or even improve the outcomes of retreatment [193, 194].

6.3.4.3 Monoblocks

Gutta-percha does not bond to dentine. A search for simpler methods of filling canals, their ramifications, and dentinal tubules led to investigations of low-viscosity unfilled BISGMA composite resins in the late 1970s [195]. These adapted well to the canal walls and could offer a way of filling canals without applying pressure. Much later, Resilon, a polycaprolactone thermoplastic material, was developed as an alternative core material with similar handling to gutta-percha. Alongside a UDMA-based sealer (e.g. Epiphany), it was intended to form a 'monoblock', a single interface between the dentine and the core [196]. With the smear layer removed, a primer was applied, the dual-cured sealer was coated on to the dentine wall, and the

core was placed. Many factors inform the effectiveness of these systems, including any smear layer present, the effects of irrigants, dentine tubule permeability, the surface area available for bonding, sealer thickness, and polymerization shrinkage.

A review in 2011 indicated that methacrylate-based obturation systems required further development [197], and the product was discontinued a few years later. The polycaprolactone may be susceptible to enzymatic hydrolysis by endodontic bacteria and fungi. It might also be that unknown voids were present in some canals, as the material was promoted as being more radiopaque than gutta-percha. Recent work has revealed that these materials behave very poorly in clinical situations. It was shown [198] that Resilon had a 5.7 times greater odds ratio of failure compared to gutta-percha. In another clinical study, Resilon-treated teeth were found to be over five times more likely to have a periapical index (PAI) of 3–5 at follow-up compared to teeth filled with gutta-percha [199]. The degradation of Resilon in unhealed canals of teeth with persisting periapical disease was studied, and it was found to have degraded in 78% of cases, whereas gutta-percha had degraded in none [200]. Whilst not all cases have failed, the material was in use for almost a decade, and patients treated with it have created a recall dilemma for practitioners.

6.3.4.4 Hydrophilic Polymers

Introduced in 2007, the SmartSeal system (DRFP Ltd., Peterborough, UK), also marketed as the CPoint system (EndoTechnologies, LLC, Shrewsbury, MA, USA), uses a single master cone (SmartPoint) made of materials similar to those in intraocular and contact lenses. In root canals, these are designed to swell and self-seal the 'wet' canal. The central cores of the cones are of two polyamide (nylon) polymers covered by a hydrophilic polymer sheath of acrylonitrile/vinyl pyrolidone. A resin-based epoxyamine sealer (SmartPaste Bio), containing bioceramics, is used in conjunction with the SmartPoint cone; it too hydrates and swells to fill voids. No special equipment is required and the cones are made to match preparation instruments; oval canals may be filled with multiple cones. The polymer sheath is radiolucent and appears different to gutta-percha on radiographs. The system is claimed to be easier to handle and less technique-sensitive than other obturation methods, with cost and time savings in both preparation and obturation. SmartPoints have comparable biocompatibility to gutta-percha [201] and show a significant lateral expansion within 20 minutes when exposed to water [202]. The SmartSeal system demonstrated comparable adhesion to root dentine to gutta-percha and AH 26 when tested using a push-out strength test [203]. When it was used with SmartPaste sealer in an *in vitro* study, there was good extension of material into simulated lateral canals and comparable homogeneity of obturation compared to laterally condensed gutta-percha and AH Plus [204]. Unfortunately, a moist environment is needed with these hydophilic polymers, which runs counter to the accepted concept of ensuring that the root canals are dry before obturation.

6.4 Orifice Barrier Materials and Tooth Restoration

The seal provided in root-filled teeth was first investigated by Dow and Ingle in 1955 [205], and it was not long before concerns were raised about the efficacy of coronal seals [206]. It was once common practice to pack excess gutta-percha over the pulp chamber floor when treating molars, but this was shown to lead to leakage [207]. Gutta-percha and sealer alone is not an adequate barrier to coronal microleakage, which may adversely affect the outcome of root canal treatment [208, 209]. Therefore, attempts have been made to protect the root filling itself by placement of a barrier material. Such an orifice barrier should:

1) be easy to place;
2) bond to the tooth structure (retentive);

3) seal effectively against coronal microleakage;
4) be easily distinguishable from natural tooth structure;
5) not interfere with the final restoration of the access preparation [210]; and
6) ideally have an antimicrobial effect.

Many materials have been used as orifice barriers, including Cavit (3M ESPE), IRM (Dentsply De Trey), Super-EBA (Bosworth, Skokie, IL, USA), and MTA. The ideal material is yet to be developed. ZOE materials do not bond to dentine but do have a strong antibacterial effect, depending on the consistency of mix used [19]. GICs have a long history of use for this purpose; whilst as liners they bond to dentine, their fluoride release has minimal antibacterial effect [211]. Resin-modified GICs can be light-cured, allowing easier and more controlled placement. An experiment using a bacterial marker showed Vitrebond to be successful over a 60-day period [212]. Studies using India ink on a flowable composite resin (Tetric, Ivoclar Vivadent) over seven days showed its sealing ability to be superior to that of ProRoot MTA and Cavit [213]. As a composite resin, etching and a bonding agent are required, but this additional process could be accomplished in about two minutes.

Temporary restorations should be in place for as short a duration as possible [214], root-filled teeth requiring good-quality coronal restorations of permanent materials [215]. These are best placed during the obturation visit, provided the clinical conditions are appropriate and the technical quality of the entire endodontic procedure has been satisfactory.

6.5 Retreatment

The removal of any previous root filling material is necessary to allow nonsurgical root canal retreatment. Where there is evidence of disease, the need for retreatment is established. However, in cases of patients with an exposed root filling, this presents a conundrum [216].

A recent narrative review provides some guidance [217].

When necessary, there are many ways of mechanically removing gutta-percha, and several solvents may be used in the final stages to clean canals. With carrier-based systems, the carriers may present specific problems during retreatment [218, 219]. The lastest generation of Thermafil obturators featured a V-shaped groove in the carrier shaft to facilitate removal, and research shows that these may be removed from moderately curved canals using rotary NiTi files [173].

No mechanical device is completely able to remove all filling materials from root canals [220], so efforts have been made to investigate combinations of techniques [221]. The effectiveness of NiTi and sonic and ultrasonic systems has been compared in a micro-computed tomography (CT) study of oval canals [222], which found ProTaper Next and Reciproc to be equally effective, whilst additional cleaning methods did not significantly improve removal. Most often, it is sealer that remains in the root canal after retreatment [223]. One early study, which included Ketac Endo GIC sealer [224], assessed debris scores following hand or ultrasonic removal of gutta-percha and sealers (Roth's 801 and AH 26). Most debris remained in the apical third of the roots examined. Hand removal of GIC the slowest method. The conclusion was that ultrasound was significantly faster, and that whilst the GIC sealer could be satisfactorily removed ultrasonically, the amount of debris remaining suggested that it bonded to dentine [224].

The removal of HCSC- and epoxy resin-based sealers has also been compared [225], and the results, using Gates Glidden drills and ProFiles (Dentsply Maillefer) to remove EndoSequence BC and AH Plus, showed no significant difference in terms of retreatment time or debris remaining at different levels within the root. Neither material could be removed completely. Sealer penetration depth was significantly higher with AH Plus.

HCSCs are hard once set, and there is concern over retreatment following their use. Some studies have found that root canals obturated using these sealers and a core material are easily retreatable with conventional techniques [226, 227], but a study found that it was impossible to completely remove the HCSC-based sealer EndoSequence BC from the mesiobuccal canals of mandibular molars using conventional retreatment techniques, heat, chloroform, rotary instruments, and hand files [228]. Sankin Apatite Root Canal Sealer could be easily removed from the canal without the use of a solvent [229]. The retreatability when MTA Fillapex is used as a sealer has been compared to that of AH Plus with regard to the amount of debris and material remaining in the canal and the time required to reach working length [230]. Interestingly, more root filling material was left in the AH Plus group, and the time taken to reach working length and achieve dentine removal was also highest with this material [230]. Studying the removal of MTA Fillapex, Totalfill BC, and AH Plus sealers, it was demonstrated that Totalfill was the most difficult to remove and AH Plus was the easiest; the authors used D-RaCe (FKG) and XP-endo Finisher R files (FKG) and no solvents [231]. The XP-endo Finisher R file was also efficient in removing HCSC sealer, even when combined with the ProTaper system [232]. It has been reported that the application of chloroform may help patency reestablishment if MTA Fillapex is used as the root filling [233]. The use of supplemental irrigant agitation also helped reduce the quantity of sealer left in the canal [234]. Targeted chemical removal of sealer with formic acid achieved over 95% retreatability with reestablishment of apical patency [235]. Clinicians must be mindful that the reality of performing retreatment in canals that have been filled using bioceramic sealers may be challenging, and it is inevitable that dentine will be removed during the process.

In addition to being challenging to fill, the retreatment of oval canals presents a special difficulty; a recent paper using micro-CT to investigate the removal of gutta-percha and AH Plus sealer via three motor-driven devices found that none left the canals completely free of filling materials [236].

6.6 Conclusion

Do root fillings strengthen teeth?

A recent study has shown that there is a tendency for dentine to decrease in strength as it increases in age [237]. Dentine is removed during canal preparation, and the strength of the root tissue is further reduced by other treatment processes, with root treated teeth more likely to undergo vertical root fracture than unrestored and healthy ones. Gutta-percha is incapable of bonding to the walls of root canals. Root filling materials with a proven ability to strengthen roots would thus represent a Holy Grail of endodontics. In 1992, Trope and Ray [238] found that the GIC sealer Ketac Endo significantly strengthened roots compared to prepared but unobturated ones and to those obturated with gutta-percha and Roth's 801 sealer. They speculated that the only reason for using a single cone of gutta-percha with Ketac Endo as a root filling was to allow retreatment, if required.

A review which systematically investigated and analysed relevant publications concluded that the use of a root canal sealer might increase the fracture resistance of a root-filled tooth, and that no particular sealer appeared superior in this respect [239]. Much of the evidence collected was conflicting. For instance, twelve studies supported a reinforcing effect of epoxy resin-based sealers, whilst five did not. Five studies on GIC sealers showed they positively affected fracture strength, whilst three did not. No study compared the effects of GIC and HCSC sealers on resistance to root fracture. A major problem with all such investigations is the heterogeneity in the methods used by researchers in this field. In one well-controlled experiment, White ProRoot MTA placed manually into canals and used alone resulted in teeth which were significantly more resistant to vertical root fracture after one and six months [189]. This technique may have particular application in overinstrumented or otherwise weakened teeth.

The Future

Certain canal shapes, particularly oval ones, remain difficult to obturate adequately, so further research and innovation are required. The quest continues for new materials with improved clinically reliability, better dentinal tubule penetration, slight expansion, resistance to degradation, and an enhanced ability to adhere to dentine irrespective of root canal conditions.

References

1 American Association of Endodontists (2016). Canal preparation and obturation: an updated view of the two pillars of nonsurgical endodontics. Available from https://www.aae.org/specialty/newsletter/canal-preparation-obturation-updated-view-two-pillars-nonsurgical-endodontics/ (accessed 10 August 2020).

2 Tronstad, L., Asbjørnsen, K., Døving, L. et al. (2000). Influence of coronal restorations on the periapical health of endodontically treated teeth. *Endod. Dent. Traumatol.* 16: 218–221.

3 Craveiro, M.A., Fontana, C.E., de Martin, A.S. et al. (2015). Influence of coronal restoration and root canal filling quality on periapical status: clinical and radiographic evaluation. *J. Endod.* 41: 836–840.

4 Ricucci, D., Russo, J., Rutberg, M. et al. (2011). A prospective cohort study of endodontic treatments of 1,369 root canals: results after

5 years. *Oral Surg. Oral Med. Oral Pathol. Oral Radiol. Endod.* 112: 825–842.

5 Violich, R. and Chandler, N.P. (2010). The smear layer in endodontics- a review. *Int. Endod. J.* 43: 2–15.

6 Wu, M.K. and Wesselink, P.R. (1993). Endodontic leakage studies reconsidered. Part I. Methodology, application and relevance. *Int. Endod. J.* 26: 37–43.

7 Ørstavik, D. (2005). Materials used for root canal obturation: technical, biological and clinical testing. *Endod. Top.* 12: 25–38.

8 Chandler, N. and Chellappa, D. (2019). Lubrication during root canal treatment. *Aust. Dent. J.* 45: 106–110.

9 Anbu, R., Nandini, S., and Velmurugan, N. (2009). Volumetric analysis of root fillings using spiral computed tomography: an in vitro study. *Int. Endod. J.* 43: 64–68.

10 Trope, M., Bunes, A., and Debelian, G. (2015). Root filling materials and techniques: bioceramics a new hope? *Endod. Top.* 32: 86–96.

11 Elyassi, Y., Moinzadeh, A.T., and Kleverlaan, C.J. (2019). Characterization of leachates from 6 root canal sealers. *J. Endod.* 45: 623–627.

12 Sousa, C.J.A., Montes, C.R.M., Pascon, E.A. et al. (2006). Comparison of the intraosseous biocompatibility of AH Plus, EndoREZ, and Epiphany root canal sealers. *J. Endod.* 32: 656–662.

13 Lacey, S., Pitt Ford, T.R., Watson, T.F., and Sherriff, M. (2005). A study of the rheological properties of endodontic sealers. *Int. Endod. J.* 38: 499–504.

14 Lacey, S., Pitt Ford, T.R., Yuan, X.F. et al. (2006). The effect of temperature on viscosity of root canal sealers. *Int. Endod. J.* 39: 860–866.

15 International Organization for Standardization (2012). ISO 6876:2012, Dentistry – Root canal sealing materials. Available from https://www.iso.org/standard/45117.html (accessed 10 August 2020).

16 Stamos, D.E., Gutmann, J.L., and Gettleman, B.H. (1995). In vitro evaluation of root canal sealer distribution. *J. Endod.* 21: 177–179.

17 Camilleri, J. (2015). Sealers and warm gutta-percha obturation techniques. *J. Endod.* 41: 72–78.

18 Rickert, U. and Dixon, C. (1933). The control of root surgery. *Transactions of the 8th International Dental Congress*, Section IIIA, No. 9.20:1458.

19 Heling, I. and Chandler, N.P. (1996). The antimicrobial effect within dentinal tubules of four root canal sealers. *J. Endod.* 22: 257–259.

20 Johnson, W., Kulild, J.C., and Tay, F. (2016). Obturation of the cleaned and shaped root canal system. In: Cohen's Pathways of the Pulp, 11e (eds. K.M. Hargreaves, L.H. Berman and I. Rotstein), 280–322. St Louis, MO: Elsevier.

21 Michaud, R.A., Burgess, J., Barfield, R.D. et al. (2008). Volumetric expansion of gutta-percha in contact with eugenol. *J. Endod.* 34: 1528–1532.

22 Desai, S.V. and Chandler, N.P. (2009). Calcium hydroxide-based root canal sealers: a review. *J. Endod.* 35: 475–480.

23 Tronstad, L., Barnett, F., and Flax, M. (1988). Solubility and biocompatibility of calcium hydroxide-containing root canal sealers. *Dent. Traumatol.* 4: 152–159.

24 Jacobsen, E.L., BeGole, E.A., Vitkus, D.D. et al. (1987). An evaluation of two newly formulated calcium hydroxide cements: a leakage study. *J. Endod.* 13: 164–169.

25 Wilson, A.D. and Kent, B.E. (1971). The glass-ionomer cement: a new translucent dental filling material. *J. Appl. Chem. Biotech.* 21: 313–318.

26 Pitt Ford, T.R. (1979). The leakage of root fillings using glass ionomer cement and other materials. *Br. Dent. J.* 146: 273–278.

27 Ray, H. and Seltzer, S. (1991). A new glass ionomer root canal sealer. *J. Endod.* 17: 598–603.

28 Saunders, W.P., Saunders, E.M., Herd, D. et al. (1992). The use of glass ionomer as a

root canal sealer – a pilot study. *Int. Endod. J.* 25: 238–244.

29 De Gee, A.J., Wu, M.-K., and Wesselink, P.R. (1994). Sealing properties of Ketac-Endo glass ionomer cement and AH26 root canal sealers. *Int. Endod. J.* 27: 239–244.

30 Friedman, S., Löst, C., Zarrabian, M. et al. (1995). Evaluation of success and failure after endodontic therapy using a glass ionomer cement sealer. *J. Endod.* 21: 384–390.

31 Timpawat, S., Harnirattisai, C., and Senawongs, P. (2001). Adhesion of a glass-ionomer root canal sealer to the root canal wall. *J. Endod.* 27: 168–171.

32 Lee, K.-W., Williams, M.C., Camps, J.J. et al. (2002). Adhesion of endodontic sealers to dentin and gutta-percha. *J. Endod.* 28: 684–688.

33 Herrera, M., Carrion, P., Baca, P. et al. (2001). In vitro antibacterial activity of glass-ionomer cements. *Microbios* 104: 141–148.

34 Patel, V., Santerre, J.P., and Friedman, S. (2000). Suppression of bacterial adherence by experimental root canal sealers. *J. Endod.* 26: 20–24.

35 Thom, D., Davies, J., Santerre, J. et al. (2003). The hemolytic and cytotoxic properties of a zeolite-containing root filling material in vitro. *Oral Surg. Oral Med. Oral Pathol. Oral Radiol. Endod.* 95: 101–108.

36 Silva Almeida, L.H., Moraes, R.R. et al. (2017). Are premixed calcium silicate-based endodontic sealers comparable to conventional materials? A systematic review of in vitro studies. *J. Endod.* 43: 527–535.

37 Marciano, M.A., Camilleri, J., Lia Mondelli, R.F. et al. (2015). Potential dental staining of root canal sealers with formulations containing bismuth oxide and formaldehyde. *Endo (Lond. Engl.)* 9: 39–45.

38 Versiani, M.A., Carvalho-Junior, J.R., Padilha, M.I. et al. (2006). A comparative study of physicochemical properties of AH Plus and Epiphany root canal sealants. *Int. Endod. J.* 39: 464–471.

39 Ersahan, S. and Aydin, C. (2010). Dislocation resistance of iRoot SP, a calcium silicate-based sealer, from radicular dentine. *J. Endod.* 36: 2000–2002.

40 Vilanova, W.V., Carvalho-Junior, J.R., Alfredo, E. et al. (2012). Effect of intracanal irrigants on the bond strength of epoxy resin-based and methacrylate resin-based sealers to root canal walls. *Int. Endod. J.* 45: 42–48.

41 Zhou, H.M., Shen, Y., Zheng, W. et al. (2013). Physical properties of 5 root canal sealers. *J. Endod.* 39: 1281–1286.

42 Borges, R.P., Sousa-Neto, M.D., Versiani, M.A. et al. (2012). Changes in the surface of four calcium silicate-containing endodontic materials and an epoxy resin-based sealer after a solubility test. *Int. Endod. J.* 45: 419–428.

43 Kim, T.G., Lee, Y.H., Lee, N.H. et al. (2013). The antioxidant property of pachymic acid improves bone disturbance against AH Plus-induced inflammation in MC-3T3 E1 cells. *J. Endod.* 39: 461–466.

44 Hergt, A., Hulsmann, M., and Rodig, T. (2015). AH Plus root canal sealer – an updated literature review. *ENDO (Lond. Engl.)* 9: 245–265.

45 Viapiana, R., Guerreiro-Tanomaru, J.M., Tanomaru-Filho, M. et al. (2014). Investigation of the effect of sealer use on the heat generated at the external root surface during root canal obturation using warm vertical compaction technique with System B heat source. *J. Endod.* 40: 555–561.

46 Viapiana, R., Baluci, C.A., Tanumaro-Filho, M. et al. (2015). Investigation of chemical changes in sealers during application of the warm vertical compaction technique. *Int. Endod. J.* 48: 16–27.

47 Donnermeyer, D., Vahdat-Pajouh, N., Schäfer, E., and Dammaschke, T. (2019). Influence of the final irrigation solution on the push-out bond strength of calcium silicate-based, epoxy resin-based and silicone-based endodontic sealers. *Odontology* 107: 231–236.

48 Raina, R., Loushine, R.J., Weller, R.N. et al. (2007). Evaluation of the quality of the apical seal in Resilon/Epiphany and gutta-percha/AH Plus-filled root canals by using a fluid filtration approach. *J. Endod.* 33: 944–947.

49 Kataoka, H., Yoshioka, T., Suda, H. et al. (2000). Dentin bonding and sealing ability of a new root canal resin sealer. *J. Endod.* 26: 230–235.

50 Imai, Y. and Komabayashi, T. (2003). Properties of a new injectable type of root canal filling resin with adhesiveness to dentin. *J. Endod.* 29: 20–23.

51 Wu, M.-K., Tigos, E., and Wesselink, P.R. (2002). An 18-month longitudinal study on a new silicon-based sealer, RSA RoekoSeal: a leakage study in vitro. *Oral Surg. Oral Med. Oral Pathol. Oral Radiol. Endod.* 94: 499–502.

52 Miletic, I., Devcic, N., Anic, I. et al. (2005). The cytotoxicity of RoekoSeal and AH Plus compared during different setting periods. *J. Endod.* 31: 307–309.

53 Da Silva, E.J.N.L., Santos, C.C., and Zaia, A.A. (2013). Long-term cytotoxic effects of contemporary root canal sealers. *J. Appl. Oral Sci.* 21: 43–47.

54 Zielinski, T.M., Baumgartner, J.C., and Marshall, J.G. (2008). An evaluation of GuttaFlow and gutta-percha in the filling of lateral grooves and depressions. *J. Endod.* 34: 295–298.

55 De-Deus, G., Brandão, M.C., Fidel, R.A.S. et al. (2007). The sealing ability of GuttaFlow in oval-shaped canals: an *ex vivo* study using a polymicrobial leakage model. *Int. Endod. J.* 40: 794–799.

56 Vasiliadis, L., Kodonas, K., Economides, N. et al. (2010). Short- and long-term sealing ability of Gutta-flow and AH-Plus using an *ex vivo* fluid transport model. *Int. Endod. J.* 43: 377–381.

57 Camilleri, J., Montesin, F.E., Brady, K. et al. (2005). The constitution of mineral trioxide aggregate. *Dent. Mater.* 21: 297–303.

58 Camilleri, J. (2008). Characterization of hydration products of mineral trioxide aggregate. *Int. Endod. J.* 41: 408–417.

59 Kebudi Benezra, M., Schembri Wismayer, P., and Camilleri, J. (2017). Influence of environment on testing of hydraulic sealers. *Sci. Rep.* 7: 17927.

60 Guerreiro-Tanomaru, J.M., Duarte, M.A.H., Gonçalves, M., and Tanomaru-Filho, M. (2009). Radiopacity evaluation of root canal sealers containing calcium hydroxide and MTA. *Braz. Oral Res.* 23: 119–123.

61 Gandolfi, M.G., Iacono, F., Agee, K. et al. (2009). Setting time and expansion in different soaking media of experimental accelerated calcium-silicate cements and ProRoot MTA. *Oral Surg. Oral Med. Oral Pathol. Oral Radiol. Endod.* 108: e39–e45.

62 Loushine, B.A., Bryan, T.E., Looney, S.W. et al. (2011). Setting properties and cytotoxicity evaluation of a premixed bioceramic root canal sealer. *J. Endod.* 37: 673–677.

63 Camilleri, J. and Mallia, B. (2011). Evaluation of the dimensional changes of mineral trioxide aggregate sealer. *Int. Endod. J.* 44: 416–424.

64 Zhang, H., Shen, Y., Ruse, N.D. et al. (2009). Antibacterial activity of endodontic sealers by modified direct contact test against *Enterococcus faecalis*. *J. Endod.* 35: 1051–1055.

65 Jefferies, S. (2014). Bioactive and biomimetic restorative materials: a comprehensive review. Part I. *J. Esthet. Rest. Dent.* 26: 14–26.

66 Camilleri, J. (2011). Characterization and hydration kinetics of tricalcium silicate cement for use as a dental biomaterial. *Dent. Mat.* 27: 836–844.

67 Sarkar, N.K., Caicedo, R., Ritwik, P. et al. (2005). Physicochemical basis of the biologic properties of mineral trioxide aggregate. *J. Endod.* 31: 97–100.

68 Richardson, I.G. (2008). The calcium silicate hydrates. *Cem. Concr. Res.* 38: 137–158.

69 Hench, L.L. and Wilson, J. (1984). Surface-active biomaterials. *Science* 226: 630–636.

70 Reyes-Carmona, J.F., Felippe, M.S., and Felippe, W.T. (2009). Biomineralization ability and interaction of mineral trioxide aggregate and white portland cement with dentin in a phosphate-containing fluid. *J. Endod.* 35: 731–736.

71 Xuereb, M., Vella, P., Damidot, D. et al. (2015). In situ assessment of the setting of tricalcium silicate-based sealers using a dentin pressure model. *J. Endod.* 41: 111–124.

72 Dreger, L.A., Felippe, W.T., Reyes-Carmona, J.F. et al. (2012). Mineral trioxide aggregate and portland cement promote biomineralization *in vivo*. *J. Endod.* 38: 324–329.

73 Taccio, G., Corriera, T.C., Duarte, M. et al. (2012). Evaluation of radiopacity, pH release of calcium ions and flow of a bioceramic root canal sealer. *J. Endod.* 38: 842–845.

74 Scarparo, R.K., Haddad, D., Acasigua, G.A. et al. (2010). Mineral trioxide aggregate-based sealer: analysis of tissue reactions to a new endodontic material. *J. Endod.* 36: 1174–1178.

75 Guerreiro-Tanomaru, J.M., Duarte, M.A.H., Gonçalves, M. et al. (2013). Radiopacity evaluation of root canal sealers containing calcium hydroxide and MTA. *Braz. Oral Res.* 23: 119–123.

76 Gomes-Filho, J.E., Moreira, J.V., Watanabe, S. et al. (2012). Sealability of MTA and calcium hydroxide-containing sealers. *J. Appl. Oral Sci.* 20: 347–351.

77 Assmann, E., Scarparo, R.K., Böttcher, D.E. et al. (2012). Dentin bond strength of two mineral trioxide aggregate-based and one epoxy resin-based sealers. *J. Endod.* 38: 219–221.

78 Mohammadi, Z., Giardino, L., Palazzi, F. et al. (2012). Antibacterial activity of a new mineral trioxide aggregate-based root canal sealer. *Int. Dent. J.* 62: 70–73.

79 Bramante, C.M., Kato, M.M., Assis, G.F. et al. (2013). Biocompatibility and setting time of CPM-MTA and white Portland cement clinker with or without calcium sulfate. *J. Appl. Oral Sci.* 21: 32–36.

80 Weller, R.N., Tay, K.C., Garrett, L.V. et al. (2008). Microscopic appearance and apical seal of root canals filled with gutta-percha and ProRoot Endo Sealer after immersion in a phosphate-containing fluid. *Int. Endod. J.* 11: 977–986.

81 Huffman, B.P., Mai, S., Pinna, L. et al. (2009). Dislocation resistance of ProRoot Endo Sealer, a calcium silicate-based root canal sealer, from radicular dentine. *Int. Endod. J.* 42: 34–46.

82 Bernardes, R.A., de Amorim Campelo, A., Junior, D.S. et al. (2010). Evaluation of the flow rate of 3 endodontic sealers: Sealer 26, AH Plus, and MTA Obtura. *Oral Surg. Oral Med. Oral Pathol. Oral Radiol. Endod.* 109: e47–e49.

83 de Vasconcelos, B.C., Bernardes, R.A., Duarte, M.A.H. et al. (2011). Apical sealing of root canal fillings performed with five different endodontic sealers: analysis by fluid filtration. *J. Appl. Oral Sci.* 19: 324–328.

84 Viapiana, R., Flumignan, D.L., Guerreiro-Tanomaru, J.M. et al. (2014). Physicochemical and mechanical properties of zirconium oxide and niobium oxide modified Portland cement-based experimental endodontic sealers. *Int. Endod. J.* 47: 437–448.

85 Morgental, R.D., Vier-Pelisser, F.V., Oliveira, S.D. et al. (2011). Antbacterial activity of two MTA-based root canal sealers. *Int. Endod. J.* 44: 1128–1133.

86 Siboni, F., Taddei, P., Zamparini, F. et al. (2017). Properties of BioRoot RCS, a tricalcium silicate endodontic sealer modified with povidone and polycarboxylate. *Int. Endod. J.* 50: e120–e136.

87 Silva, E.J.N.L., Rosa, T.P., Herrera, D.R. et al. (2013). Evaluation of cytotoxicity and physiochemical properties of calcium silicate-based endodontic sealer MTA Fillapex. *J. Endod.* 39: 274–277.

88 Torres, F.F.E., Guerreiro-Tanomaru, J.M., Bosso-Martelo, R. et al. (2019). Solubility, porosity, dimensional and volumetric change of endodontic sealers. *Braz. Dent. J.* 30: 368–373.

89 Razavian, H., Barekatain, B., Shadmehr, E. et al. (2014). Bacterial leakage in root canals

filled with resin-based and mineral trioxide aggregate-based sealers. *Dent. Res. J.* 11: 599–603.

90 Ioannidis, K., Mistakidis, I., Beltes, P. et al. (2013). Spectrophotometric analysis of crown discoloration induced by MTA- and ZnOE-based sealers. *J. Appl. Oral Sci.* 21: 138–144.

91 Bin, C.V., Valera, M.C., Camargo, S.E.A. et al. (2012). Cytotoxicity and genotoxicity of root canal sealers based on mineral trioxide aggregate. *J. Endod* 38: 495–500.

92 Gomes-Filho, J.E., Watanabe, S., Lodi, C.S. et al. (2012). Rat tissue reaction to MTA Fillapex. *Dent. Traumatol.* 28: 452–456.

93 Tavares, C.O., Böttcher, D.E., Assmann, E. et al. (2013). Tissue reactions to a new mineral trioxide aggregate-containing endodontic sealer. *J. Endod.* 39: 653–657.

94 Assmann, E., Böttcher, D.E., Hoppe, C.B. et al. (2015). Evaluation of bone tissue response to a sealer containing mineral trioxide aggregate. *J. Endod.* 41: 62–66.

95 da Silva, E.J., Zaia, A.A., and Peters, O.A. (2017). Cytocompatibility of calcium silicate-based sealers in a three-dimensional cell culture model. *Clin. Oral Investig.* 21: 1531–1536.

96 Rodríguez-Lozano, F.J., García-Bernal, D., Oñate-Sánchez, R.E. et al. (2017). Evaluation of cytocompatibility of calcium silicate-based endodontic sealers and their effects on the biological responses of mesenchymal dental stem cells. *Int. Endod. J.* 50: 67–76.

97 Collado-González, M., Tomás-Catalá, C.J., Oñate-Sánchez, R.E. et al. (2017). Cytotoxicity of GuttaFlow, Bioseal, GuttaFlow2, MTA Fillapex, and AH plus on human periodontal ligament stem cells. *J. Endod.* 43: 816–822.

98 Victoria-Escandell, A., Ibañez-Cabellos, J.S., De Cantunda, S.B. et al. (2017). Cellular responses in human dental pulp stem cells treated with three endodontic materials. *Stem Cells Int.* 2017 (1): 1–14.

99 López-García, S., Pecci-Lloret, M.R., Guerrero-Gironés, J. et al. (2019).

Comparative cytocompatibility and mineralization potential of Bio-C Sealer and TotalFill BC Sealer. *Materials (Basel)* 12: pii:E3087.

100 López-García, S., Lozano, A., García-Bernal, D. et al. (2019b). Biological effects of new hydraulic materials on human periodontal ligament stem cells. *J. Clin. Med.* 8: pii: E1216.

101 Zordan-Bronzel, C.L., Esteves Torres, F.F., Tanomaru-Filho, M. et al. (2019). Evaluation of physicochemical properties of a new calcium silicate-based sealer, Bio-C Sealer. *J. Endod.* 45: 1248–1252.

102 Reszka, P., Nowicka, A., Lipski, M. et al. (2016). A comparative chemical study of calcium silicate-containing and epoxy resin-based root canal sealers. *Biomed. Res. Int.* 2016: 9808432.

103 Viapiana, R., Moinzadeh, A.T., Camilleri, L. et al. (2016). Porosity and sealing ability of root fillings with gutta-percha and BioRoot RCS or AH Plus sealers. Evaluation by three ex vivo methods. *Int. Endod. J.* 49: 774–782.

104 Loison-Robert, L.S., Tassin, M., Bonte, E. et al. (2018). In vitro effects of two silicate-based materials, Biodentine and BioRoot RCS, on dental pulp stem cells in models of reactionary and reparative dentinogenesis. *PLoS One* 13: e0190014.

105 Dimitrova-Nakov, S., Uzunoglu, E., Ardila-Osorio, H. et al. (2015). In vitro bioactivity of BioRoot RCS, via A4 mouse pulpal stem cells. *Dent. Mat.* 31: 1290–1297.

106 Prüllage, R.K., Urban, K., Schäfer, E. et al. (2016). Material properties of a tricalcium silicate-containing, a mineral trioxide aggregate-containing, and an epoxy resin-based root canal sealer. *J. Endod.* 42: 784–788.

107 Long, J., Kreft, J.U., and Camilleri, J. (2020). Antimicrobial and ultrastructural properties of root canal filling materials exposed to bacterial challenge. *J. Dent.* 93: 103283.

108 Arias-Moliz, M.T. and Camilleri, J. (2016). The effect of the final irrigant on the antimicrobial activity of root canal sealers. *J. Dent.* 52: 30–36.

109 Koch, K.A., Brave, D.G., and Nasseh, A.A. (2010a). Bioceramic technology: closing the endo-restorative circle, part I. *Dent. Today* 29: 100–105.

110 Koch, K.A., Brave, G.D., and Nasseh, A.A. (2010b). Bioceramic technology: closing the endo-restorative circle, part 2. *Dent. Today* 29: 98–105.

111 Agarwal, R. and Nikhil, V. (2016). The comparison of physicochemical properties of new and established root canal sealers. *Endodontology* 28: 97–101.

112 Topçuoglu, H.S., Tuncay, Ö., Karatas, E. et al. (2013). In vitro fracture resistance of roots obturated with epoxy-resin-based, mineral trioxide-based, and bioceramic root canal sealers. *J. Endod.* 39: 1630–1633.

113 Chen, B., Haapasalo, M., Mobuchon, C. et al. (2020). Cytotoxicity and the effect of temperature on physical properties and chemical composition of a new calcium silicate-based root canal sealer. *J. Endod.* 46: 531–538.

114 Atmeh, A.R., Hadis, M., and Camilleri, J. (2020). Real-time chemical analysis of root filling materials with heating: guidelines for safe temperature levels. *Int. Endod. J.* 53: 698–708.

115 Zhang, W., Li, Z., and Peng, B. (2010). *Ex vivo* cytotoxicity of a new calcium silicate-based canal filling material. *Int. Endod. J.* 43: 769–774.

116 Baraba, A., Pezelj-Ribaric, S., Roguljić, M. et al. (2016). Cytotoxicity of two bioactive root canal sealers. *Acta Stomatol. Croatica* 50: 8–13.

117 Ghoneim, A.G., Lutfy, R.A., Sabet, N.E. et al. (2011). Resistance to fracture of roots obturated with novel canal-filling systems. *J. Endod.* 37: 1590–1592.

118 Akcay, M., Arslan, H., Durmus, N. et al. (2016). Dentinal tubule penetration of AH Plus, iRoot SP, MTA Fillapex and GuttaFlow Bioseal root canal sealers after different final irrigation procedures: a confocal microscopic study. *Lasers Surg. Med.* 48: 70–76.

119 Nagas, E., Uyanik, M.O., Eymirli, A. et al. (2012). Dentin moisture conditions affect adhesion of root canal sealers. *J. Endod.* 38: 240–244.

120 Kim, J.S., Baek, S.H., and Bae, K.S. (2004). In vivo study on the biocompatibility of newly developed calcium phosphate-based root canal sealers. *J. Endod.* 30: 708–711.

121 Kashaba, R.M., Moussa, M.M., Chutkan, N.B., and Borke, J.L. (2011). The response of subcutaneous connective tissue to newly developed calcium phosphate-based root canal sealers. *Int. Endod. J.* 44: 342–352.

122 Krastl, G., Allgayer, N., Lenherr, P. et al. (2013). Tooth discoloration induced by endodontic materials: a literature review. *Dent. Traumatol.* 29: 2–7.

123 Jasper, E.A. (1941). Adaptation and tissue tolerance of silver root canal fillings. *J. Dent. Res.* 20: 355–360.

124 Seltzer, S., Green, D.B., Weiner, N. et al. (1972). A scanning electron microscope examination of silver cones removed from endodontically treated teeth. *Oral Surg. Oral Med. Oral Pathol.* 33: 589–605.

125 Brady, J.M. and del Rio, C.E. (1975). Corrosion of endodontic silver cones in humans: a scanning electron microscope and X-ray microprobe study. *J. Endod.* 1: 205–210.

126 Schilder, H., Goodman, A., and Aldrich, W. (1974a). The thermomechanical properties of gutta-percha. I. The compressibility of gutta-percha. *Oral Surg. Oral Med. Oral Pathol.* 37: 946–953.

127 Goodman, A., Schilder, H., and Aldrich, W. (1974). The thermomechanical properties of gutta-percha. II. The history and molecular chemistry of gutta-percha. *Oral Surg. Oral Med. Oral Pathol.* 37: 954–961.

128 Schilder, H., Goodman, A., and Aldrich, W. (1974b). The thermomechanical properties of gutta-percha. III. Determination of phase transition temperatures for gutta-percha. *Oral Surg. Oral Med. Oral Pathol.* 38: 109–114.

129 Schilder, H., Goodman, A., and Aldrich, W. (1981). The thermomechanical properties of gutta-percha. Part IV. A thermal profile of the warm gutta-percha packing procedure. *Oral Surg. Oral Med. Oral Pathol.* 51: 544–551.

130 Schilder, H., Goodman, A., and Aldrich, W. (1985). The thermomechanical properties of gutta-percha. Part V. Volume changes in bulk gutta-percha as a function of temperature and its relationship to molecular phase transformation. *Oral Surg. Oral Med. Oral Pathol.* 59: 285–296.

131 Ingle, J.I. (1961). A standardized endodontic technique utilizing newly designed instruments and filling materials. *Oral Surg. Oral Med. Oral Pathol.* 14: 83–91.

132 Gutmann, J.L. and Manjarrés, V. (2019). Disinfection of gutta-percha cones prior to obturation: a smattering of historical perspectives with a focus on contemporary considerations. *ENDO (Lond. Engl.)* 13: 191–206.

133 Torabinejad, M., Ung, B., and Kettering, J.D. (1990). In vitro bacterial penetration of coronally unsealed endodontically treated teeth. *J. Endod.* 16: 566–569.

134 Rose, K. and Steinbüchel, A. (2005). Biodegradation of natural rubber and related compounds: recent insights into a hardly understood catabolic capability of microorganisms. *Appl. Environ. Microbiol.* 71: 2803–2812.

135 Fransen, J.N., He, J., Glickman, G.N. et al. (2008). Comparative assessment of ActiV GP/glass ionomer sealer, Resilon/Epiphany, and gutta-percha/AH Plus obturation: a bacterial leakage study. *J. Endod.* 34: 725–727.

136 Osiri, S., Banomyong, D., Sattabanasuk, V. et al. (2018). Root reinforcement after obturation with calcium silicate-based sealer and modified gutta-percha cone. *J. Endod.* 44: 1843–1848.

137 Byström, A., Sundqvist, G., and Claesson, R. (1985). The antibacterial effect of camphorated paramonochlorophenol, camphorated phenol and calcium hydroxide in the treatment of infected root canals. *Endod. Dent. Traumatol.* 1: 170–175.

138 Haapasalo, M. and Ørstavik, D. (1987). In vitro infection and disinfection of dentinal tubules. *J. Dent. Res.* 66: 1375–1379.

139 Podbielski, A., Boeckh, C., and Haller, B. (2000). Growth inhibitory activity of gutta-percha points containing root canal medications on common endodontic bacterial pathogens as determined by an optimized quantitative in vitro assay. *J. Endod.* 26: 398–403.

140 Lui, J.N., Sae-Lim, V., Song, K.P. et al. (2004). In vitro antimicrobial effect of chlorhexidine-impregnated gutta percha points on *Enterococcus faecalis*. *Int. Endod. J.* 37: 105–113.

141 Szep, S., Grumann, L., Ronge, K. et al. (2003). In vitro cytotoxicity of medicated and nonmedicated gutta-percha points in cultures of gingival fibroblasts. *J. Endod.* 29: 36–40.

142 Wang, D., Wang, Z., and Gao, J. (2003). The development and in vitro release rate determination of controlled-release delivery gutta-percha point containing metronidazole compound (Chinese). *Hua Xi Kou Qiang Yi Xue Za Zhi.* 21: 361–363.

143 Gazelius, B., Olgart, L., and Wrangsjo, K. (1986). Unexpected symptoms to root filling with gutta-percha – a case report. *Int. Endod. J.* 19: 202–204.

144 Boxer, M., Grammer, L., and Orfan, N. (1994). Gutta-percha allergy in a health care worker with latex allergy. *J. Allergy Clin. Immunol.* 93: 943–944.

145 Costa, G.E., Johnson, J.D., and Hamilton, R.G. (2001). Cross-reactivity studies of gutta-percha, gutta-balata and natural rubber latex (*Hevea brasiliensis*). *J. Endod.* 27: 584–587.

146 Kang, P., Vogt, K., Gruninger, S. et al. (2007). The immuno cross-reactivity of gutta percha points. *Dent. Mater.* 23: 380–384.

147 Augsburger, R.A. and Peters, D.D. (1990). Radiographic evaluation of extruded obturation materials. *J. Endod.* 16: 492–497.

148 Gordon, M.P.J., Love, R.M., and Chandler, N.P. (2005). An evaluation of .06 tapered gutta-percha cones for filling of .06 taper prepared curved root canals. *Int. Endod. J.* 38: 87–96.

149 Blum, J.-Y., Machtou, P., and Micallef, J.-P. (1998). Analysis of forces developed during obturations. Wedging effect: part II. *J. Endod.* 24: 223–228.

150 Madison, S. and Zakariasen, K.L. (1984). Linear and volumetric analysis of apical leakage in teeth prepared for posts. *J. Endod.* 10: 422–427.

151 Eltair, M., Pitchika, V., Hickel, R. et al. (2018). Evaluation of the interface between gutta-percha and two types of sealers using scanning electron microscopy (SEM). *Clin. Oral Investig.* 22: 1631–1639.

152 Wang, Y., Liu, S., and Dong, Y. (2018). *In vitro* study of dentinal tubule penetration and filling quality of bioceramic sealer. *PLoS One* 13: e0192248.

153 Celikten, B., Uzuntas, C.F., Orhan, A.I. et al. (2016). Evaluation of root canal sealer filling quality using a single-cone technique in oval shaped canals: an *in vitro* Micro-CT study. *Scanning* 38: 133–140.

154 Moinzadeh, A.T., Zerbst, W., Boutsioukis, C. et al. (2015). Porosity distribution in root canals filled with gutta percha and calcium silicate cement. *Dent. Mater.* 31: 1100–1108.

155 Celikten, B., Tufenkci, P., Misirli, M.K., and Orhan, K. (2015). Micro-CT assessment of the sealing ability of three root canal filling techniques. *J. Oral Sci.* 57: 361–366.

156 Kim, S., Park, J.W., Jung, I.Y., and Shin, S.J. (2017). Comparison of the percentage of voids in the canal filling of a calcium silicate-based sealer and gutta percha cones using two obturation techniques. *Materials (Basel)* 10: 1170–1179.

157 Kim, J.A., Hwang, Y.C., Rosa, V. et al. (2018). Root canal filling quality of a premixed calcium silicate endodontic sealer applied using gutta-percha cone-mediated ultrasonic activation. *J. Endod.* 44: 133–138.

158 Chybowski, E.A., Glickman, G.N., Patel, Y. et al. (2018). Clinical outcome of non-surgical root canal treatment using a single-cone technique with Endosequence Bioceramic Sealer: a retrospective analysis. *J. Endod.* 44: 941–945.

159 Gençoglu, N., Garip, Y., Bas, M. et al. (2002). Comparison of different gutta-percha root filling techniques: Thermafil, Quick-fill, System B, and lateral condensation. *Oral Surg. Oral Med. Oral Pathol. Oral Radiol. Endod.* 93: 333–336.

160 Gutmann, J.L. (1993). Adaptation of injected thermoplasticized gutta-percha in the absence of the dentinal smear layer. *Int. Endod. J.* 26: 87–92.

161 Ordinola-Zapata, R., Bramante, C.M., Graeff, M.S.Z. et al. (2009). Depth and percentage penetration of endodontic sealers into dentinal tubules after root canal obturation using lateral compaction technique: a confocal laser scanning micrsocopy study. *Oral Surg. Oral Med. Oral Pathol. Oral Radiol. Endod.* 108: 450–457.

162 Schilder, H. (1967). Filling root canals in three dimensions. *Dent. Clin. N. Am.* 11: 723–744.

163 Wong, M., Peters, D.D., and Lorton, L. (1981). Comparison of gutta-percha filling techniques, compaction (mechanical), vertical (warm), and lateral condensation techniques, part 1. *J. Endod.* 7: 551–558.

164 Zmener, O. and Banegas, G. (1999). Clinical experience of root canal filling by ultrasonic condensation of gutta-percha. *Endod. Dent. Traumatol.* 15: 57–59.

165 Buchanan, L.S. (1994). The Buchanan continuous wave of condensation technique. A convergence of conceptual and procedural advances in obturation. *Dent. Today* 13: 80–85.

166 Chang, H.S., Park, S.H., Cho, K.M., and Kim, J.W. (2018). Plugger temperature of cordless heat carriers according to the time elapsed. *Restor Dent. Endod.* 43: e12.

167 Ahmed, H., Cathro, P.R., and Chandler, N.P. (2017). Effect of an additional application of sealer during continuous wave of condensation obturation. *Int. Endod. J.* 50 (Suppl. 1): 34.

168 Donnermeyer, D., Schäfer, E., and Bürklein, S. (2018). Real-time intracanal temperature measurement during different obturation techniques. *J. Endod.* 44: 1832–1836.

169 Qu, W., Bai, W., Liang, Y.-H. et al. (2016). Influence of warm vertical compaction technique on physical properties of root canal sealers. *J. Endod.* 42: 1829–1833.

170 von Schroeter, C. (2008). Thermafil obturation technique: an overview from the practitioner's point of view. *Endo (Lond. Engl.)* 2: 43–54.

171 Somma, F., Cretella, G., Carotenuto, M. et al. (2011). Quality of thermoplasticized and single point root fillings assessed by micro-computed tomography. *Int. Endod. J.* 44: 362–369.

172 Soo, W.K.M., Thong, Y.L., and Gutmann, J.L. (2015). A comparison of four gutta-percha filling techniques in simulated C-shaped canals. *Int. Endod. J.* 48: 736–746.

173 Royzenblat, A. and Goodell, G.G. (2007). Comparison of removal times of Thermafil plastic obturators using ProFile rotary instruments at different rotational speeds in moderately curved canals. *J. Endod.* 33: 256–258.

174 Beasley, R.T., Williamson, A.E., Justman, B.C. et al. (2013). Time required to remove GuttaCore, Thermafil Plus and thermoplasticized gutta-percha from moderately curved root canals with ProTaper files. *J. Endod.* 39: 125–128.

175 Li, G., Niu, L., Selem, L.C. et al. (2014). Quality of obturation achieved by an endodontic core-carrier system with crosslinked gutta-percha carrier in single-root canals. *J. Dent.* 42: 1124–1134.

176 Wu, M.-K., Kast'akova, A., and Wesselink, P.R. (2001). Quality of cold and warm gutta-percha fillings in oval canals in mandibular premolars. *Int. Endod. J.* 34: 485–491.

177 Keles, A., Alcin, H., Kamalak, A. et al. (2014). Micro-CT evaluation of root filling quality in oval-shaped canals. *Int. Endod. J.* 47: 1177–1184.

178 Pagavino, G., Giachetti, L., Nieri, M. et al. (2006). The percentage of gutta-percha-filled area in simulated curved canals when filled using Endo Twinn, a new heat device source. *Int. Endod. J.* 39: 610–615.

179 McSpadden, J. (1980). Self-Study Course for the Thermatic Condensation of Gutta-Percha. York, PA: Dentsply.

180 Tagger, M., Tamse, A., Katz, A., and Korzen, B.H. (1984). Evaluation of apical seal produced by a hybrid root canal filling method combining lateral condensation and thermatic compaction. *J. Endod.* 10: 299–303.

181 Sargenti, A. and Richter, S.L. (1965). Rationalized Root Canal Treatment. New York: AGSA.

182 Witherspoon, D.E., Small, J.C., Regan, J.D. et al. (2008). Retrospective analysis of open apex teeth obturated with mineral trioxide aggregate. *J. Endod.* 34: 1171–1176.

183 Mente, J., Hage, N., Pfefferle, T. et al. (2009). Mineral trioxide aggregate apical plugs in teeth with open apical foramina: a retrospective analysis of treatment outcome. *J. Endod.* 35: 1354–1358.

184 Desai, S. and Chandler, N. (2009). The restoration of permanent immature teeth, root filled using MTA: a review. *J. Dent.* 37: 652–657.

185 Naseri, M., Eftekhar, L., Gholami, F. et al. (2019). The effect of calcium hydroxide and nano-calcium hydroxide on microhardness and superficial chemical structure of root canal dentin: an *ex vivo* study. *J. Endod.* 45: 1148–1154.

186 Bogen, G., Lawaty, I., and Chandler, N.P. (2013). MTA root canal obturation. In:

Mineral Trioxide Aggregate: Properties and Clinical Applications (ed. M. Torabinejad), 207–249. Hoboken, NJ: Wiley Blackwell.

187 EL-Ma'aita, A.M., Qualtrough, A.J.E., and Watts, D.C. (2012). A micro-computed tomography evaluation of mineral trioxide aggregate root canal fillings. *J. Endod.* 38: 670–672.

188 Basturk, F.B., Nekoofar, M.H., Gunday, M. et al. (2015). Effect of varying water-to-powder ratios and ultrasonic placement on the compressive strength of mineral trioxide aggregate. *J. Endod.* 41: 531–534.

189 EL-Ma'aita, A.M., Qualtrough, A.J.E., and Watts, D.C. (2014). Resistance to vertical fracture of MTA-filled roots. *Dent. Traumatol.* 30: 36–42.

190 Sawyer, A.N., Nikonov, S.Y., Pancio, A.K. et al. (2012). Effects of calcium silicate-based materials on the flexural properties of dentin. *J. Endod.* 38: 680–683.

191 Lamb, E.L., Loushine, R.J., Weller, R. et al. (2003). Effect of root resection on the apical sealing ability of mineral trioxide aggregate. *Oral Surg. Oral Med. Oral Pathol. Oral Radiol. Endod.* 95: 732–735.

192 Boutsioukis, C., Noula, G., and Lambrianidis, T. (2008). Ex vivo study of the efficiency of two techniques for the removal of mineral trioxide aggregate used as a root canal filling material. *J. Endod.* 34: 1239–1242.

193 Yoo, J.S., Chang, S.-W., Oh, S.R. et al. (2014). Bacterial entombment by intratubular mineralization following orthograde mineral trioxide aggregate obturation: a scanning electron microscope study. *Int. J. Oral Sci.* 6: 227–232.

194 Russell, A.A., Friedlander, L.T., and Chandler, N.P. (2018). Sealer penetration and adaptation in root canals with the butterfly effect. *Aust. Endod. J.* 44: 225–234.

195 Tidmarsh, B.G. (1978). Acid-cleansed and resin-sealed root canals. *J. Endod.* 4: 117–121.

196 Tay, F.R. and Pashley, D.H. (2007). Monoblocks in root canals: a hypothetical or a tangible goal. *J. Endod.* 33: 391–398.

197 Shanahan, D.J. and Duncan, H.F. (2011). Root canal filling with Resilon: a review. *Br. Dent. J.* 211: 81–88.

198 Barborka, B.J., Woodmansey, K.F., Glickman, G.N. et al. (2017). Long-term clinical outcome of teeth obturated with Resilon. *J. Endod.* 43: 556–560.

199 Strange, K.A., Tawil, P.Z., Phillips, C. et al. (2019). Long-term outcomes of endodontic treatment performed with Resilon/Epiphany. *J. Endod.* 45: 507–512.

200 Payne, L.A., Tawil, P.Z., Phillips, C. et al. (2019). Resilon: assessment of degraded filling material in nonhealed cases. *J. Endod.* 45: 691–695.

201 Eid, A.A., Nikonov, S.Y., Looney, S.W. et al. (2013). *In vitro* biocompatibility evaluation of a root canal filling material that expands on water sorption. *J. Endod.* 39: 883–888.

202 Didato, A., Eid, A.A., Levin, M.D. et al. (2013). Time-based lateral hygroscopic expansion of a water-expandable endodontic obturation point. *J. Dent.* 41: 796–801.

203 Economides, N., Gogos, C., Kodonas, K. et al. (2012). An ex vivo comparison of the push-out bond strength of a new endodontic filling system (Smartseal) and various gutta-percha techniques. *Odontology* 100: 187–191.

204 Arora, S. and Hegde, V. (2014). Comparative evaluation of a novel smart-seal obturating system and its homogeneity of using cone beam computed tomography: In vitro simulated lateral canal study. *J. Conserv. Dent.* 17: 364–368.

205 Dow, P.R. and Ingle, J.I. (1955). Isotope determination of root canal failure. *Oral Surg. Oral Med. Oral Pathol.* 8: 1100–1104.

206 Marshall, F.J. and Massler, M. (1961). The sealing of pulpless teeth evaluated with radioisotopes. *J. Dent. Med.* 16: 172–184.

207 Saunders, W.P. and Saunders, E.M. (1990). Assessment of leakage in the restored pulp chamber of endodontically treated multirooted teeth. *Int. Endod. J.* 23: 28–33.

208 Saunders, W.P. and Saunders, E.M. (1994). Coronal leakage as a cause of failure in root canal therapy: a review. *Endod. Dent. Traumatol.* 10: 105–108.

209 Mannocci, F., Innocenti, M., Bertelli, E. et al. (1999). Dye leakage and SEM study of roots obturated with Thermafil and dentin bonding agent. *Endod. Dent. Traumatol.* 15: 60–64.

210 Wolcott, J.F., Hicks, M.L., and Himel, V.T. (1999). Evaluation of pigmented intraorifice barriers in endodontically treated teeth. *J. Endod.* 25: 589–592.

211 Chandler, N.P. and Heling, I. (1995). Efficacy of three cavity liners in eliminating bacteria from infected dentinal tubules. *Quintessence Int.* 26: 655–659.

212 Chailertvanitkul, P., Saunders, W.P., Saunders, E.M. et al. (1997). An evaluation of microbial coronal leakage in the restored pulp chamber of root-canal treated multirooted teeth. *Int. Endod. J.* 30: 318–322.

213 Jenkins, S., Kulild, J., Williams, K. et al. (2006). Sealing ability of three materials in the orifice of root canal systems obturated with gutta-percha. *J. Endod.* 32: 225–227.

214 Naoum, H.A. and Chandler, N.P. (2002). Temporization for endodontics. *Int. Endod. J.* 35: 964–978.

215 Ng, Y.-L., Mann, V., and Gulabivala, K. (2011). A prospective study of the factors affecting outcomes of nonsurgical root canal treatment: part 1: periapical health. *Int. Endod. J.* 44: 583–609.

216 Chong, B.S. (2017). The five-second rule. *ENDO (Lond. Engl.)* 11: 3.

217 Keinan, D., Moshonov, J., and Smidt, A. (2011). Is endodontic re-treatment mandatory for every relatively old temporary restoration? *J. Am. Dent. Assoc.* 142: 391–396.

218 Wilcox, L.R. (1993). Thermafil retreatment with and without chloroform solvent. *J. Endod.* 19: 563–566.

219 Wilcox, L.R. and Juhlin, J.J. (1994). Endodontic retreatment of Thermafil versus laterally condensed gutta-percha. *J. Endod.* 20: 115–117.

220 Duncan, H.F. and Chong, B.S. (2011). Removal of root filling materials. *Endod. Top.* 19: 33–57.

221 Duncan, H.F. and Chong, B.S. (2010). Non-surgical retreatment: experimental studies on the removal of root filling materials. *ENDO (Lond. Engl.)* 4: 111–126.

222 Martins, M.P., Duarte, M.A.H., Cavenago, B. et al. (2017). Effectiveness of the ProTaper Next and Reciproc systems in removing root canal filling material with sonic or ultrasonic irrigation: a micro-computed tomographic study. *J. Endod.* 43: 467–471.

223 Wilcox, L.R., Krell, K.V., Madison, S. et al. (1987). Endodontic retreatment: evaluation of gutta-percha and sealer removal and canal reinstrumentation. *J. Endod.* 13: 453–457.

224 Friedman, S., Moshonov, J., and Trope, M. (1992). Efficacy of removing glass ionomer cement, zinc oxide eugenol, and epoxy resin sealers from retreated root canals. *Oral Surg. Oral Med. Oral Pathol.* 73: 609–612.

225 Kim, H., Kim, E., Lee, S.-J. et al. (2015). Comparisons of the retreatment efficiency of calcium silicate and epoxy resin-based sealers and residual sealer in tubules. *J. Endod.* 41: 2025–2030.

226 Koch, K. and Brave, D. (2009). Bioceramic technology- the game changer in endodontics. *Endocr. Pract.* 2: 14–17.

227 Malhotra, S., Hegde, M.N., and Shetty, C. (2014). Bioceramic technology in endodontics. *Br. J. Med. Med. Res.* 4: 2446–2454.

228 Hess, D., Solomon, E., Spears, R. et al. (2011). Retreatability of a bioceramic root canal sealing material. *J. Endod.* 37: 1547–1549.

229 Erdemir, A., Adanir, N., and Belli, S. (2003). *In vitro* evaluation of the dissolving effect of solvents on root canal sealers. *J. Oral Sci.* 45: 123–126.

230 Neelakantan, P., Grota, D., and Sharma, S. (2013). Retreatability of 2 mineral trioxide aggregate-based root canal sealers: a cone-beam computed tomography analysis. *J. Endod.* 39: 893–896.

231 Kontogiannis, T.G., Kerezoudis, N.P., Kozyrakis, K. et al. (2019). Removal ability of MTA-, bioceramic-, and resin-based sealers from obturated root canals, following XP-Endo Finisher R File: an *ex vivo* study. *Saudi Endod. J.* 9: 8–13.

232 Aksel, H., Küçükkaya Eren, S., Askerbeyli Örs, S. et al. (2019). Micro-CT evaluation of the removal of root fillings using the ProTaper Universal Retreatment system supplemented by the XP-Endo Finisher file. *Int. Endod. J.* 52: 1070–1076.

233 Carpenter, M.T., Sidow, S.J., Lindsey, K.W. et al. (2014). Regaining apical patency after obturation with gutta-percha and a sealer containing mineral trioxide aggregate. *J. Endod.* 40: 588–590.

234 Pedullà, E., Abiad, R.S., Conte, G. et al. (2019). Retreatability of two hydraulic calcium silicate-based root canal sealers using rotary instrumentation with supplementary irrigant agitation protocols: a laboratory-based micro-computed tomographic analysis. *Int. Endod. J.* 52: 1377–1387.

235 Garrib, M. and Camilleri, J. (2020). Retreatment efficacy of hydraulic calcium silicate sealers used in single cone obturation. *J. Dent.* 98: 103370.

236 De-Deus, G., Belladonna, F.G., Zuolo, A.S. et al. (2019). 3-dimensional ability assessment in removing root filling material from pair-matched oval-shaped canals using thermal-treated instruments. *J. Endod.* 45: 1135–1141.

237 Yan, W., Montoya, C., Øilo, M. et al. (2019). Contribution of root canal treatment to the fracture resistance of dentin. *J. Endod.* 45: 189–193.

238 Trope, M. and Ray, H.L. (1992). Resistance to fracture of endodontically treated roots. *Oral Surg. Oral Med. Oral Pathol.* 73: 99–102.

239 Uzunoglu-Özyürek, E., Eren, S.K., and Karahan, S. (2018). Effect of root canal sealers on the fracture resistance of endodontically treated teeth: a systematic review of in vitro studies. *Clin. Oral Investig.* 22: 2475–2485.

7

Root-End Filling and Perforation Repair Materials and Techniques

Josette Camilleri[1] and Christof Pertl[2,3]

[1] *School of Dentistry, Institute of Clinical Sciences, College of Medical and Dental Sciences, University of Birmingham, Birmingham, UK*
[2] *Department of Dental Medicine and Oral Health, Medical University of Graz, Austria*
[3] *Harvard School of Dental Medicine, Boston, MA, USA*

7.1 Introduction

Corrective or apical surgery is undertaken when management of primary disease fails or problems are encountered during root canal therapy. The prognosis of apical surgery has changed with the adoption of microsurgical approaches (i.e. using a microscope, ultrasonic tips, and new materials). However, a review of the effects of surgical and nonsurgical therapy in the retreatment of teeth with apical periodontitis and of surgical root-end resection employing various conditions, materials, devices, and techniques found no clear evidence of superiority for either with regard to healing at 1-, 4- or 10-year follow-up, although the results were of very low quality [1]. Only two random controlled clinical trials have found that healing rates can be higher in cases treated surgically as compared to nonsurgically, at least in the short term. A single trial reported that, in the medium to long term, healing rates for the two procedures were very similar. There is presently little evidence for a sound decision-making process amongst alternatives for the retreatment of cases presenting with periradicular pathosis. More well-designed random controlled trials should be performed, with a follow-up of at least four years and a consistent sample size, in order to detect the true difference in the long term between the outcomes of the two approaches, if any exists [2].

Apical surgery is necessary when there is persistent active periodontitis at the root end of the tooth. Corrective or reparative surgery is required to seal off perforations connecting the root canal system to the periodontal ligament space along the tooth root and surrounding bone. Perforation repair can be performed through the root canal or surgically. The challenges with nonsurgical repair of perforations include the inability to properly assess the size of the defect, difficulty in gaining access, difficulty in controlling the amount of material extruded to the periodontium and subsequently in removing this excess, and difficulty in controlling bleeding, which might affect the material used to seal the perforation.

For both corrective and apical surgery, a material is required to block the pathway from the canal to the periapical area or the exit created along the root during perforation. Several materials have been used for this purpose. The major advances in this field have been the introduction of the operative microscope and microsurgery, the use of piezo-sonics for root-end canal preparation, and the development of the hydraulic silicate cements.

7.2 The Surgical Environment

Access to the apical area, or the root face which needs repair, is gained by raising a flap and possibly removing overlying bone. Flap design is dependent on the anatomy of the area, the number and location of roots, and whether the flap is in an aesthetically sensitive region. Usually, sulcular incisions with either mesial or distal vertical releasing incisions (Figure 7.1a), or both, are performed. The vertical part of the incision should extend from the alveolar mucosa to the attached gingiva and end in a line perpendicular to the gingival margin (Figure 7.1b). Vertical releasing incisions allow easier mobilization of the flap for better visibility (Figure 7.1c). The releasing incisions of a palatal flap must be rather short (4–6 mm) to avoid trauma to the palatal artery (Figure 7.1d) A submarginal flap design (Figure 7.2) avoids touching the critical gingival margin but creates a risk of unpleasant postoperative scarring along the incision line.

Once incisions are made and the flap is raised, the root end or area of perforation often needs to be accessed by removal of the overlying bone (Figure 7.2a), although in some cases there is none as it has been resorbed during the disease process (Figure 7.3a). For perforation repair, the intervention is similar.

With apical surgery, once the flap is raised, the root apex is exposed, and root-end

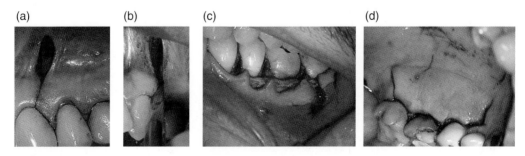

(a)   (b)   (c)   (d)

Figure 7.1 Flap outline showing (a) sulcular triangular flap with a mesial vertical incision; (b) guiding of the releasing incision from the alveolar mucosa, proceeding to the attached gingiva; (c) flap retraction to expose the surgical site of a full-thickness flap with a distal vertical incision; (d) sulcular palatal flap with two short releasing incisions. *Source:* Christof Pertl.

(a) (b) (c)

(d) (e)

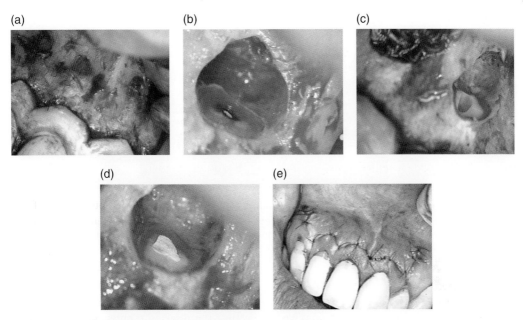

Figure 7.2 (a) Raised submarginal flap and buccal bone perforation around the root apices of affected teeth, caused by pathological inflammatory processes. (b) After apical resection, the black discolouration of the root canal indicates bacterial contamination. (c) Retrograde preparation of the root canal. (d) Root-end filling. (e) Suture placement. *Source:* Christof Pertl.

(a) (b) (c)

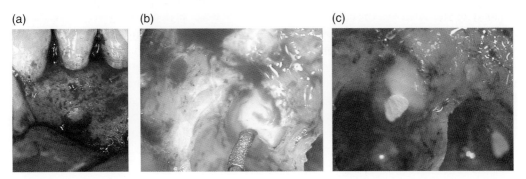

Figure 7.3 Details of an apical surgical procedure following incision and raising of a flap. (a) Surgical site, showing the cystic lesion having eroded the buccal plate. (b) Root-end cavity preparation with ultrasonic tip. (c) Placement of root-end filling material. *Source:* Christof Pertl.

resection follows (Figure 7.2b); the clinical implications and management of this have been thoroughly discussed [3]. Root-end resection is necessary to remove any pathology, such as root resorption, fractured root tips, cysts, granulomata, tissues, and infected cementum and dentine at the root apex. It further allows removal of anatomical variations such as root curvatures, lateral and accessory canals, apical deltas, and calcifications. Other indications include the avoidance of operator errors in canal preparation, likely improvement in the removal of a soft tissue lesion, and the need for access to the canal system. The root end should not be significantly bevelled buccally; a rather perpendicular resection angle reduces the number of exposed dentinal tubules and facilitates an anatomically correct class I retrograde ultrasonic preparation. Still, the angles of resection used will be affected by

(a) (b) (c) (d)

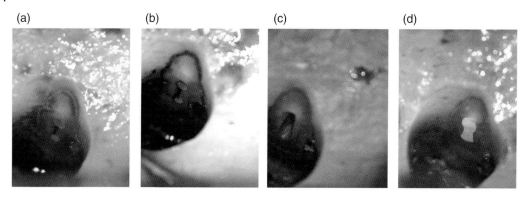

Figure 7.4 Root-end resection, preparation, and filling. (a) Resected root end of a lower first molar mesial root, showing two canals filled with gutta-percha, joined by an isthmus which has been left unobturated. (b) Use of methylene blue to differentiate the isthmus region and the dentine from the surrounding bone. (c) Root-end cavity preparation. (d) Filled root end. *Source:* Christof Pertl.

the root inclination and curvature, number of roots, thickness of bone, and position of the root in the bone and arch. Root-end resection is best performed with a fissure bur under water spray.

The appearance of the root face following root-end resection will vary depending upon the type of bur used, external root anatomy, anatomy of the canal system exposed at the particular angle of resection chosen, and nature and density of the root canal filling material. Once the root tip is removed, it is necessary to check for isthmuses (Figure 7.4a), as these will be a continuous source of infection. Methylene blue is used to delimit the dentine from the surrounding bone and to expose any untreated canal anatomy present (Figure 7.4b).

Microscopically, dentinal tubules will now be exposed to the periradicular tissues. Cementum can reform over such resected tubules and a periodontal encapsulation, with a variable degree of fibre attachment, can occur [4]. Another problem with exposed dentinal tubules is the risk of reinfection of the periradicular tissues by bacteria entrapped inside them. However, no correlation has been found between the presence of microrganisms in the dentinal tubules and the degree of periradicular inflammation [4]. The prepared dentine surface also has a potentially infected smear layer, which may serve as a source of

irritation to the periradicular tissues, primarily preventing the intimate layering of cementum against the resected tubules. The smear layer may block these tubules and serve as a source of obturation of the potential avenues of communication, especially with tubules contaminated with bacteria or exposed to oral fluids over long periods of time. Experiments designed to evaluate these aspects are essential, as there are no unequivocal data to guide the proper management of such a smear layer.

A root-end cavity is prepared in order to enable an adequate seal against potential avenues of communication from the resected root end to the canal system (Figures 7.2c and 7.4c). This preparation should be performed with ultrasonic tips (Figure 7.3b), and its design made to suit the material to be used to make the seal. The use of ultrasonic tips allows apical preparations along the long axis of the root after minimal root-end resection. Dentine demineralization, and thus exposure of collagen by smear-layer removal, is debatable. Ideally, the area should not be irritated. The prepared end is filled (Figures 7.2d, 7.3c, and 7.4d), the site irrigated, and the flap repositioned and sutured (Figures 7.2e). A similar procedure is used for perforation repair (Figure 7.5).

The cavity design for adhesive materials is essentially a simple concave shape, as the materials can be bonded. Other material types,

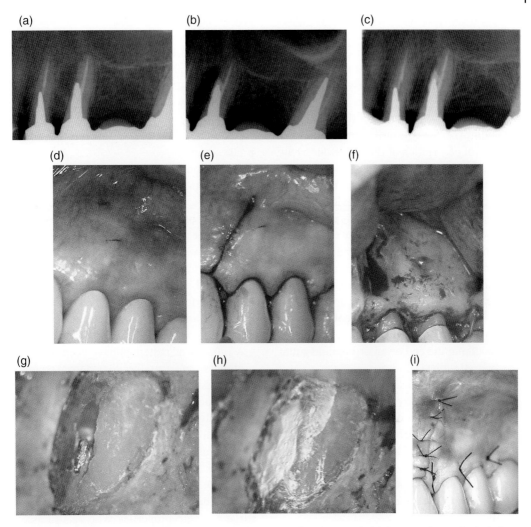

Figure 7.5 Clinical case showing the procedure for root perforation repair. (a) Preoperative periapical view, showing a mesial mid-root perforation by a metal post, part of a crown used as a bridge abutment on tooth 25, and a pier abutment for a four-unit bridge replacing tooth 26. (b) Postoperative radiograph. (c) Recall radiograph taken two years later, showing complete healing and bone formation in the defect. (d) Clinical photograph of the site. (e) Flap design showing a sulcular flap with a mesial relieving incision. (f) Flap raised and surgical site exposed. (g) Exposed root surface showing perforation. (h) After repair. (i) Flap repositioned and sutured. *Source:* Christof Pertl.

such as hydraulic calcium silicate cements (HCSCs) and zinc oxide-eugenol (ZOE), require a deeper retentive cavity. The use of high magnification in the preparation of shallow and concave root-end cavities for bonded resin-based root-end filling materials, as compared with endodontic microsurgery with the use of high-magnification, ultrasonic root-end preparation, and root-end filling with Super EBA, intermediate restorative material (IRM), and HCSC, has been reviewed [5]. The root-end cavities prepared for ZOE and HCSC had a higher probability of success compared with shallow cavity preparation and placement of a resin-based material.

In terms of surgical protocol, there is some evidence that using a papilla base incision may be beneficial for the preservation of the interdental papilla compared with complete papilla mobilization, with no evidence of less pain in the papilla base-incision group at day 1 post-surgery [1]. However, suturing of the flap to a small papilla fragment may lead to poor healing in practice. Using more modern techniques, such as by modifying the method of osteotomy (i.e. the type of instrument used) or the type of preparation of the retrograde cavity (apicoectomy angle, instruments used for root-end preparation), resulted in better healing [6]. Although there is very little evidence that ultrasonic devices for root-end preparation improve healing at one year after retreatment as compared with the use of a traditional bur, in practice such burs are not much used nowadays, as the dedicated ultrasonic tips allow better access. One study showed evidence of better healing at one year when root ends were filled with an HCSC rather than being treated by smoothing the end of an orthograde gutta-percha root filling [1].

The use of magnification helps the clinical procedure, and is today accepted as best practice. The type of optics used seems to be important: an operating microscope provided 94.9% successful healing, whereas loupes gave only 90.6%. Endoscopic devices have been advocated in order to improve visibility [7]. No difference in outcome is shown with the treatment of different arches [8].

The correlation between clinical outcome and material type is not very clear. However, a longitudinal assessment of the prognosis of apical microsurgery at five years was 8% poorer compared to assessment at one year, and material choice was shown to affect this rate [7]. ProRoot MTA had a better outcome than either Super EBA [7] or amalgam [6] at five years.

7.3 Materials for Endodontic Surgery

The environment in which endodontic surgery is performed – specifically, where root-end filling and perforation repair materials are placed – is shown in Figures 7.1–7.5. For convenience, nonsurgical perforation repair is included here too, as the intent, context, and materials are all the same. However, when the materials are used in the coronal aspect, which is the only location where nonsurgical repair is possible, they may be subject to a different environment. This will be noted in the appropriate sections.

A root-end filling material must be adapted to preexisting gutta-percha and sealer as well as to the exposed, cut dentine surface, which potentially has exposed dentinal tubules and a smear layer (Figures 7.3 and 7.4). The area is inherently wet and will get blood over it within a few minutes. These conditions are very particular and very adverse. The materials used for root perforation offer other challenges, too (e.g. for the irrigation protocol and the material used to restore the tooth after repair).

A number of materials have been used for root-end filling, usually adopted from restorative dentistry and not specifically designed for this purpose. Such materials have included dental silver amalgam and ZOE cements, as well as filled (composite) resins (FRs) and glass ionomer cement (GICs). The properties of these materials will be discussed in Section 7.3.1. In the mid-1990s, HCSCs were specifically developed for use in endodontic surgery. Their properties will be discussed separately in Section 7.3.2.

To date, there are no standards for testing endodontic surgery materials. The only ISO standard for endodontics-related procedures is that for root canal sealer [9]. Otherwise, the conventional materials used in this context are tested according to their own respective standards [10–14]. As yet, there is no standard for HCSCs.

7.3.1 Conventional Materials

A wide range of types of materials have been used clinically for root-end filling. These include gold foil, polycarboxylate cement, gutta-percha (both cold and injectable), silver amalgam, GIC, and various ZOE-based cements. In this chapter, only the most common and most researched materials will be discussed. Although historically dental silver amalgam was used as a root-end filling material, it will not be included here due to the European directive to limit its use [15]. This directive was based on environmental pollution concerns rather than for any toxicity issues.

The chemistry, mixing, and physical and biological properties of each material type will be discussed, with special attention given to clinical applications and particular clinical interactions. There is no evidence of any leakage technique which shows the superiority of any one material compared to another, never mind of the clinical relevance of leakage [16]. Any reference to sealing ability in this chapter is related to the interaction of the material with dentine.

7.3.1.1 Zinc Oxide-Eugenol Cements

ZOE-based materials have a variety of uses in dentistry. Commercial formulations also contain zinc acetate dihydrate as an accelerator, which furnishes the water required to initiate the setting reaction. Reinforced versions have been used for root-end cavity restoration. These include Super EBA (Bosworth Co., Skokie, IL, USA) and IRM (Dentsply Caulk, Milford, DE, USA). Although these are often grouped together, they exhibit slightly different characteristics and properties.

7.3.1.1.1 Chemistry and Physical Properties

Super EBA is a cement whose liquid is a mixture of 32% eugenol and 68% ortho-ethoxybenzoic acid (EBA). This kind of material was first suggested for root-end filling in 1978 [17]. The chelating agent is EBA, which leads to a material with high water solubility, although this is reduced by the addition of hydrogenated rosin [18]. The mechanical properties can be improved by the addition of substances such as monocalcium phosphate, fused quartz, or aluminium oxide. In fact, the commercial product also has an 'alumina-reinforced' version.

IRM includes polymer particles in the powder, an idea first suggested by Curtis [19]. For root-end fillings, a high powder-to-liquid ratio (P:L) is recommended. High P:L has other advantages, such as ease of placement and decreased setting time, toxicity, and solubility [20].

ZOE materials set through the formation of the salt zinc eugenolate, a weak five-membered ring chelate, as a matrix embedding unreacted zinc oxide, whilst Super EBA forms zinc ortho-ethoxybenzoate, a stronger six-membered ring chelate.

The properties of Super EBA and IRM are listed in Table 7.1 [21, 22]. Super EBA was stable with no weight changes over a period of storage in water, whilst IRM showed a reduction in weight over three weeks [23]. Reinforced ZOE cements have a radiopacity of between 5 and 8 mm Al/mm, which is similar to that of a filled gutta-percha, at about 6.1 mm Al/mm [24]. It is thus difficult to distinguish such a root-end filling material from the obturating material.

Although leakage studies are not being taken into consideration here, it is worth mentioning the marginal adaptation of these materials.

Table 7.1 Properties of ZOE-based root-end filling materials.

Property	Super EBA	IRM	Reference
Setting time (min)	9	6	[21]
Compressive strength after setting (MPa)	60	52.2	[21]
Compressive strength after three weeks (MPa)	78.1	57.4	[21]
Tensile strength (MPa)	–	4.1	[22]

IRM exhibits the largest gaps and poorest adaptation compared with both Super EBA and amalgam [23]. Using a high-speed bur to finish and contour hardened Super EBA preserves the marginal adaptation [25].

7.3.1.1.2 Biological Properties

The biological activity of root-end filling materials is important, particularly their interaction with the periodontium and bone. This interaction has been studied at the cellular level, assessing toxicity in contact with human periodontal ligament cells and osteoblast-like cells. In one study, both IRM and Super EBA cement were found to be less toxic than amalgam [26]. In another, later study, however, both freshly mixed and set amalgam were found to be significantly less toxic than Super EBA or IRM [27]. Compared with the HCSCs developed later, IRM has been shown to be more cytotoxic [28]. In other work, modified ZOE cements induced cell death in both periodontal ligament cells [29, 30] and gingival fibroblasts, even after their surfaces had been washed to remove eluate [30]. Both material composition and surface texture affect cellular adhesion and morphology. The contradictory data obtained could be due to variations in the test method and the cell culture system used. It has been reported that the choice of end point and the cell culture system affect the results of cytotoxicity experiments on dental materials [31]. Neither IRM nor Super EBA is mutagenic, as determined by the Ames Test [32].

Reactions to implanted IRM and Super EBA include the formation of granulation tissue [33] and the production of a fibrous mass. When set materials were used as implants, the EBA-containing cement was always less irritating than ZOE ones [34]. An initial inflammatory reaction was observed, which subsided over time. Furthermore, when there was no inflammation, healing progressed by formation of connective tissue [35]. There was no evidence of inhibition of dentoalveolar or osseous wound healing associated with these materials [36].

When used as a root-end filling material in dogs, IRM showed a better interaction than Super EBA. Both materials were associated with the formation of new root cementum on the resected dentine surface [37].

It has recently been shown that application of enamel matrix derivatives on denuded root dentine promotes periodontal regeneration. Enamel matrix derivatives were shown to adhere to the etched dentin, but their adherence to IRM was significantly less than that to dentine or FR [38].

7.3.1.1.3 Antimicrobial Properties

The antimicrobial properties of these materials have not been extensively studied for this specific application. There is no literature on these properties in perforation repair. Using *Enterococcus faecalis* bacterial cultures, IRM was found to be adequately antimicrobial initially, but to be significantly less so after seven days [39]. It also showed a three-hour delay before any antimicrobial activity manifested. The set material completely inhibited *Pseudomonas aeruginosa* and delayed or limited the growth of *Staphylococcus aureus* and *E. faecalis* [40]. In contact with *S. aureus*, *E. faecalis*, and *Streptococcus mutans*, the minimum bactericidal concentration of IRM was higher than that of HCSC. Both materials were reported to show adequate antimicrobial properties [41].

7.3.1.1.4 Clinical Technique

For root-end surgery, after raising the flap and exposing the surgical site, the materials must be prepared and placed *in situ* as described in Section 7.1. For perforation repair, depending on the level of the perforation, either a flap can be raised or the repair can be effected through the access cavity. In either case, the dentine will be prepared and a smear layer, potentially packed with bacteria, will be formed. There are no reports of the effect of smear-layer removal on the performance of reinforced ZOE cements.

Super EBA and IRM are both presented in a powder and liquid form (Figure 7.6). Super

(a)

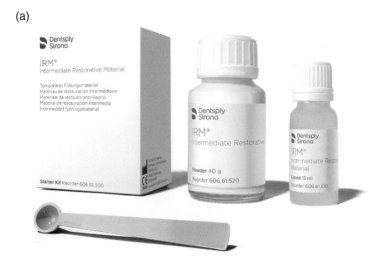

(b)

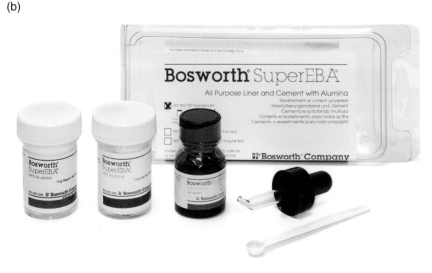

Figure 7.6 Presentation of (a) IRM (*Source:* Courtesy of Dentsply Sirona) and (b) Super EBA (*Source:* Keystone Industries) as both a powder and a liquid.

EBA cement provides good handling characteristics when properly mixed. However, mixing is difficult, requiring more effort and practice than most other root-end filling materials. The cement is well suited for conservative ultrasonic root-end preparations and may be placed through the use of the convex surface of a small spoon excavator and packed with appropriately-sized instruments [42]. IRM behaves best when handled correctly.

A thick mixture improves the ease of root-end placement. Because it does not adhere well to itself, it should be inserted as a single mass and packed in place rather than being placed incrementally [42].

Both materials are mixed on a glass slab by adding increments of powder to the liquid until the mixture is not sticky and can be rolled into a ball. The postoperative healing of root-end surgery performed using IRM has been reported to be similar to that of HCSCs at around three to five hours, and still to be so even 48 hours after the procedure [43].

7.3.1.1.5 Environmental Interactions For all endodontic surgery materials, the environmental interactions include that with dentine and that with blood and tissue fluids. For perforation repair materials, the interactions with the irrigating solutions and subsequently the restorative materials must additionally be considered.

There has not been much research on the interaction of ZOE cements with dentine. Any 'bond' is purely a result of mechanical key, although its failure has been said to be 'mixed adhesive and cohesive' [44]. However, the bond 'strength' when the material is used as a root-end filling material is lower than that of HCSCs [44]. Super EBA was shown to have a very good sealing ability, although this deteriorated with time [45]. The use of irrigating solutions affected the bond strength and sealing ability of these materials when they were used for perforation repair. Either sodium hypochlorite irrigation or no irrigation was better than irrigation with chelating agents such as ethylene diamine tetra-acetic acid (EDTA), which led to reduced sealing ability [46]. Hypochlorite irrigation did not affect the bond strength of IRM [47, 48], whilst Super EBA lost strength when exposed to sodium hypochlorite and other oxidizing agents used in tooth bleaching [47].

For both procedures, washout behaviour is important, both during the irrigation of the site prior to flap repositioning and in the long term via natural interaction with blood in the area. IRM exhibited low washout, similar to amalgam and lower than for HCSCs [49, 50]. The importance to the long-term success of the procedure arises because if washout is fast, the area may be recolonized by bacteria, leading to treatment failure.

7.3.1.1.6 Clinical Evaluation Although a number of studies evaluating material properties have included reinforced ZOE cements as perforation repair materials, there is no clinical evidence of their suitability for this specific purpose. No clinical study has ever reported success in such an application, notwithstanding long clinical use.

Both IRM and Super EBA had a successful outcome when used as root-end filling materials. Radiologic and clinical examination indicated a success rate of 91% for IRM and of 82% for Super-EBA after 12 months [51]. Similarly, an 85% success rate has been found for IRM, although this is lower than the 90% recorded for gutta-percha [52]. IRM used in cavities prepared ultrasonically exhibited an 80% success rate overall; this was highest for incisors (100%) and lowest for molars and premolars (78 and 69%, respectively) [53]. When IRM was used as a retrograde filling material, the clinical success rate was similar to that of an HCSC [54, 55]. Super EBA gave a similar outcome [56], even at four years [57].

7.3.1.2 Glass Ionomer Cements

Both conventional and resin-based GICs will be discussed in this section, although the latter are less popular for use in perforation repair and root-end filling. The main material characteristic of interest is dentine bonding through chemical interaction (chelation), but attention has also been given to ion leaching, particularly of fluoride.

7.3.1.2.1 Chemistry and Physical Properties GICs are composed of an acid-reactive calcium fluoroaluminosilicate glass powder mixed with a polyacrylic acid solution. The material properties are dependent on the glass composition. Various compositions have been used, and aluminium-free formulations containing strontium [58–60], zinc [59, 61, 62], or both have been developed for use as bone cements. The partial substitution of calcium oxide by strontium, magnesium, or zinc enhances the cement's mechanical properties [63], improves its antimicrobial characteristics [64], and reduces the available aluminium.

The chemical composition and properties of GICs are well documented in a series of articles by Crisp and Wilson published between 1974 and 1977 [65–73]. The polyacrylic acid solution is modified by the addition of tartaric and maleic acids, which improve the material's handling and setting.

GICs undergo various stages of setting and maturation, which may be described as dissolution, gelation, and hardening. The acidic liquid attacks and dissolves the glass surface, leaching predominantly calcium early in the reaction, followed by the slower release of aluminium (and further calcium); these ions form the salt matrix. At the same time, a hydrated silica gel is formed. Fluoride and sodium are also released in the long term. Initial set (gelation) is due to the cross-linking of the polymeric acid by calcium ions. Hardening occurs when the calcium is subsequently displaced by aluminium ions. The gelation stage is the most susceptible to contamination and drying out. Hardening can take up to seven days.

In part, the tartaric acid binds the calcium ions released early in the reaction and so controls the working and setting times. The rate of formation of aluminium cross-links is also increased, with a resultant reduction in setting time.

GICs have been modified by sintering with silver or by the addition of a resin (i.e. a light-curing polymer component), for so-called 'cermets' and resin-modified GICs (rmGICs), respectively. Cermets are not very popular in endodontic practice. The ability to command-cure by light makes rmGICs useful for various clinical applications, although they release less fluoride than the non-resin-modified cements. The resin improves working and setting times, strength, toughness, and resistance to acid attack and desiccation. These materials are dual-cure: light activation leads to polymerization of the monomer, whilst the conventional GIC acid–base reaction proceeds at a slightly slower pace than in unmodified cements.

7.3.1.2.2 Biological Properties

The biocompatibility of GICs used as root-end filling materials and for the repair of root perforations has been assessed both at the cellular level and following implantation in test animals. The reported cellular interaction is not clear, with studies showing dense and confluent cells [74], poor cellular attachment [75], or periodontal ligament cell apoptosis [76, 77], indicating that the material does not preserve the integrity of the periodontal tissues [78]. The leachate has been found to be worse than that from Super EBA, amalgam, and mineral trioxide aggregate (MTA) in inhibiting cell proliferation [31]. The resin-based cements were cytotoxic to primary human gingival fibroblast cultures, inhibiting cell growth and proliferation [79]. Their eluates were also toxic. In contrast, Geristore, an rmGIC, exhibited enhanced biological behaviour for human periodontal ligament cells and superior biocompatibility in comparison with MTA and conventional GIC [80]. On this basis, it can be suggested as a material of choice for root resorption, perforations, and root-end filling. Both material and time affected cell viability with rmGICs, showing less cell-inhibitory effect initially when compared with dental silver amalgam; at 48 and 72 hours, however, all materials exhibited a similar, slightly inhibitory effect [81].

Intraosseous implantation of GIC resulted in connective tissue infiltration with plasma cells and a reaction similar to that induced by ZOE-based materials [82, 83]. The tissue response to rmGIC was shown to be similar to that with ZOE: a mild inflammation initially, which subsided with time – much better than the response to amalgam [84].

7.3.1.2.3 Antimicrobial Properties

The antibacterial effect of GICs is related to their acidity [85], since adjustment of the liquid to pH 5 resulted in a decrease in activity [86]. Furthermore, fluoride concentration has been linked with antimicrobial activity, with no such activity reported when the fluoride release was lowered [87]. The effect of fluoride will not have a great impact in GICs used in endodontic surgery, however, since fluoride recharge is necessary for continuous fluoride release. The antibacterial activity of GICs increases with topical applications of fluoride toothpaste and gels [87].

7.3.1.2.4 Clinical Technique

GICs are marketed according to their particular use in dentistry. For endodontic surgery, the ordinary restorative materials are employed. For these purposes, several brands are available, and further material developments have been undertaken to improve their properties. The restorative GICs require a specific clinical technique which involves the removal of the smear layer from the dentine by treatment with polyacrylic acid solution. There is no literature on the effectiveness of this cavity 'conditioning' on the bonding of GICs to root dentine in the present context.

Conventional GICs are powder–liquid systems. The polyacrylic acid may be present in solution, as is the case with Fuji IX (GC Europe, Leuven, Belgium; Figure 7.7a), or incorporated in the powder (when the cement is to be mixed with water), as in Chemfil (Dentsply, DeTrey, Konstanz, Germany; Figure 7.7b). The mixing ratio is critical to the outcome. The scoop provided to dose the powder must be used, and the liquid must be properly measured by a dropper. The conventional GICs are also available in pre-dosed capsules, to be mixed by mechanical shaking, which therefore require a nozzle and a special applicator in order to facilitate clinical application (Figure 7.7c), even though the P:L ratio is adjusted lower to enable this approach. The rmGICs have various presentations: both powder–liquid systems and syringeable pastes which can be placed directly at the site (Figure 7.7d). The mixing of powder–liquid systems is done on a paper pad supplied for the purpose, in proportions specified by the manufacturer. The root-end cavity may be a simple saucer shape prepared by ultrasonic instrumentation. GIC can also be placed as a retrograde filling material without a root-end cavity preparation. A resin-modified version in particular exhibited good adaptation to the root canal walls [88]. The placement of GIC at the surgical site is carried out by the use of a 'flat plastic' instrument, and it is packed with a plugger or burnisher.

7.3.1.2.5 Environmental Interactions

The ordinary restorative clinical use of GICs includes dentine 'conditioning' to enable adhesion, and a varnish over the material to minimize water sorption and early ion leaching, both of which result in poorer cross-linking and deterioration of strength. This behaviour has not been investigated in the context of surgery and perforation repair. GICs show very good interaction with coronal but not with radicular dentine. The quality of the seal is debatable. It has been shown to be comparable to that of amalgam in one study [89] but not in others [90, 91]. Debatable findings are also reported for the rmGICs compared with the plain acid–base version. Whilst larger gaps were found on a scanning electron microscope (SEM) for resin-modified cements at the root end [92], dye leakage with methylene blue was less than with conventional GICs [93]. In more recent studies, GIC root-end filling materials exhibited large marginal gaps compared with HCSCs [94, 95], but again this result is debatable as good marginal adaptation was observed for GICs when measured both directly and on resin replicas [96] and when using capillary-flow porometry [97].

The bond strength of GICs to root dentine has only been reported for perforation repair materials; blood contamination results in a drop in value [98]. Neither the effect of irrigating solutions nor washout appears to have been investigated for GICs in the present context.

7.3.1.2.6 Clinical Evaluation

Although GICs have been used for endodontic applications for a number of years, clinical studies assessing their performance are scarce. A review of the literature showed that GIC appeared to be

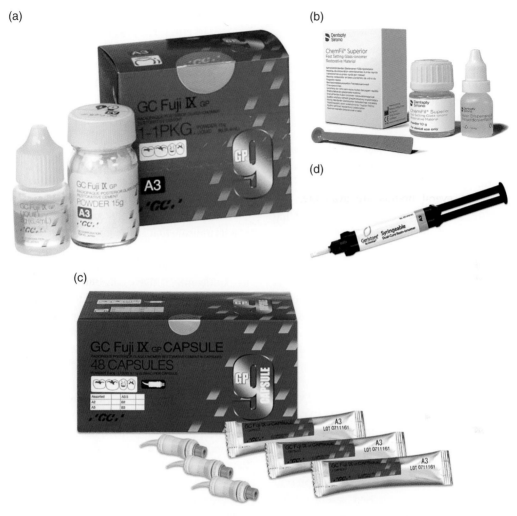

Figure 7.7 Various presentations of glass ionomer cement. (a) Fuji IX. *Source:* Courtesy of GC Europe. (b) Chemfil. *Source:* Courtesy of Dentsply Sirona. Both (a) and (b) are examples of conventional hand-spatulated cements. (c) Fuji IX capsules (a dentine conditioner is also supplied). *Source:* Courtesy of GC Europe. (d) Geristore, a resin-modified glass ionomer. *Source:* Denmat.

equivalent to amalgam [99], with amalgam being the worst root-end filling material studied.

7.3.1.3 Filled Resin and Dentine Bonding Systems

The use of a dentine bonding system (DBS), with or without the use of FR, is another example of a material (and technique) borrowed from restorative dentistry and adapted to endodontic surgery. Creation of a leak-resistant apical seal is possible with this approach, although

such use is technique-sensitive. A dry field is necessary for the dentine bonding agent and FR root-end filling, although some such fills may be less sensitive to moisture. The popularity of the approach lies in the ability to bond to dentine and thus (presumably) seal off the freshly exposed dentinal tubules following root resection. FRs and DBSs as used in restorative dentistry for coronal restoration can be employed, although a number of products have been developed especially for root-end filling;

one such is Retroplast (Retroplast Trading, Roervig, Denmark). For the repair of root perforations, the use of a restorative material does not pose much difficulty except in the need to maintain a dry field during application. In nonsurgical repair of root perforations, the tooth can be restored by bulk filling with FR.

7.3.1.3.1 Chemistry and Mechanical Properties

FRs used for restorative procedures are classified according to the filler particle size. They consist of an organic polymeric matrix with an inorganic filler bonded to it by a silane coupling agent. The initially fluid but viscous monomer is converted into a rigid polymer by free radical-addition polymerization, now commonly light-activated. Conceptually, the base monomer is the very high-viscosity bisphenol A-glycidyl methacrylate (bis-GMA). Its high molecular weight helps minimize polymerization shrinkage. However, low-viscosity monomers must be incorporated to make the filled system workable (e.g. methyl methacrylate (MMA), ethylene glycol dimethacrylate (EDMA), or triethylene glycol dimethacrylate (TEGDMA)). An activator–initiator system is present to allow command set, but polymerization inhibitors such as hydroquinone must be included to provide a useful storage life. The filler is present for many reasons: increased strength and stiffness, reduced polymerization shrinkage, water sorption and thermal expansion, control of optical appearance, and provision of radiopacity.

Retroplast was developed specifically for root-end filling and uses ytterbium trifluoride as its principal filler. The original formulation included silver to increase its radiopacity, but this led to discolouration [100].

7.3.1.3.2 Biological Properties

The release of unpolymerized monomer in contact with periapical tissues is of particular concern. Various possible resin components have been found to suppress macrophage mitochondrial activity, with TC_{50} values at 24 hours reported as follows: HEMA, $10\,000\,\mu$mol/l; 4-META, $3800\,\mu$mol/l; Bis-GMA, $130\,\mu$mol/l; UDMA, $110\,\mu$mol/l [101]. The effect is time-dependent, and residual effects were observed for all resins [101]. Macrophage cytokine secretion has also been investigated [102]. All dentine bonding components completely suppressed lipopolysaccharide (LPS)-induced interleukin-1β (IL-1β) and tumour necrosis factor alpha (TNF-α) secretion at concentrations that suppressed mitochondrial activity by 50%. In addition, 4-methacryloxyethyl trimellitic anhydride induced secretion of IL-1β, but not TNF-α, without the LPS challenge. These results indicate that DBS components may alter normal macrophage-directed inflammatory responses if the macrophages are exposed to sufficiently high concentrations [102]. Polymerized DBSs can also alter the viability of monocytes, decreasing it with time [103].

The biological activity of root-end filling materials has been assessed at the relevant local cellular level using gingival fibroblasts, periodontal ligament, and bone cells. Retroplast in contact with fibroblasts and macrophages resulted in cell death and no cytokine production, particularly early in incubation [104]. Conversely, leachates from Retroplast were less cytotoxic than those from Super EBA cement [105]. Reactions at the tissue level were assessed by connective tissue interactions in test animals. FRs caused moderate to severe inflammatory reactions in the first seven days, but these decreased by 60 and 90 days, performing as well as amalgam [106]. Although most materials were considered to be biocompatible when first tested, compared with more recent developments they actually performed poorly. In fact, cellular attachment to Retroplast was shown to be very poor compared with MTA [75].

7.3.1.3.3 Antimicrobial Properties

The antimicrobial properties of FRs and DBSs used for root-end filling have been assessed using the direct-contact test, which is independent of the solubility of the materials and so gives more predictive and quantitative data. These materials are not as antimicrobial as MTA or IRM [40].

7.3.1.3.4 *Clinical Technique*

Use of a DBS and FR permits conservative root-end preparation. A slightly concave preparation (rather than a conventional deep cavity) followed by resin bonding to the entire resected root end is suggested. This has the advantage of sealing exposed dentinal tubules as well as the main canal(s). All polymerizing resins leave an uncured oxygen-inhibited surface layer that may interfere with initial healing and should therefore be removed with a cotton swab before wound closure [107], although this is likely to be an incomplete process.

7.3.1.3.5 *Environmental Interactions*

The effect of blood contamination has been investigated for DBSs by evaluating their leakage. Although leakage has been shown to be a very limited and essentially useless test, it is used very frequently. A number of systems tested did not leak, and blood contamination did not adversely affect their performance [108]. The use of a DBS enhances the retention of composites and reduces leakage [109].

7.3.1.3.6 *Clinical Evaluation*

An excellent long-term clinical success rate (90%) with the use of Retroplast FR and Gluma (Bayer AG) DBS has been reported [100]. A clinical study comparing modified Retroplast with the original formulation containing silver at one year showed 80% complete healing, 2% scar tissue, 12% uncertain healing, and 6% failure. No significant difference in this healing pattern was found between the two formulations. When the outcome was uncertain at one year, a roughly two- to four-year follow-up showed improved outcomes [100]. Retroplast also gave a very good outcome in another clinical study [110], where based on radiographic evaluation the healing of treated roots was characterized as complete (77%), incomplete (5%), uncertain (7%), or unsatisfactory (11%). Some 95% of roots classified as completely

healed at the one-year control were also completely healed at the final examination at four years. Long-term study therefore suggests that Retroplast can be used for root-end filling with a successful treatment outcome [110]. However, Retroplast also gave less predictable healing compared with MTA, with lower success rates, and did not perform as well in all tooth types, especially mandibular premolars and molars [111]. Five-year follow-up showed that MTA had a higher success rate in the long term [112].

7.3.1.4 Other Materials and Techniques

Besides the conventional materials used in restorative dentistry, other materials and agents have also been employed with a view to enhancing healing potential and thus clinical success. Enamel matrix derivatives adhere to dentine, but also very well to FRs used as root-end filling materials [38]. Bone cement has been tested as an alternative to restorative materials, but with no apparent benefit – although the testing was limited to that for leakage [113].

7.3.2 Hydraulic Cements

HCSCs were first introduced in 1993, specifically for root-end surgery and repair of root perforations. The first two papers published on hydraulic cements described the sealing ability of so-called 'mineral trioxide aggregate' (MTA), used to repair lateral root perforations [114] and as a root-end filling material [115]. MTA is essentially composed of Portland cement and bismuth oxide, and this formulation was patented – the grey version in 1993 and 1995 [116, 117], the white in 2002 [118, 119]; all patents are now expired.

The invention was based on the hydraulic nature of Portland cement, used in the construction industry as a binder for concrete. Bismuth oxide (Bi_2O_3) was added as a radio-opacifier [24]. The first product was Grey MTA, marketed by Dentsply Tulsa in 1998, followed shortly by White MTA. These were the only

Table 7.2 Classification of hydraulic cements based on their composition.

Type	Cement	Radiopacifier	Additives	Water
1	Portland cement	✓ / ✗	✗	✓
2	Portland cement	✓	✓	✓
3	Portland cement	✓	✓	✗
4	Tricalcium/dicalcium silicate	✓	✓	✓
5	Tricalcium/dicalcium silicate	✓	✓	✗

such products available until MTA Angelus was launched in 2001 by Brazilian company Angelus. Being a trade name, 'MTA' should only be used as such for relevant branded products: mixtures of Portland cement-like materials and bismuth oxide. The term 'MTA-like' is sometimes used to describe other formulations, but it is improper to use 'MTA' generically. The term that describes this type of material precisely is 'hydraulic silicate cement' [120]; in this book, the abbreviation 'HCSC' is used, as it stresses the calcium content. Such materials are distinct from all other types of dental material in that they interact chemically with the environment they are placed in as a result of their hydraulic nature; that is, the setting reaction can in part (at least) involve water from the site. A classification of hydraulic cements was proposed in Chapter 1, and the different subtypes based on the material composition are summarized in Table 7.2. In this chapter, only the subtypes used in reparative and corrective procedures will be discussed. A complete classification of the hydraulic cements has been published in the literature [121].

7.3.2.1 Portland Cement-Based Hydraulic Cements: Types 1–3

7.3.2.1.1 Chemistry and Mechanical Properties
The Type 1–3 materials include Portland cement as the main cementitious and active system. The most well characterized of these is the first product to have been sold: ProRoot MTA (Dentsply). Type 2 materials include additives to enhance their performance. The Type 3 materials are provided in ready to use

syringes and are not mixed with water. They hydrate by interaction with the environmental fluids. One type of commercial material is Bio C-Repair by Angelus.

MTA Chemistry
The essential compounds of the original products called 'MTA' are di- and tricalcium silicates, plus small amounts of tricalcium aluminate, which make up the Portland cement portion, along with a little calcium sulphate added to control setting and 20% bismuth oxide for radiopacity [122, 123]. Grey MTA also contains tetracalcium aluminoferrite [21]. The initial reports were somewhat confused, indicating the presence of oxides and phosphates [21, 114, 115], which is apparently what prompted the label 'mineral trioxide aggregate'.

An HCSC such as MTA is mixed and reacts with water to form hydrated calcium silicate and calcium hydroxide. Tricalcium aluminate reacts with sulphate (from the added calcium sulphate) and rapidly forms a so-called 'high' sulphate or sulphoaluminate known as ettringite, which decomposes to a 'low' sulphate or sulphoaluminate (monosulphate) when the sulphate ions are depleted in solution by the first reaction [124, 125]. This controls the rate of the setting process. The overall progress of the reaction with water is quite complex, having four stages [126–129]. In the pre-induction stage (first few minutes), rapid ion dissolution occurs and the tricalcium silicate reacts to form calcium hydroxide and calcium silicate hydrate gel, deposited at the cement particle surface. Very little dicalcium silicate reacts in the initial stages. The tricalcium aluminate also hydrolyses rapidly, forming ettringite, again on the cement particle surface. A halo of reaction products can be seen to form around the cement particles (Figure 7.8). Pre-induction is followed by the induction or dormant stage (1–2 hours), in which the hydration reaction progresses very slowly because the first products form a diffusive barrier. In this stage, the cement is plastic and workable. Setting proper commences when the barrier coating ruptures and solid reaction products gradually replace the liquid phase. The acceleration stage follows (some 3~12 hours after mixing), when the rate of hydration increases again, controlled by the nucleation and growth of the reaction products. At this stage, the dicalcium silicate reaction commences, forming more calcium silicate hydrate gel and calcium hydroxide. Finally, in the post-acceleration stage, the hydration rate slows gradually as the amount of unreacted material declines and diffusion becomes more difficult.

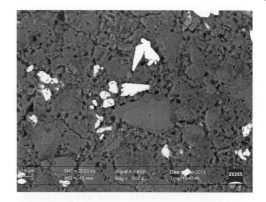

Figure 7.8   Scanning electron micrograph of hydrated MTA, showing the microstructural components. *Source:* Reprinted with permission from Camilleri, J. Composition and setting reaction. Chapter 2 in *Mineral Trioxide Aggregate in Dentistry: From Preparation to Application.* Springer; 2014. ISBN 978-3-642-55157-4.

The hydration reactions are outlined as follows:

$$2(3CaO.SiO_2) \;+\; 6H_2O \;\rightarrow\; 3CaO.2SiO_2.3H_2O \;+\; 3Ca(OH)_2$$

tricalcium silicate   water   calcium silicate hydrate   calcium hydroxide

$$2(2CaO.SiO_2) \;+\; 4H_2O \;\rightarrow\; 3CaO.2SiO_2.3H_2O \;+\; Ca(OH)_2$$

dicalcium silicate   water   calcium silicate hydrate   calcium hydroxide

$$3CaO.Al_2O_3 \;+\; CaSO_4 \;+\; H_2O \;\rightarrow\; 3CaO.Al_2O_3.3CaSO_4.31H_2O$$

tricalcium aluminate   calcium sulphate   water   ettringite

The phases present before and after hydration are listed in Table 7.3, which also compares the hydration products of MTA and Portland cement (the hydrated silicate compositions are 'ideal'; much variation occurs).

The interaction of bismuth oxide with the Portland cement system is still unclear. It has always been assumed to be inert, but as indicated in Table 7.2, some reaction appears to have occurred in that the amount of crystalline oxide detected has been diminished. Only a small amount can have been lost by direct leaching, because of its very slight solubility

(Table 7.4) [125], but the leaching of calcium is substantial, leading to marked material porosity (Figure 7.9).

MTA Properties

For endodontic surgery materials, the most important properties include handling, setting, radiopacity, solubility, dimensional stability, and washout, in addition to colour stability and microhardness for perforation repair materials in particular. The poor handling of the Type 1 materials is their main shortcoming. MTA products are particularly noted as

Table 7.3 Proportions of phases detected in unreacted and set MTA and Portland cement, from Rietveld-refined XRD data.

	Weight fractions			
	Unhydrated cement		Hydrated cement	
Phases	OPC	MTA	OPC	MTA
Tricalcium silicate	74.7	53.1	8.2	10.6
Dicalcium silicate	7.4	22.5	0	14.9
Tetracalcium alumino ferrite	0	0	0	0
Tricalcium aluminate	3.6	0	0	0
Gypsum	1.1	0	0	0
Hemi-hydrate	1.1	0.7	0	0
Anhydrite	2.7	1.5	0	0
Calcium hydroxide	2.1	1.0	15.7	14.4
Calcium carbonate	5.0	1.4	3.2	0
Bismuth oxide	0	21.6	0	8.4
Ettringite	0	0	7.5	2.1
Calcium silicate hydrate	0	0	62.2	49.5

OPC, ordinary Portland cement; MTA, mineral trioxide aggregate.
Source: From Camilleri, J. (2008), Characterization of hydration products of mineral trioxide aggregate. *International Endodontic Journal*, 41: 408–417. DOI:10.1111/j.1365-2591.2007.01370.x. Reproduced with the permission of John Wiley & Sons.

Table 7.4 Leaching of calcium and bismuth form Portland cement and MTA over a period of five weeks.

	MTA		Portland cement	
	Bismuth (μg/g)	Calcium (μg/g)	Bismuth (μg/g)	Calcium (μg/g)
Week 1	3.62	12368.00	0.68	9692.83
Week 2	7.23	8534.64	<0.68	4436.86
Week 3	13.74	5858.53	<0.68	3481.23
Week 4	10.13	3833.36	<0.68	2935.15
Week 5	16.64	2459.13	<0.68	1911.26

Source: From Camilleri, J. (2008), Characterization of hydration products of mineral trioxide aggregate. *International Endodontic Journal*, 41: 408–417. DOI:10.1111/j.1365-2591.2007.01370.x. Reproduced with the permission of John Wiley & Sons.

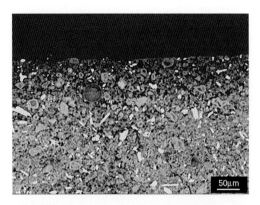

Figure 7.9 Scanning electron micrograph of hydrated MTA, showing porosity resulting from ion leaching. *Source:* Reprinted with permission from Camilleri, J. Characterization of hydration products of mineral trioxide aggregate. *Int. Endod. J.* 2008 May;41(5):408–17.

having a sandy consistency and as being very difficult to place, especially at the root end. This was one of the reasons prompting the development of the newer materials.

Setting

The setting time of MTA has been reported to be more than two hours [21]. Whilst when MTA is used as a root-end filling material the setting time is not crucial, failure to set implies slow hydration; this affects the properties of the material, which are dependent on the release of calcium hydroxide, namely the high pH and thus the antimicrobial and biological properties, which will be discussed later. MTA fails to set in the presence of phosphates from physiological solutions [130–132] and human blood [133, 134], which may be detrimental in a root-end filling material.

Setting time can be important for perforation repair materials if a restorative material is to immediately be placed on the MTA. Additives in the modified materials have improved the setting time of HCSCs.

Radiopacity

The radiopacity of Portland cement is approximately equivalent to 3 mm Al/mm [135, 136]. ProRoot MTA has been reported to have a radiopacity of approximately 6 mm Al/mm [21, 136, 137].

Solubility

The solubility of MTA was said to be negligible in the original study of its chemistry and physical properties [21, 138, 139], but other studies showed it to be alarmingly high (22~31%), depending on the P:L ratio [140, 141] – the addition of more mixing water increased the solubility [140–142]. The differences in results may be attributable to differences in the methods used. For example, if the material is dried in air, calcium carbonate is formed, increasing the mass of the test piece, which may account for the reports of negligible solubility. The ISO method [9] was developed for conventional sealers, which do not interact with components of the environment. An alternative has been used: plastic roots with root-end filling materials in place are examined using micro-computed tomography (μCT) to measure changes in void volume, on the assumption that this represents dissolution [142]. This method is closer to the clinical scenario than the ISO standard method. The role of the solution used to test the solubility should not be understated: MTA solubility depends on the medium [143–145].

Dimensional Stability

The dimensional stability of endodontic surgery materials is important mostly because any shrinkage leads to a gap between the material and the tooth, which may allow possible microbial recolonization, whilst expansion may lead to root fracture. There are no specific standardized tests for this. ISO 6876 [9] used to specify testing for dimensional stability by change in length, but the most recent version (2012) excludes this test.

MTA has been reported to be dimensionally stable even when the P:L ratio is varied [146], but this is in contrast to other data showing that the cement shrinks, particularly in the early stages of setting, and that physiologically-based solutions affect setting [147]. The ISO standard method [9] allows unrestrained changes that are measured in one direction. Other, more precise methods – such as using a linear variable differential transformer measuring a horizontally restrained test piece – have been said to give more meaningful results [143].

Washout

Resistance to washout is an important characteristic of endodontic surgery materials. Once again, no standard method exists for this. The challenge may be short-term, where the area in which the material is placed is irrigated prior to flap closure or where a final restoration is placed, or it may be long-term, involving the action of body fluids.

A number of methods for measuring washout have been proposed [49, 148, 149]; all calculate it as material loss over time. The washout resistance of MTA has been shown to be low [49, 149], but this is improved in formulations using an 'antiwashout gel' [49, 150], such as MTA Plus or Neo MTA Plus (NuSmile, Houston, TX, USA).

Colour Stability

MTA is not colour-stable [151, 152], but this has very little clinical impact when it is used as a root filling material or in the repair of root perforations, as most such procedures are subgingival. Colour stability is discussed in detail in Chapter 2.

Hardness

Hardness is not important for root-end filling materials, but it is for perforation repair materials, particularly where the sealer is going to be layered immediately with a (more conventional) restorative material. It has been reported as ~40 H_V [138]. Hardness may be compromised when root canal therapy is undertaken after sealing a perforation, since instrumentation and the use of the various irrigants can affect the surface chemistry. Surface protection (using materials such as GIC, cyanoacrylate, and castor oil bean cement) has been shown not to improve

hardness [153]. The effect of the environment on MTA properties and microstructure will be discussed later.

Properties of Type 2 Materials

There are a number of Type 2 materials available. One is MTA Angelus (Angelus, Londrina, Brazil), but although this retains the label 'MTA', it has a number of distinct features compared to standard MTA. It is Portland cement-based but shows very low trace-element contamination [154], and it includes 8% calcium oxide to enhance early calcium ion release and reaction rate [155]. The concentration of trace elements is due to the in-house production of the material (Figure 7.10). The bismuth oxide originally used in its formulation has recently been replaced with calcium tungstate, according to the material safety data sheet – although the date when this change took place is not noted. The radiopacity of MTA Angelus with bismuth oxide has been reported to be similar to that of ProRoot MTA [155, 156]. However, since most publications reporting this do not characterize the materials, it is not clear which radiopacifier was used.

Other additives in various formulations include calcium carbonate and calcium chloride, the latter as an accelerator (MM MTA; Coltène MicroMega, Besançon, France); hydroxyapatite (Bio MTA+; Cerkamed, Stalowa Wola, Poland); calcium oxide and zinc oxide (CEM; Bionique Dent, Tehran, Iran); and microsilica filler (Bioaggregate, Verio Dental, Vancouver, Canada). Although such additions may have a specific declared role, they might also modify the chemistry and consequentially other properties. The Type 2 materials address handling difficulties, setting time, physical properties, and biocompatibility through such additives.

Handling properties are improved in materials with added polymers, such as MTA HP (Angelus), MTA Flow (Ultradent), and MTA Plus and Neo MTA Plus (NuSmile). The polymer addition in MTA HP improves the

(a)

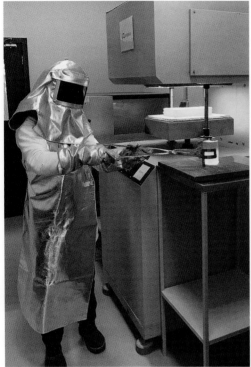

(b)

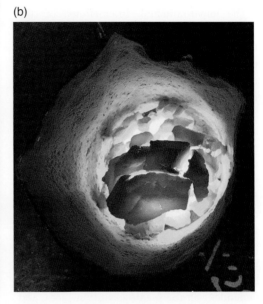

Figure 7.10 In-house manufacturing process of MTA Angelus, showing the furnace where the clinker is formed (left) and the clinker just out of the furnace (right). *Source:* Courtesy of Angelus.

material's compressive strength but increases the setting time. The biological characteristics and calcium ion release of MTA HP [157] and MTA Flow [158] are similar to those of MTA Angelus. Products with an anti-washout gel (MTA Plus, Neo MTA) exhibit lower levels of calcium ions in solution and reduced fluid uptake in the early stages of reaction. The anti-washout gel reduces the setting time and enhances the compressive strength [150].

The setting time of Type 2 cements is controlled by the use of calcium chloride, as in MM MTA (Coltene MicroMega) [159]. Additives such as calcium phosphate in Bio MTA+ (Cerkamed) are meant to enhance bioactivity by making phosphate ions available in solution.

There is no literature to substantiate many of these claims. The behaviour of these additives has not been well documented; most materials in clinical use are not well characterized in any case. However, such additives conceivably could interfere with the hydration reaction. It has been suggested that calcium carbonate might affect the formation of ettringite with substitutions [159], but this requires substantiation. Even so, addition of calcium carbonate to MTA has been shown to alter its properties, reducing setting time, dimensional change, and compressive strength and increasing solubility [160], whilst calcium chloride reduces both setting time and solubility [161] and may increase pH very slightly in the early stages [162].

7.3.2.1.2 Biological Properties The biological properties of MTA are very well investigated using cells, animal models, and molecular methods. The calcium hydroxide formed on setting has been indicated as the basis of the biocompatibility that is reported for MTA. Thus, anything that inhibits or otherwise affects the hydration reactions will potentially affect the biological properties of the material.

The environmental interactions of the cement also play a role in the assessment of the biological properties as the translation of the results of laboratory methods to *in vivo* material interactions is important. The environmental *in vivo* interactions are discussed in Section 7.3.2.1.5. In laboratory tests, the calcium hydroxide has been shown to react with atmospheric carbon dioxide, converting to calcium carbonate [163]. Furthermore, since it is very reactive, the medium used for cell cultures can be expected to affect the chemistry. A recent study on the chemical interactions of medical-grade Portland cement with various physiological solutions showed that its chemistry is dependent on the solution used [164]. The solubility of hydraulic cements is also dependent on the soaking solution [165], and it is this solubility that is responsible for their biological characteristics. In fact, a comparison of cell growth and proliferation over MTA and MTA leachate shows that the cells preferentially grew over the extracts better than on the material surface [166].

Due to this material reactivity, which cannot be translated to *in vivo* conditions, all experimental methods using SEM to assess cell growth and proliferation will be excluded from discussion here, since they involve material processing and thus changes in material microstructure which affect the results of biological testing [167, 168]. Other methods that assess cell viability and enzyme activity on cells native to the area are thus preferred. The cells used to test materials have ranged from fibroblasts, both human and animal [30, 169–171], to human periodontal ligament cells [30, 170–172], peripheral lymphocytes [173], macrophages [104], human alveolar bone cells [104, 174, 175], and cell lines [176]. The most frequently used marker of biocompatible

behaviour is an assessment of cell metabolic activity by 3-(4,5-dimethylthiazol-2-yl)-2,5-di-phenyltetrazolium bromide (MTT) assay [30, 104, 169, 170, 172, 177], where the enzymes in viable cells reduce the MTT to its insoluble formazan, which is purple in colour and can be read by colourimetry.

Cell interactions have been studied using Alamar blue [178], trypan blue [179], and XTT [180] assays. Other methods used have been for inflammatory mediators expressed in response to MTA employed as a root-end filling material using quantitative real-time polymerase chain reaction (PCR) analysis [30], alkaline phosphatase expression [180–182], Western blot analysis for Runt-related transcription factor [104], and enzyme-linked immunosorbent assay (ELISA) [175, 182]. The products have been tested using freshly mixed material, where they were found to be cytotoxic [30, 104, 170, 174], or aged material [169, 172], where the reactions were mixed, with one product giving more favourable results than another [179]. Besides the materials themselves, their leachates have also been assessed [28, 179], which may be more indicative of tissue toxicity as the results did not depend on the surface characteristics of the material and its interaction with the fluids used for testing.

MTA in contact with periradicular tissues led to the expression of inflammatory mediators and cytokines [176, 182, 183]. More advanced testing using a zebra fish model has been used based on survivability and hatching. Mechanistic and comparative analysis of toxicity was performed by oxidative stress analysis, with molecular investigation at the protein level carried out via a computational approach using *in silico* molecular docking and pathway analysis [184]. A significant reduction was shown in hatching and survivability, along with morphological malformations, which increased with leachate concentration [184]. 3D models with *in situ* fibroblast growth at the root apex [185] showed MTA to be similar to Biodentine (Septodont), a Type 4 material, whilst another 3D model using osteoblastic differentiation [186] showed it to perform worse than Endosequence Root Repair Material (Brasseler; Type 5). MTA has been shown to be neurotoxic [187], but no genotoxicity has been detected [173, 188, 189].

Tissue reactions have also been assessed using a variety of animals via subcutaneous and intraosseous implantation. Although the former is a popular method, it is not very indicative of the interactions of materials *in vivo* when used in endodontic surgery, since there is no hard tissue involvement. An inflammatory reaction has been found that involves the deposition of amyloid-like protein and an increase in the mast cell population. Later, areas of mononuclear cell aggregation, abscess formation, and necrosis were observed, with formation of a thick fibrous capsule [190]. With subcutaneously implanted dentine tubes, mineralization was shown in relation to MTA, initially at the cement–dentine interface and eventually even in the interior of the dentine tubules [191]. The biological process involved in this mineralization seems to be the induction of a time-dependent proinflammatory cytokine upregulation with upregulated expression of myeloperoxidase, nuclear factor-kappa B (NF-κβ), activating protein-1 (AP-1), cyclooxygenase-2 (COX-2), inducible nitric oxide synthase (iNOS), and vascular endothelial growth factor (vEGF). The formation of apatite-like clusters on collagen fibrils over the surface of tubes containing MTA was also found, which was shown to increase with time. Thus, MTA induced a proinflammatory and pro-wound-healing environment. The biomineralization process at the material–dentin tissue interface occurred simultaneously with the acute inflammatory response [192].

Subcutaneous interactions differ from those occurring with intraosseous implantation. Subcutaneous implantation initially elicited severe reactions with coagulation necrosis and dystrophic calcification; most, however, subsided to 'moderate' with time. Osteogenesis was not observed for this implantation, indicating that MTA is not osteoinductive.

Reactions to intraosseous implants are similar to – but less intense than – reactions to subcutaneous ones, in that an initial severe inflammatory reaction occurs, which subsides with time [193, 194].

For root-end filling in dogs, less periradicular inflammation and more fibrous capsule formation have been found adjacent to MTA compared with amalgam. In addition, the formation of cementum on the surface of the MTA is a frequent finding [195]. In one study, MTA led to complete sealing of root perforations, with the formation of mineralized tissue with greater thickness and area. No bone resorption in the furcation region, fewer inflammatory cells, and greater RUNX2 immunostaining intensity were observed in comparison with gutta-percha [196]. No inflammation could be detected, but cementum deposition was observed [197]. The presence of infection and bacteria led to compromised healing in cases of root perforation. There were a larger number of cases of complete or partial biologic seal in noncontaminated compared with contaminated groups. It might be concluded that lateral root perforations sealed with MTA after contamination gave poorer repair than did noncontaminated, immediately-sealed perforations. Temporary filling with a bactericidal agent such as a calcium hydroxide-based paste did not improve the repair of perforations exposed to contamination [197].

Systemic diseases such as diabetes mellitus [199] and hypertension [200, 201] have been associated with an increase in inflammatory infiltrate and reduction in the biocompatibility and biomineralization of subcutaneously implanted MTA. However, such interactions cannot be extrapolated to the clinical use of MTA for endodontic surgery.

Subcutaneous implantation of MTA has been found to lead to a local, self-limited, inflammatory reaction, but systemically there were adverse and persistent inflammatory reactions in the liver and kidneys, with elevated liver enzyme activity [202]. Such effects do not appear to have been permanent [203].

Transfer of aluminium from the surgical site to the plasma and liver of test animals [204] has been shown, causing oxidative stress in the brain [205]. Chromium and magnesium levels in internal organs have been reported to be raised [206]. These effects are of some concern and need to be investigated further.

Neo MTA Plus exhibited mineralized nodule formation in contact with osteosarcoma cells at a higher rate than did MTA Angelus [207].

7.3.2.1.3 Antimicrobial Properties

When root-end surgery is undertaken, the root tip – which is the path of communication between the bacteria in the root canal system and the periradicular tissues, through which bacterial contamination occurs – is removed. Thus, the antimicrobial properties of root-end filling materials, although important, are not as crucial as for root canal sealers. Perforation repair materials need to be more antimicrobial as they are in contact with contaminated dentine. Most of the research work undertaken on this has used bacteria to measure leakage at the tooth apex. However, measurement of leakage is not considered here for the reasons outlined earlier.

Various bacteria have been used to test anti-microbial effects, including facultative anaerobes: *Streptococcus faecalis, Streptococcus mitis, Streptococcus mutans, Streptococcus salivarius, Lactobacillus* spp., *Streptococcus aureus, Staphylococcus epidermidis, Bacillus subtilis,* and *Escherichia coli* B; and strict anaerobes: *Prevotella* (*Bacteroides*) *buccae, Prevotella* (*Bacteroides*) *intermedia, Prevotella* (*Bacteroides*) *melaninogenica, Bacteroides fragilis, Fusobacterium necrophorum, Fusobacterium nucleatum,* and *Peptostreptococcus anaerobius* [208]. The agar diffusion method, which measures the effect of diffusion of leachate from discs of the test material and thus the killing capacity from the zones of inhibition, has been very popular [208]. However, the direct-contact test [40] is more reliable and does not depend on the diffusion process in agar. The most clinically relevant method is that of tubule infection, as

this uses a dentine substrate and relies on bacterial growth in dentine tubules [39].

MTA exhibits antimicrobial properties when both fresh and set, although these vary with the strain of bacteria used [40]. The minimum bactericidal effect against *S. aureus* and *E. faecalis* is said to be adequate [41]. The antimicrobial effect of MTA is stable even when using the intratubular infection method [39], so it would appear that the dentine does not affect this. The presence of blood contamination has a buffering effect on MTA; ProRoot MTA was shown to be less antimicrobial when in contact with blood [209], which it always is in the case of root-end filling.

7.3.2.1.4 Clinical Technique

The earlier formulations of MTA (ProRoot; Angelus) are presented as a powder in sachets (ProRoot) or air-tight bottles (Angelus) and supplied with a pre-dosed ampoule or container filled with water (Figure 7.11a,b). The Type 2 cements are available in a variety of presentations: MTA HP (Angelus) comes in a pre-dosed capsule with an air-tight seal (Figure 7.11c), to be mixed with the liquid provided; Harvard Opticaps (Harvard Dental International, Hoppegarten, Germany) is also available in a capsule (Figure 7.11d), but to be activated and mixed in an automatic mixer; whilst MTA Flow (Ultradent), although presented as a bulk powder and liquid (Figure 7.11e), similar to MTA, comes in the form of a 'gel', and the kit offers the ability to mix in three consistencies, depending on the clinical application. This product can thus be used in any relevant clinical context.

Since variation of the P:L ratio results in changes in material properties [135, 210], care must be taken when dispensing powder and liquid to keep this ratio accurate. The loose MTA powder and the liquid, from pre-dosed sachets and ampoules, are to be mixed on a glass slab using a spatula, and losses must be avoided. There have been reports of inaccurate dosing of liquid in the ampoule [211]. The capsule presentation should provide more

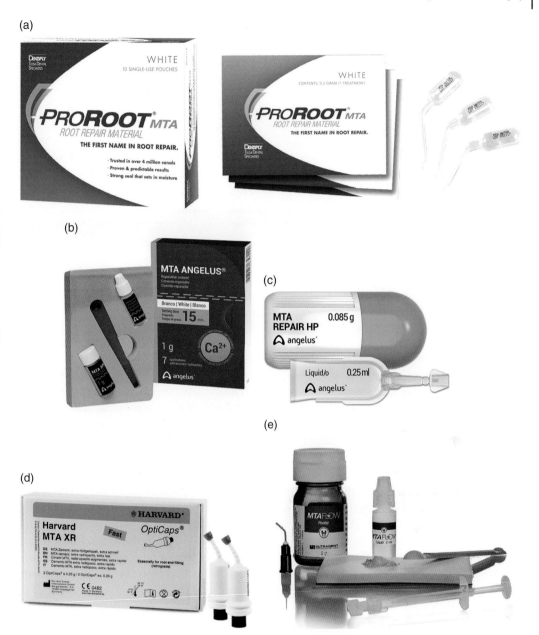

Figure 7.11 (a) ProRoot MTA (Dentsply). *Source:* Courtesy of Dentsply Sirona. (b) MTA Angelus (Angelus). *Source:* Courtesy of Angelus. (c) MTA HP (Angelus). *Source:* Courtesy of Angelus. (d) Harvard Opticaps capsules (Harvard). *Source:* Harvard Dental International. (e) MTA Flow (Ultradent). *Source:* Courtesy of Ultradent.

precision in mixing ratio, and mechanical mixing has been shown to enhance properties [212, 213].

Because the handling of the Type 1 materials is difficult, a number of delivery systems have

been invented to help get them to the surgical site (Figure 7.12a–c). These include the MTA 'gun', consisting of a long flexible titanium tip attached to a syringe, which delivers the material directly to the site, and the MTA block,

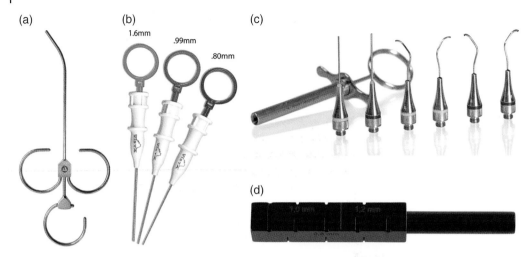

Figure 7.12 Various MTA carrier systems developed to aid in dispensing material at the surgical site. (a) Carrier system by Angelus. *Source:* Courtesy of Angelus. (b) Disposable plastic carriers of different sizes. *Source:* Courtesy of Vista-Dental. (c) Selection of tips with different angles for optimal delivery. *Source:* Courtesy of Produits Dentaire. (d) MTA block. *Source:* Courtesy of Brasseler USA.

which includes indentations (Figure 7.12d) into which the mixed material is pressed to form small cylindrical pellets that can be applied directly to the surgical site. The additives in the Type 2 materials aid in their placement, particularly the polymers added to improve handling; these allow the material to be placed at the surgical site with a 'flat plastic' instrument. In all cases, the material must be packed with long-shank pluggers.

Agitation by ultrasonic tips [214] and the application of high packing pressure [215] have been shown to give improved properties. However, the validity or usefulness of these methods when using MTA for endodontic surgery is questionable due to the limited access.

7.3.2.1.5 Environmental Interactions The
MTA used for endodontic surgery comes into contact with root dentine, blood, and tissue fluids. That used to manage perforations in the coronal region in a tooth that needs to be restored comes into contact with other materials, such as GIC and ZOE cement, as well as acid-etching and bonding systems. These environmental interactions are discussed in Chapter 2, particularly in the

context of HCSCs used as dentine replacement materials. However, it is worth noting some specific interactions here. Layering of MTA placed over a perforation with ZOE and GIC results in microstructural changes that may be detrimental to the MTA. ZOE causes a layer of unhydrated MTA as zinc ions inhibit its reaction. Furthermore, GIC disrupts the MTA microstructure due to its acidity [216]. When placing an FR over MTA, the use of a bonding agent is important to avoid changes at the interface [217]. Due to the long setting time of MTA, it has been recommended that its surface be covered with a moist barrier prior to tooth restoration [218].

The preparation and treatment of dentine prior to the placement of MTA is not well documented, especially for these specific clinical uses. EDTA and sodium hypochlorite [219–221] affect MTA's chemistry and hardness and are used routinely in root canal therapy, such that when MTA is used for perforation repair, they will come into contact with the set material.

Although MTA is hydraulic and wetting with water should not affect its properties, contact with blood and tissue fluids – as in ordinary clinical use – has been shown to adversely affect its material characteristics, because of their solutes. Thus, blood contamination affects its mechanical properties, dimensional stability, and colour. Similar effects have been reported with foetal bovine serum [130] and synthetic tissue fluids. Indeed, blood [132, 222, 223] and tissue fluids [130] inhibit the hydration reaction due to precipitates from the reaction of calcium with phosphate [224]. Retardation results from the formation of insoluble hydroxides in the alkaline liquid of the material coating the cement particles. MTA in contact with tissue fluids undergoes expansion [143, 225]; in contact with blood, it undergoes severe discolouration [226, 227].

The formation of phosphates has been called 'bioactivity' [228–231]. This deposition is implicated in increasing the push-out bond resistance resulting from interaction with dentine [232]. Clinically, there is limited free phosphate in blood and tissue fluids. However, it has been shown that calcium carbonate forms on the surface of MTA in contact with subcutaneous tissue [226], the carbonate coming from carbon dioxide in the blood. The limited ability of *in vitro* studies to provide any meaningful information related to clinical interaction of these materials has been highlighted [233]. Such deposits may reduce the surface pH, and this has clinical implications, including the weakening of antimicrobial properties [209].

7.3.2.1.6 Clinical Evaluation There is very limited information on the clinical performance of MTA used for root perforation repair, there being only one report on this subject [234]. MTA used as a root-end filling material accompanied by microsurgery showed an 88% success rate [235]. This was higher than the rate for simple smoothing of the gutta-percha [236, 237], indicating the importance of placing a root-end filling material. However, despite its hydraulic nature and claimed superior properties, this use of MTA produced clinical outcomes similar to those with

IRM [54, 55] and Super EBA cement [56], even in the long term [57]. Nonetheless, MTA had a better outcome than Retroplast [111, 112].

In one study, MTA showed a success rate of 84% healed cases after 12 months, rising to 92% at two years [54], although there were lower rates in anterior teeth at one week, three months, and one year [55]. Similarly, another study found success rates of 94% for MTA and 93% for Super EBA, with no appreciable difference between the two materials [56]. Postoperative healing after root-end surgery using MTA was similar to that for IRM at 3–5 hours and even 48 hours after the procedure [43].

7.3.2.2 Tricalcium Silicate Cement-Based Hydraulic Cements: Types 4 and 5

Tricalcium silicate-based materials may be formulated to be mixed with water (Type 4), or they may be supplied as a paste or putty in a syringe and so not require mixing (Type 5). Tricalcium silicate has a reaction chemistry similar to that of Portland cement and can be used successfully to replace it [238]. Biodentine (Septodont) is a Type 4 material, but although it is tricalcium silicate-based, it was developed for use as a dentine replacement material. For that reason, it will not be considered here, but instead is discussed under the materials used for pulp protection in Chapter 2.

Type 5 materials are labelled 'premixed' but use a vehicle other than water to suspend the powder. Examples include the products Endosequence (Brasseler, Savannah GA, USA), Totalfill (FKG Dentaire, La Chaux-de-Fonds, Switzerland), and IRoot (Veriodent, Vancouver, Canada), all of which were specifically developed for endodontic surgery. The differently labelled presentations for what are otherwise identical materials may indicate regional licencing. At the time of writing, a number of other 'premixed' products are appearing on the market; this presentation improves the ease of use, particularly for surgical procedures. Since there is as yet limited scientific evidence on these new materials, they are not covered here. The Endosequence/Totalfill/Iroot product group is referred to by its manufacturers as 'bioceramic' root repair materials (BC-RRMs), but this terminology is not scientifically based, as discussed in Chapter 1.

7.3.2.2.1 Chemistry and Physical Properties

The main feature of this material type is its 'premixed' condition (although this label is again misleading; see Chapter 1). Thus, the hydration reaction requires moisture from the environment. The first group of such products sold specifically as root repair materials was Endosequence BC putty and paste, followed later by a fast-set paste. Tantalum oxide is used

as the radiopacifier, with monobasic calcium phosphate as an additive said to enhance the material properties. (The first such material was Type 4, with similar components, but mixed with water (Bioaggregate, Verio Dental, Vancouver, Canada), but as this is no longer available, it was not discussed alongside the Type 4 materials earlier.) The components of a BC-RRM – cement, additive, and radiopacifier – are readily distinguishable (Figure 7.13).

The BC-RRM products are currently the only 'premixed' materials with reported studies. They have the advantage of using tricalcium silicate and an alternative radiopacifier. The calcium phosphate is claimed to

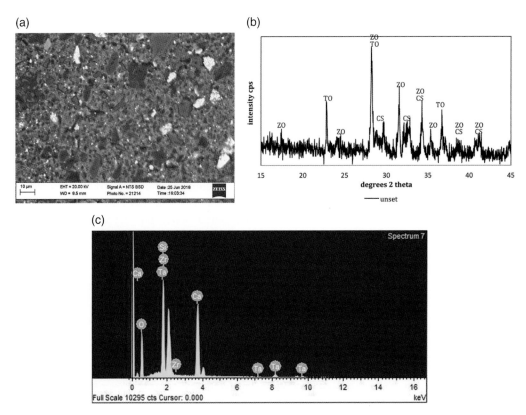

Figure 7.13 Characterization of BC-RRM, showing the material microstructure. (a) Back-scatter scanning electron micrograph showing the various components (×2000). *Source:* Josette Camilleri. (b) Phase analysis showing the main phases present. CS, calcium silicate; TO, tantalum oxide; ZO, zirconium oxide. *Source:* From Moinzadeh, A.T., Aznar Portoles, C., Schembri Wismayer, P., Camilleri, J. Bioactivity potential of EndoSequence BC RRM Putty. *J. Endod.* 2016 Apr;42(4):615–21 © 2016. Reproduced with the permission of Elsevier. (c) Elemental analysis. *Source:* Modified from Moinzadeh, A.T., Aznar Portoles, C., Schembri Wismayer, P., Camilleri, J. Bioactivity potential of EndoSequence BC RRM Putty. *J. Endod.* 2016 Apr;42(4):615–21.

provide free phosphate ions in solution, facilitating the formation of hydroxyapatite on the material surface in contact with tissue fluids. An investigation of the setting of tricalcium silicate with added monobasic calcium phosphate or hydroxyapatite indicated that the overall reaction outcome was affected by the extra ions [239]: the less calcium hydroxide formed, the lower the pH. The biological properties were also altered, giving reduced cell proliferation [239]. Thus, some of the properties of such products as Endosequence BC may be a result of their additives.

The setting time of these materials is not modified but retarded when in contact with blood or a culture medium (to simulate body fluid) [240]. The fast-set version has a shorter setting time than either the 'regular' version or MTA, but it also has an intense exothermic reaction [241]. The pH of BC-RRM is lower than that of MTA [242]. The hardness is also lower than that of MTA in the initial stages of the reaction, but the compressive strength is higher [241] – although this is not affected by immersion in foetal bovine serum [243]. BC-RRM does not induce tooth discolouration [244], even in the presence of blood [245].

7.3.2.2.2 *Biological Properties*   BC-RRM exhibits good cell viability, comparable to that of MTA [177, 242], except in the early stages when it is lower [177]. Dermal fibroblasts showed a negative interaction with BC-RRM [246]. Osteoblast differentiation was affected: expression of osteoblastic genes and ALP staining were increased significantly [247]. The leachate also showed good cell viability [248], but this depended on its dilution and age; BC-RRM had reduced viability early on compared with MTA Angelus [249].

Tissue interactions after apical microsurgery in dogs have also been investigated. Minimal or no inflammatory tissue response was observed in the periapical area using both MTA and BC-RRM. Histologically, BC-RRM adjacent to the resected root-end surface had the better tissue healing response. This superior healing tendency could be detected by cone-beam microcomputed tomography (CBCT) and μCT, but not by periapical radiography [249].

7.3.2.2.3 *Antimicrobial Properties*   BC-RRM exhibits antimicrobial activity against a number of strains, including *Candida albicans* [250], with a roughly two- to fivefold reduction in viable counts (not affected by the preincubation period) using the direct-contact method [251].

7.3.2.2.4 *Clinical Technique*   The paste version (Figure 7.14a) is syringeable using disposable tips and is thus very easy to apply directly to the site. The putty version, which is of higher viscosity, may nonetheless also be

(a)   (b)   (c)

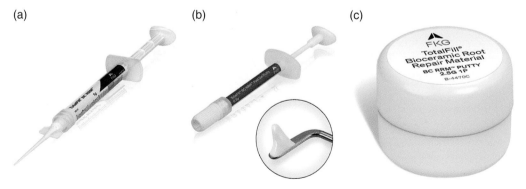

Figure 7.14   Presentation of BC-RRM (Totalfill; FKG Dentaire, Switzerland): (a) syringe with paste, including a tip for easy delivery; (b) syringe with putty; (c) container with putty. *Source:* Illustration FKG: © FKG Dentaire SA, all rights reserved.

dispensed from a syringe (Figure 7.14b) or from a jar (Figure 7.14c) using microsurgery application tips.

7.3.2.2.5 Environmental Interactions Regardless of the inclusion of calcium phosphate, supposedly to enable the formation of hydroxyapatite, only calcium carbonate has been found on material retrieved from a failed root-end surgery clinical case [252]. Likewise, in contact with blood, calcium carbonate is preferentially formed, as with MTA [226].

Better push-out strength was reported for BC-RRM than for MTA in ultrasonically prepared concave retrograde cavities [253]. When used to repair root perforations, the presence of sodium hypochlorite increased this value [254].

7.3.2.2.6 Clinical Evaluation BC-RRM has shown over 90% success rate in use as a root-end filling material [255–257], comparable to MTA [255, 256]. This rate was higher when scored on periapical radiographs than when using CBCT [256].

7.4 Conclusion

The development of better instruments for microsurgery, better visualization and magnification, and new materials has enhanced clinical success rates for endodontic surgical procedures, whilst the introduction of hydraulic cements specifically developed for endodontic surgery has led to a number of changes to the procedures used, with better clinical outcomes. Although much is now known, a better understanding of the material interactions is necessary in order to develop better clinical protocols, specific to the material employed, so that full benefit can be obtained.

Acknowledgements

The following need to be thanked for their proofreading: Professor Brian Darvell and Professor Pierre Machtou. Professor Saulius Drukteinis is thanked for his help with the nonclinical images.

References

1 Del Fabbro, M., Corbella, S., Sequeira-Byron, P. et al. (2016). Endodontic procedures for retreatment of periapical lesions. *Cochrane Database Syst. Rev.* (10): CD005511.

2 Del Fabbro, M., Taschieri, S., Testori, T. et al. (2007). Surgical versus non-surgical endodontic re-treatment for periradicular lesions. *Cochrane Database Syst. Rev.* (3): CD005511.

3 Gutmann, J.L. and Pitt Ford, T.R. (1993). Management of the resected root end: a clinical review. *Int. Endod. J.* 26 (5): 273–283.

4 Andreasen, J.O. and Rud, J. (1972). A histobacteriologic study of dental and periapical structures after endodontic surgery. *Int. J. Oral Max. Surg.* 1: 272–281.

5 Kohli, M.R., Berenji, H., Setzer, F.C. et al. (2018). Outcome of endodontic surgery: a meta-analysis of the literature – part 3: comparison of endodontic microsurgical techniques with 2 different root-end filling materials. *J. Endod.* 44 (6): 923–931.

6 Tortorici, S., Difalco, P., Caradonna, L., and Tetè, S. (2014). Traditional endodontic surgery versus modern technique: a 5-year controlled clinical trial. *J. Craniofac Surg.* 25 (3): 804–807.

7 von Arx, T., Jensen, S.S., Hänni, S., and Friedman, S. (2012). Five-year longitudinal assessment of the prognosis of apical microsurgery. *J. Endod.* 38 (5): 570–579.

8 Taschieri, S., Del Fabbro, M., Testori, T. et al. (2006). Endodontic surgery using 2 different magnification devices: preliminary results of a randomized controlled study. *J. Oral Maxillofac. Surg.* 64 (2): 235–242.

9 International Standards Organization (2012). Dentistry – root canal sealing materials. ISO 6876:2012.

10 International Standards Organization (2011). Dentistry – zinc oxide/eugenol cements and zinc oxide/non-eugenol cements. ISO 3107:2011.

11 International Standards Organization (2007). Dentistry – water-based cements – Part 1: Powder/liquid acid-base cements. ISO 9917-1:2007.

12 International Standards Organization (2010). Dentistry – water-based cements – Part 2: Resin-modified cements. ISO 9917-2:2010.

13 International Standards Organization (2009). Dentistry – polymer-based restorative materials. ISO 4049:2009.

14 International Standards Organization (2015). Dentistry – dental amalgam. ISO 24234:2015.

15 European Union (2017). Regulation (EU) 2017/852 of the European Parliament and of the Council of 17 May 2017 on mercury, and repealing Regulation (EC) No 1102/2008.

16 Wu, M.K. and Wesselink, P.R. (1993). Endodontic leakage studies reconsidered. Part I. Methodology, application and relevance. *Int. Endod. J.* 26 (1): 37–43.

17 Oynick, J. and Oynick, T. (1978). A study of a new material for retrograde fillings. *J. Endod.* 4: 203–206.

18 Brauer, G.M., Simon, L., and Sangermano, L. (1962). Improved zinc oxide-eugenol type cements. *J. Dent. Res.* 41: 1096.

19 Curtis, D. (1946). US patent 2413294.

20 Crooks, W.G., Anderson, R.W., Powell, B.J., and Kimbrough, W.F. (1994). Longitudinal evaluation of the seal of IRM root end fillings. *J. Endod.* 20 (5): 250–252.

21 Torabinejad, M., Hong, C.U., McDonald, F., and Pitt Ford, T.R. (1995). Physical and chemical properties of a new root-end filling material. *J. Endod.* 21 (7): 349–353.

22 Jendresen, M.D., Phillips, R.W., Swartz, M.L., and Norman, R.D. (1969). A comparative study of four zinc oxide and eugenol formulations as restorative materials. Part I. *J. Proth. Dent.* 21 (2): 176–183.

23 Torabinejad, M., Smith, P.W., Kettering, J.D., and Pitt Ford, T.R. (1995). Comparative investigation of marginal adaptation of mineral trioxide aggregate and other commonly used root-end filling materials. *J. Endod.* 21 (6): 295–299.

24 Shah, P.M., Chong, B.S., Sidhu, S.K., and Ford, T.R. (1996). Radiopacity of potential root-end filling materials. *Oral Surg. Oral Med. Oral Pathol. Oral Radiol. Endod.* 81 (4): 476–479.

25 Fitzpatrick, E.L. and Steiman, H.R. (1997). Scanning electron microscopic evaluation of finishing techniques on IRM and EBA retrofillings. *J. Endod.* 23: 423–427.

26 Zhu, Q., Safavi, K.E., and Spangberg, L.S. (1999). Cytotoxic evaluation of root-end filling materials in cultures of human osteoblast-like cells and periodontal ligament cells. *J. Endod.* 25 (6): 410–412.

27 Torabinejad, M., Hong, C.U., Pitt Ford, T.R., and Kettering, J.D. (1995). Cytotoxicity of four root end filling materials. *J. Endod.* 21 (10): 489–492.

28 Mozayeni, M.A., Milani, A.S., Marvasti, L.A., and Asgary, S. (2012). Cytotoxicity of calcium enriched mixture cement compared with mineral trioxide aggregate and intermediate restorative material. *Aust. Endod. J.* 38 (2): 70–75.

29 Balto, H. and Al-Nazhan, S. (2003). Attachment of human periodontal ligament fibroblasts to 3 different root-end filling materials: scanning electron microscope observation. *Oral Surg. Oral Med. Oral Pathol. Oral Radiol. Endod.* 95 (2): 222–227.

30 Bonson, S., Jeansonne, B.G., and Lallier, T.E. (2004). Root-end filling materials alter fibroblast differentiation. *J. Dent. Res.* 83 (5): 408–413.

31 Souza, N.J., Justo, G.Z., Oliveira, C.R. et al. (2006). Cytotoxicity of materials used in perforation repair tested using the V79 fibroblast cell line and the granulocyte-macrophage progenitor cells. *Int. Endod. J.* 39 (1): 40–47.

32 Kettering, J.D. and Torabinejad, M. (1995). Investigation of mutagenicity of mineral

trioxide aggregate and other commonly used root-end filling materials. *J. Endod.* 21 (11): 537–542.

33 Torabinejad, M., Ford, T.R., Abedi, H.R. et al. (1998). Tissue reaction to implanted root-end filling materials in the tibia and mandible of Guinea pigs. *J. Endod.* 24 (7): 468–471.

34 Coleman, J.M. and Kirk, E.E.J. (1965). An assessment of a modified zinc oxide-eugenol cement. *Brit. Dent. J.* 118: 482.

35 Yildirim, T., Gençoğlu, N., Firat, I. et al. (2005). Histologic study of furcation perforations treated with MTA or Super EBA in dogs' teeth. *Oral Surg. Oral Med. Oral Pathol. Oral Radiol. Endod.* 100 (1): 120–124.

36 Harrison, J.W. and Johnson, S.A. (1997). Excisional wound healing following the use of IRM as a root-end filling material. *J. Endod.* 23 (1): 19–27.

37 Wälivaara, D.Å., Abrahamsson, P., Isaksson, S. et al. (2012). Periapical tissue response after use of intermediate restorative material, gutta-percha, reinforced zinc oxide cement, and mineral trioxide aggregate as retrograde root-end filling materials: a histologic study in dogs. *J. Oral Maxillofac. Surg.* 70 (9): 2041–2047.

38 Safavi, K., Kazemi, R., and Watkins, D. (1999). Adherence of enamel matrix derivatives on root-end filling materials. *J. Endod.* 25 (11): 710–712.

39 Prestegaard, H., Portenier, I., Ørstavik, D. et al. (2014). Antibacterial activity of various root canal sealers and root-end filling materials in dentin blocks infected ex vivo with *Enterococcus faecalis*. *Acta Odontol. Scand.* 72 (8): 970–976.

40 Eldeniz, A.U., Hadimli, H.H., Ataoglu, H., and Orstavik, D. (2006). Antibacterial effect of selected root-end filling materials. *J. Endod.* 32 (4): 345–349.

41 Koçak, M.M., Koçak, S., Oktay, E.A. et al. (2013). In vitro evaluation of the minimum bactericidal concentrations of different root-end filling materials. *J. Contemp. Dent. Pract.* 14 (3): 371–374.

42 Gartner, A. and Dorn, S.O. (1992). Advances in endodontic surgery. *Dent. Clin. N. Am.* 36: 364–373.

43 Chong, B.S. and Pitt Ford, T.R. (2005). Postoperative pain after root-end resection and filling. *Oral Surg. Oral Med. Oral Pathol. Oral Radiol. Endod.* 100 (6): 762–766.

44 Vivan, R.R., Guerreiro-Tanomaru, J.M., Bosso-Martelo, R. et al. (2016). Push-out bond strength of root-end filling materials. *Braz. Dent. J.* 27 (3): 332–335.

45 Weldon, J.K. Jr., Pashley, D.H., Loushine, R.J. et al. (2002). Sealing ability of mineral trioxide aggregate and super-EBA when used as furcation repair materials: a longitudinal study. *J. Endod.* 28 (6): 467–470.

46 Uyanik, M.O., Nagas, E., Sahin, C. et al. (2009). Effects of different irrigation regimens on the sealing properties of repaired furcal perforations. *Oral Surg. Oral Med. Oral Pathol. Oral Radiol. Endod.* 107 (3): e91–e95.

47 Loxley, E.C., Liewehr, F.R., Buxton, T.B., and McPherson, J.C. 3rd (2003). The effect of various intracanal oxidizing agents on the push-out strength of various perforation repair materials. *Oral Surg. Oral Med. Oral Pathol. Oral Radiol. Endod.* 95 (4): 490–494.

48 Guneser, M.B., Akbulut, M.B., and Eldeniz, A.U. (2013). Effect of various endodontic irrigants on the push-out bond strength of biodentine and conventional root perforation repair materials. *J. Endod.* 39 (3): 380–384.

49 Formosa, L.M., Mallia, B., and Camilleri, J. (2013). A quantitative method for determining the antiwashout characteristics of cement-based dental materials including mineral trioxide aggregate. *Int. Endod. J.* 46 (2): 179–186.

50 Grech, L., Mallia, B., and Camilleri, J. (2013). Investigation of the physical properties of tricalcium silicate cement-based root-end filling materials. *Dent. Mater.* 29 (2): e20–e28.

51 Wälivaara, D.Å., Abrahamsson, P., Fogelin, M., and Isaksson, S. (2011). Super-EBA and IRM as root-end fillings in periapical surgery with ultrasonic preparation: a prospective randomized clinical study of 206 consecutive teeth. *Oral Surg. Oral Med. Oral Pathol. Oral Radiol. Endod.* 112 (2): 258–263.

52 Wälivaara, D.A., Abrahamsson, P., Sämfors, K.A., and Isaksson, S. (2009). Periapical surgery using ultrasonic preparation and thermoplasticized gutta-percha with AH Plus sealer or IRM as retrograde root-end fillings in 160 consecutive teeth: a prospective randomized clinical study. *Oral Surg. Oral Med. Oral Pathol. Oral Radiol. Endod.* 108 (5): 784–789.

53 Wälivaara, D.A., Abrahamsson, P., Isaksson, S. et al. (2007). Prospective study of periapically infected teeth treated with periapical surgery including ultrasonic preparation and retrograde intermediate restorative material root-end fillings. *J. Oral Maxillofac. Surg.* 65 (5): 931–935.

54 Lindeboom, J.A., Frenken, J.W., Kroon, F.H., and van den Akker, H.P. (2005). A comparative prospective randomized clinical study of MTA and IRM as root-end filling materials in single-rooted teeth in endodontic surgery. *Oral Surg. Oral Med. Oral Pathol. Oral Radiol. Endod.* 100 (4): 495–500.

55 Chong, B.S., Pitt Ford, T.R., and Hudson, M.B. (2003). A prospective clinical study of mineral trioxide aggregate and IRM when used as root-end filling materials in endodontic surgery. *Int. Endod. J.* 36 (8): 520–526.

56 Song, M. and Kim, E. (2012). A prospective randomized controlled study of mineral trioxide aggregate and super ethoxy-benzoic acid as root-end filling materials in endodontic microsurgery. *J. Endod.* 38 (7): 875–879.

57 Kim, S., Song, M., Shin, S.J., and Kim, E. (2016). A randomized controlled study of mineral trioxide aggregate and super ethoxybenzoic acid as root-end filling materials in endodontic microsurgery: long-term outcomes. *J. Endod.* 42 (7): 997–1002.

58 Crowley, C.M., Doyle, J., Towler, M.R. et al. (2007). Influence of acid washing on the surface morphology of ionomer glasses and handling properties of glass ionomer cements. *J. Mater. Sci. Mater. Med.* 18 (8): 1497–1506.

59 Gomes, F.O., Pires, R.A., and Reis, R.L. (2013). Aluminum-free glass-ionomer bone cements with enhanced bioactivity and biodegradability. *Mater. Sci. Eng. C Mater. Biol. Appl.* 33 (3): 1361–1370.

60 Kim, D.A., Abo-Mosallam, H.A., Lee, H.Y. et al. (2014). Development of a novel aluminum-free glass ionomer cement based on magnesium/strontium-silicate glasses. *Mater. Sci. Eng. C Mater. Biol. Appl.* 42: 665–671.

61 Dickey, B.T., Kehoe, S., and Boyd, D. (2013). Novel adaptations to zinc-silicate glass polyalkenoate cements: the unexpected influences of germanium based glasses on handling characteristics and mechanical properties. *J. Mech. Behav. Biomed. Mater.* 23: 8–21.

62 Zhang, X., Werner-Zwanziger, U., and Boyd, D. (2015). Composition–structure–property relationships for non-classical ionomer cements formulated with zinc-boron germanium-based glasses. *J. Biomater. Appl.* 29 (9): 1203–1217.

63 Kim, D.A., Abo-Mosallam, H., Lee, H.Y. et al. (2015). Biological and mechanical properties of an experimental glass-ionomer cement modified by partial replacement of CaO with MgO or ZnO. *J. Appl. Oral Sci.* 23 (4): 369–375.

64 Saxena, S. and Tiwari, S. (2016). Energy dispersive X-ray microanalysis, fluoride release, and antimicrobial properties of glass ionomer cements indicated for atraumatic restorative treatment. *J. Int. Soc. Prev. Community Dent.* 6 (4): 366–372.

65 Crisp, S. and Wilson, A.D. (1974). Reactions in glass ionomer cements: I. Decomposition of the powder. *J. Dent. Res.* 53 (6): 1408–1413.

66 Crisp, S., Pringuer, M.A., Wardleworth, D., and Wilson, A.D. (1974). Reactions in glass

ionomer cements: II. An infrared spectroscopic study. *J. Dent. Res.* 53 (6): 1414–1419.

67 Wilson, A.D., Crisp, S., and Ferner, A.J. (1976). Reactions in glass-ionomer cements: IV. Effect of chelating comonomers on setting behavior. *J. Dent. Res.* 55 (3): 489–495.

68 Crisp, S., Lewis, B.G., and Wilson, A.D. (1976). Glass ionomer cements: chemistry of erosion. *J. Dent. Res.* 55 (6): 1032–1041.

69 Crisp, S. and Wilson, A.D. (1976). Reactions in glass ionomer cements: V. Effect of incorporating tartaric acid in the cement liquid. *J. Dent. Res.* 55 (6): 1023–1031.

70 Crisp, S., Ferner, A.J., Lewis, B.G., and Wilson, A.D. (1975). Properties of improved glass-ionomer cement formulations. *J. Dent.* 3 (3): 125–130.

71 Crisp, S., Lewis, B.G., and Wilson, A.D. (1976). Characterization of glass-ionomer cements. 2. Effect of the powder: liquid ratio on the physical properties. *J. Dent.* 4 (6): 287–290.

72 Crisp, S., Lewis, B.G., and Wilson, A.D. (1977). Characterization of glass-ionomer cements. 3. Effect of polyacid concentration on the physical properties. *J. Dent.* 5 (1): 51–56.

73 Wilson, A.D., Crisp, S., and Abel, G. (1977). Characterization of glass-ionomer cements. 4. Effect of molecular weight on physical properties. *J. Dent.* 5 (2): 117–120.

74 Lee, B.N., Son, H.J., Noh, H.J. et al. (2012). Cytotoxicity of newly developed ortho MTA root-end filling materials. *J. Endod.* 38 (12): 1627–1630.

75 Al-Hiyasat, A.S., Al-Sa'Eed, O.R., and Darmani, H. (2012). Quality of cellular attachment to various root-end filling materials. *J. Appl. Oral Sci.* 20 (1): 82–88.

76 Lin, C.P., Chen, Y.J., Lee, Y.L. et al. (2004). Effects of root-end filling materials and eugenol on mitochondrial dehydrogenase activity and cytotoxicity to human periodontal ligament fibroblasts. *J. Biomed. Mater. Res. B. Appl. Biomater.* 71 (2): 429–440.

77 Vajrabhaya, L.O., Korsuwannawong, S., Jantarat, J., and Korre, S. (2006). Biocompatibility of furcal perforation repair material using cell culture technique: Ketac Molar versus ProRoot MTA. *Oral Surg. Oral Med. Oral Pathol. Oral Radiol. Endod.* 102 (6): e48–e50.

78 Vanni, J.R., Della-Bona, A., Figueiredo, J.A. et al. (2011). Radiographic evaluation of furcal perforations sealed with different materials in dogs' teeth. *J. Appl. Oral Sci.* 19 (4): 421–425.

79 Huang, F.M., Tai, K.W., Chou, M.Y., and Chang, Y.C. (2002). Resinous perforation-repair materials inhibit the growth, attachment, and proliferation of human gingival fibroblasts. *J. Endod.* 28 (4): 291–294.

80 Gupta, S.K., Saxena, P., Pant, V.A., and Pant, A.B. (2013). Adhesion and biologic behavior of human periodontal fibroblast cells to resin ionomer Geristore: a comparative analysis. *Dent. Traumatol.* 29 (5): 389–393.

81 Makkawy, H.A., Koka, S., Lavin, M.T., and Ewoldsen, N.O. (1998). Cytotoxicity of root perforation repair materials. *J. Endod.* 24 (7): 477–479.

82 Kolokuris, I., Beltes, P., Economides, N., and Vlemmas, I. (1996). Experimental study of the biocompatibility of a new glass-ionomer root canal sealer (Ketac-Endo). *J. Endod.* 22 (8): 395–398.

83 Tassery, H., Pertot, W.J., Camps, J. et al. (1999). Comparison of two implantation sites for testing intraosseous biocompatibility. *J. Endod.* 25 (9): 615–618.

84 Chong, B.S., Ford, T.R., and Kariyawasam, S.P. (1997). Tissue response to potential root-end filling materials in infected root canals. *Int. Endod. J.* 30 (2): 102–114.

85 Vermeersch, G., Leloup, G., Delmée, M., and Vreven, J. (2005). Antibacterial activity of glass-ionomer cements, compomers and resin composites: relationship between acidity and material setting phase. *J. Oral Rehabil.* 32 (5): 368–374.

86 DeSchepper, E.J., White, R.R., and von der Lehr, W. (1989). Antibacterial effects of glass ionomers. *Am. J. Dent.* 2 (2): 51–56.

87 Seppä, L., Forss, H., and Ogaard, B. (1993). The effect of fluoride application on fluoride release and the antibacterial action of glass ionomers. *J. Dent. Res.* 72 (9): 1310–1314.

88 Chong, B.S., Pitt Ford, T.R., and Watson, T.F. (1993). Light-cured glass ionomer cement as a retrograde root seal. *Int. Endod. J.* 26 (4): 218–224.

89 Olson, A.K., MacPherson, M.G., Hartwell, G.R. et al. (1990). An in vitro evaluation of injectable thermoplasticized gutta-percha, glass ionomer, and amalgam when used as retrofilling materials. *J. Endod.* 16 (8): 361–364.

90 Chong, B.S., Pitt Ford, T.R., and Watson, T.F. (1991). The adaptation and sealing ability of light-cured glass ionomer retrograde root fillings. *Int. Endod. J.* 24 (5): 223–232.

91 Ozata, F., Erdilek, N., and Tezel, H. (1993). A comparative sealability study of different retrofilling materials. *Int. Endod. J.* 26 (4): 241–245.

92 De Conto, F., Ericson Flores, M., Cucco, C. et al. (2014). A comparative study of materials and storage modes for human teeth in apicoectomy: scanning electron microscopy analysis. *Minerva Stomatol.* 63 (4): 95–102.

93 Chohan, H., Dewan, H., Annapoorna, B.M., and Manjunath, M.K. (2015). Comparative evaluation of sealing ability of glass ionomer-resin continuum as root-end filling materials: an in vitro study. *J. Int. Soc. Prev. Community Dent.* 5 (6): 488–493.

94 Xavier, C.B., Weismann, R., de Oliveira, M.G. et al. (2005). Root-end filling materials: apical microleakage and marginal adaptation. *J. Endod.* 31 (7): 539–542.

95 Ravichandra, P.V., Vemisetty, H., Deepthi, K. et al. (2014). Comparative evaluation of marginal adaptation of biodentine (TM) and other commonly used root end filling materials – an in vitro study. *J. Clin. Diagn. Res.* 8 (3): 243–245.

96 Costa, A.T., Post, L.K., Xavier, C.B. et al. (2008). Marginal adaptation and microleakage of five root-end filling materials: an in vitro study. *Minerva Stomatol.* 57 (6): 295–300.

97 De Bruyne, M.A., De Bruyne, R.J., Rosiers, L., and De Moor, R.J. (2005). Longitudinal study on microleakage of three root-end filling materials by the fluid transport method and by capillary flow porometry. *Int. Endod. J.* 38 (2): 129–136.

98 Singla, M., Verma, K.G., Goyal, V. et al. (2018). Comparison of push-out bond strength of furcation perforation repair materials – glass ionomer cement type II, hydroxyapatite, mineral trioxide aggregate, and biodentine: an in vitro study. *Contemp. Clin. Dent.* 9 (3): 410–414.

99 Niederman, R. and Theodosopoulou, J.N. (2003). A systematic review of in vivo retrograde obturation materials. *Int. Endod. J.* 36 (9): 577–585.

100 Rud, J., Rud, V., and Munksgaard, E.C. (1996). Retrograde root filling with dentin-bonded modified resin composite. *J. Endod.* 22 (9): 477–480.

101 Rakich, D.R., Wataha, J.C., Lefebvre, C.A., and Weller, R.N. (1998). Effects of dentin bonding agents on macrophage mitochondrial activity. *J. Endod.* 24 (8): 528–533.

102 Rakich, D.R., Wataha, J.C., Lefebvre, C.A., and Weller, R.N. (1999). Effect of dentin bonding agents on the secretion of inflammatory mediators from macrophages. *J. Endod.* 25 (2): 114–117.

103 Vahid, A., Hadjati, J., Kermanshah, H., and Ghabraei, S. (2004). Effects of cured dentin bonding materials on human monocyte viability. *Oral Surg. Oral Med. Oral Pathol. Oral Radiol. Endod.* 98 (5): 619–621.

104 Haglund, R., He, J., Jarvis, J. et al. (2003). Effects of root-end filling materials on fibroblasts and macrophages in vitro. *Oral Surg. Oral Med. Oral Pathol. Oral Radiol. Endod.* 95 (6): 739–745.

105 Al-Sa'eed, O.R., Al-Hiyasat, A.S., and Darmani, H. (2008). The effects of six root-end filling materials and their leachable components on cell viability. *J. Endod.* 34 (11): 1410–1414.

106 Ozbas, H., Yaltirik, M., Bilgic, B., and Issever, H. (2003). Reactions of connective tissue to compomers, composite and amalgam root-end filling materials. *Int. Endod. J.* 36 (4): 281–287.

107 Dorn, S.O. and Gartner, A.H. (1990). Retrograde filling materials: a retrospective success-failure study of amalgam, EBA, and IRM. *J. Endod.* 16 (8): 391–393.

108 Vignaroli, P.A., Anderson, R.W., and Pashley, D.H. (1995). Longitudinal evaluation of the microleakage of dentin bonding agents used to seal resected root apices. *J. Endod.* 21 (10): 509–512.

109 Economides, N., Kokorikos, I., Gogos, C. et al. (2004). Comparative study of sealing ability of two root-end-filling materials with and without the use of dentin-bonding agents. *J. Endod.* 30 (1): 35–37.

110 Yazdi, P.M., Schou, S., Jensen, S.S. et al. (2007). Dentine-bonded resin composite (Retroplast) for root-end filling: a prospective clinical and radiographic study with a mean follow-up period of 8 years. *Int. Endod. J.* 40 (7): 493–503.

111 von Arx, T., Hänni, S., and Jensen, S.S. (2010). Clinical results with two different methods of root-end preparation and filling in apical surgery: mineral trioxide aggregate and adhesive resin composite. *J. Endod.* 36 (7): 1122–1129.

112 von Arx, T., Hänni, S., and Jensen, S.S. (2014). 5-year results comparing mineral trioxide aggregate and adhesive resin composite for root-end sealing in apical surgery. *J. Endod.* 40 (8): 1077–1081.

113 Holt, G.M. and Dumsha, T.C. (2000). Leakage of amalgam, composite, and Super-EBA, compared with a new retrofill material: bone cement. *J. Endod.* 26 (1): 29–31.

114 Lee, S.J., Monsef, M., and Torabinejad, M. (1993). Sealing ability of a mineral trioxide

aggregate for repair of lateral root perforations. *J. Endod.* 19 (11): 541–544.

115 Torabinejad, M., Watson, T.F., and Pitt Ford, T.R. (1993). Sealing ability of a mineral trioxide aggregate when used as a root end filling material. *J. Endod.* 19 (12): 591–595.

116 Torabinejad, M. and White, J.D. (1993). Tooth filling material and method of use. Patent number: 5415547.

117 Torabinejad, M. and White, J.D. (1995). Tooth filling material and method of use. Patent number: 5769638.

118 Primus, C. (2002). Dental material. Publication number: 20030159618.

119 Primus, C. (2009). Dental material. Patent number: 7892342.

120 Darvell, B.W. and Wu, R.C. (2011). 'MTA' – an hydraulic silicate cement: review update and setting reaction. *Dent. Mater.* 27 (5): 407–422.

121 Camilleri, J. Classification of hydraulic cements used in dentistry. Frontiers in Dental Medicine - Dental Materials vol. 1, 9. https://doi.org/10.3389/fdmed.2020.00009.

122 Camilleri, J., Montesin, F.E., Brady, K. et al. (2005). The constitution of mineral trioxide aggregate. *Dent. Mater.* 21 (4): 297–303.

123 Belío-Reyes, I.A., Bucio, L., and Cruz-Chavez, E. (2009). Phase composition of ProRoot mineral trioxide aggregate by X-ray powder diffraction. *J. Endod.* 35 (6): 875–878.

124 Camilleri, J. (2007). Hydration mechanisms of mineral trioxide aggregate. *Int. Endod. J.* 40 (6): 462–470.

125 Camilleri, J. (2008). Characterization of hydration products of mineral trioxide aggregate. *Int. Endod. J.* 41 (5): 408–417.

126 Taylor, H.F.W. (1997). *Cement Chemistry*. London: Thomas Telford.

127 Odler, I. (1998). Hydration, setting and hardening of Portland cement. In: *Lea's Chemistry of Cement and Concrete* (ed. P.C. Hewlett), 241–284. London: Edward Arnold.

128 Moir, G.K. (2003). Cements. In: *Advanced Concrete Technology; Constituent Materials* (eds. J. Newman and B.S. Choo), 3–45. Oxford: Elsevier Butterworth Heinemann.

129 Winter, N.B. (2012). *Scanning Electron Microscopy of Cement and Concrete*. Woodbridge: WHD Microanalysis Consultants.

130 Camilleri, J., Formosa, L., and Damidot, D. (2013). The setting characteristics of MTA Plus in different environmental conditions. *Int. Endod. J.* 46 (9): 831–840.

131 Kim, Y., Kim, S., Shin, Y.S. et al. (2012). Failure of setting of mineral trioxide aggregate in the presence of fetal bovine serum and its prevention. *J. Endod.* 38 (4): 536–540.

132 Kang, J.S., Rhim, E.M., Huh, S.Y. et al. (2012). The effects of humidity and serum on the surface microhardness and morphology of five retrograde filling materials. *Scanning* 34 (4): 207–214.

133 Nekoofar, M.H., Davies, T.E., Stone, D. et al. (2011). Microstructure and chemical analysis of blood-contaminated mineral trioxide aggregate. *Int. Endod. J.* 44 (11): 1011–1018.

134 Song, M., Yue, W., Kim, S. et al. (2016). The effect of human blood on the setting and surface micro-hardness of calcium silicate cements. *Clin. Oral Investig.* 20 (8): 1997–2005.

135 Camilleri, J. (2010). Evaluation of the physical properties of an endodontic Portland cement incorporating alternative radiopacifiers used as root-end filling material. *Int. Endod. J.* 43 (3): 231–240.

136 Cutajar, A., Mallia, B., Abela, S., and Camilleri, J. (2011). Replacement of radiopacifier in mineral trioxide aggregate; characterization and determination of physical properties. *Dent. Mater.* 27 (9): 879–891.

137 Islam, I., Chng, H.K., and Yap, A.U. (2006). Comparison of the physical and mechanical properties of MTA and Portland cement. *J. Endod.* 32 (3): 193–197.

138 Danesh, G., Dammaschke, T., Gerth, H.U. et al. (2006). A comparative study of

selected properties of ProRoot mineral trioxide aggregate and two Portland cements. *Int. Endod. J.* 39 (3): 213–219.

139 Poggio, C., Lombardini, M., Alessandro, C., and Simonetta, R. (2007). Solubility of root-end-filling materials: a comparative study. *J. Endod.* 33 (9): 1094–1097.

140 Fridland, M. and Rosado, R. (2003). Mineral trioxide aggregate (MTA) solubility and porosity with different water-to-powder ratios. *J. Endod.* 29 (12): 814–817.

141 Fridland, M. and Rosado, R. (2005). MTA solubility: a long term study. *J. Endod.* 31 (5): 376–379.

142 Cavenago, B.C., Pereira, T.C., Duarte, M.A. et al. (2014). Influence of powder-to-water ratio on radiopacity, setting time, pH, calcium ion release and a micro-CT volumetric solubility of white mineral trioxide aggregate. *Int. Endod. J.* 47 (2): 120–126.

143 Camilleri, J. (2011). Evaluation of the effect of intrinsic material properties and ambient conditions on the dimensional stability of white mineral trioxide aggregate and Portland cement. *J. Endod.* 37 (2): 239–245.

144 Saghiri, M.A., Ricci, J., Daliri Joupari, M. et al. (2011). A comparative study of MTA solubility in various media. *Iran Endod. J.* 6 (1): 21–24.

145 Samiei, M., Shahi, S., Aslaminabadi, N. et al. (2015). A new simulated plasma for assessing the solubility of mineral trioxide aggregate. *Iran Endod. J.* 10 (1): 30–34.

146 Bortoluzzi, E.A., Cassel de Araújo, T., Carolina Corrêa Néis, A. et al. (2019). Effect of different water-to-powder ratios on the dimensional stability and compressive strength of mineral aggregate-based cements. *Eur. Oral Res.* 53 (2): 94–98.

147 Formosa, L.M., Mallia, B., and Camilleri, J. (2012). The effect of curing conditions on the physical properties of tricalcium silicate cement for use as a dental biomaterial. *Int. Endod. J.* 45 (4): 326–336.

148 Porter, M.L., Bertó, A., Primus, C.M., and Watanabe, I. (2010). Physical and chemical properties of new-generation endodontic materials. *J. Endod.* 36 (3): 524–528.

149 Choi, Y., Park, S.J., Lee, S.H. et al. (2013). Biological effects and washout resistance of a newly developed fast-setting pozzolan cement. *J. Endod.* 39 (4): 467–472.

150 Formosa, L.M., Mallia, B., and Camilleri, J. (2013). Mineral trioxide aggregate with anti-washout gel – properties and microstructure. *Dent. Mater.* 29 (3): 294–306.

151 Lenherr, P., Allgayer, N., Weiger, R. et al. (2012). Tooth discoloration induced by endodontic materials: a laboratory study. *Int. Endod. J.* 45 (10): 942–949.

152 Vallés, M., Mercadé, M., Duran-Sindreu, F. et al. (2013). Color stability of white mineral trioxide aggregate. *Clin. Oral Investig.* 17 (4): 1155–1159.

153 Camargo, C.H., Fonseca, M.B., Carvalho, A.S. et al. (2012). Microhardness and sealing ability of materials used for root canal perforations. *Gen. Dent.* 60 (6): e393–e397.

154 Camilleri, J., Kralj, P., Veber, M., and Sinagra, E. (2012). Characterization and analyses of acid-extractable and leached trace elements in dental cements. *Int. Endod. J.* 45 (8): 737–743.

155 Camilleri, J., Sorrentino, F., and Damidot, D. (2013). Investigation of the hydration and bioactivity of radiopacified tricalcium silicate cement, Biodentine and MTA Angelus. *Dent. Mater.* 29 (5): 580–593.

156 Vivan, R.R., Ordinola-Zapata, R., Bramante, C.M. et al. (2009). Evaluation of the radiopacity of some commercial and experimental root-end filling materials. *Oral Surg. Oral Med. Oral Pathol. Oral Radiol. Endod.* 108 (6): e35–e38.

157 Galarça, A.D., Da Rosa, W.L.O., Da Silva, T.M. et al. (2018). Physical and biological properties of a high-plasticity tricalcium silicate cement. *Biomed. Res. Int.* 2018: 8063262.

158 Guimarães, B.M., Vivan, R.R., Piazza, B. et al. (2017). Chemical-physical properties and apatite-forming ability of mineral trioxide aggregate flow. *J. Endod.* 43 (10): 1692–1696.

159 Khalil, I., Naaman, A., and Camilleri, J. (2015). Investigation of a novel mechanically mixed mineral trioxide aggregate (MM-MTA(™)). *Int. Endod. J.* 48 (8): 757–767.

160 Bernardi, A., Bortoluzzi, E.A., Felippe, W.T. et al. (2017). Effects of the addition of nanoparticulate calcium carbonate on setting time, dimensional change, compressive strength, solubility and pH of MTA. *Int. Endod. J.* 50 (1): 97–105.

161 Wiltbank, K.B., Schwartz, S.A., and Schindler, W.G. (2007). Effect of selected accelerants on the physical properties of mineral trioxide aggregate and Portland cement. *J. Endod.* 33 (10): 1235–1238.

162 Bortoluzzi, E.A., Broon, N.J., Bramante, C.M. et al. (2009). The influence of calcium chloride on the setting time, solubility, disintegration, and pH of mineral trioxide aggregate and white Portland cement with a radiopacifier. *J. Endod.* 35 (4): 550–554.

163 Camilleri, J. and Dummer, P.M.H. (2014). Reactivity and environmental factors. In: *Mineral Trioxide Aggregate in Dentistry: From Preparation to Application* (ed. J. Camilleri), 87–102. Philadelphia, PA: Springer.

164 Meschi, N., Li, X., Van Gorp, G. et al. (2019). Bioactivity potential of Portland cement in regenerative endodontic procedures: from clinic to lab. *Dent. Mater.* 35 (9): 1342–1350.

165 Kebudi Benezra, M., Schembri Wismayer, P., and Camilleri, J. (2017). Influence of environment on testing of hydraulic sealers. *Sci. Rep.* 7: 17927.

166 Camilleri, J., Montesin, F.E., Di Silvio, L., and Pitt Ford, T.R. (2005). The constitution and biocompatibility of accelerated Portland cement for endodontic use. *Int. Endod. J.* 38: 834–842.

167 Camilleri, J., Montesin, F.E., Papaioannou, S. et al. (2004). Biocompatibility of two commercial forms of mineral trioxide aggregate. *Int. Endod. J.* 37: 699–704.

168 Camilleri, J., Montesin, F.E., Brady, K. et al. (2005). The constitution of mineral trioxide aggregate. *Dent. Mater.* 21: 297–303.

169 Osorio, R.M., Hefti, A., Vertucci, F.J., and Shawley, A.L. (1998). Cytotoxicity of endodontic materials. *J. Endod.* 24 (2): 91–96.

170 Keiser, K., Johnson, C.C., and Tipton, D.A. (2000). Cytotoxicity of mineral trioxide aggregate using human periodontal ligament fibroblasts. *J. Endod.* 26 (5): 288–291.

171 Yan, P., Yuan, Z., Jiang, H. et al. (2010). Effect of bioaggregate on differentiation of human periodontal ligament fibroblasts. *Int. Endod. J.* 43 (12): 1116–1121.

172 Kim, E.C., Lee, B.C., Chang, H.S. et al. (2008). Evaluation of the radiopacity and cytotoxicity of Portland cements containing bismuth oxide. *Oral Surg. Oral Med. Oral Pathol. Oral Radiol. Endod.* 105 (1): e54–e57.

173 Braz, M.G., Camargo, E.A., Salvadori, D.M. et al. (2006). Evaluation of genetic damage in human peripheral lymphocytes exposed to mineral trioxide aggregate and Portland cements. *J. Oral Rehabil.* 33 (3): 234–239.

174 Al-Rabeah, E., Perinpanayagam, H., and MacFarland, D. (2006). Human alveolar bone cells interact with ProRoot and tooth-colored MTA. *J. Endod.* 32 (9): 872–875.

175 Perinpanayagam, H. and Al-Rabeah, E. (2009). Osteoblasts interact with MTA surfaces and express Runx2. *Oral Surg. Oral Med. Oral Pathol. Oral Radiol. Endod.* 107 (4): 590–596.

176 Bidar, M., Zarrabi, M.H., Tavakol Afshari, J. et al. (2011). Osteoblastic cytokine response to gray and white mineral trioxide aggregate. *Iran Endod. J.* 6 (3): 111–115.

177 Ma, J., Shen, Y., Stojicic, S., and Haapasalo, M. (2011). Biocompatibility of two novel root repair materials. *J. Endod.* 37 (6): 793–798.

178 Willershausen, I., Wolf, T., Kasaj, A. et al. (2013). Influence of a bioceramic root end material and mineral trioxide aggregates on fibroblasts and osteoblasts. *Arch. Oral Biol.* 58 (9): 1232–1237.

179 Samara, A., Sarri, Y., Stravopodis, D. et al. (2011). A comparative study of the effects of three root-end filling materials on proliferation and adherence of human periodontal ligament fibroblasts. *J. Endod.* 37 (6): 865–870.

180 Lee, B.N., Lee, K.N., Koh, J.T. et al. (2014). Effects of 3 endodontic bioactive cements on osteogenic differentiation in mesenchymal stem cells. *J. Endod.* 40 (8): 1217–1222.

181 Huang, T.H., Yang, C.C., Ding, S.J. et al. (2005). Biocompatibility of human osteosarcoma cells to root end filling materials. *J. Biomed. Mater. Res. B. Appl. Biomater.* 72 (1): 140–145.

182 Huang, T.H., Yang, C.C., Ding, S.J. et al. (2005). Inflammatory cytokines reaction elicited by root-end filling materials. *J. Biomed. Mater. Res. B. Appl. Biomater.* 73 (1): 123–128.

183 Garcia Lda, F., Huck, C., Menezes de Oliveira, L. et al. (2014). Biocompatibility of new calcium aluminate cement: tissue reaction and expression of inflammatory mediators and cytokines. *J. Endod.* 40 (12): 2024–2029.

184 Makkar, H., Verma, S.K., Panda, P.K. et al. (2018). In vivo molecular toxicity profile of dental bioceramics in embryonic zebrafish (*Danio rerio*). *Chem. Res. Toxicol.* 31 (9): 914–923.

185 Silva, E.J., Senna, P.M., De-Deus, G., and Zaia, A.A. (2016). Cytocompatibility of Biodentine using a three-dimensional cell culture model. *Int. Endod. J.* 49 (6): 574–580.

186 Rifaey, H.S., Villa, M., Zhu, Q. et al. (2016). Comparison of the osteogenic potential of mineral trioxide aggregate and Endosequence root repair material in a

3-dimensional culture system. *J. Endod.* 42 (5): 760–765.

187 Asrari, M. and Lobner, D. (2003). In vitro neurotoxic evaluation of root-end-filling materials. *J. Endod.* 29 (11): 743–746.

188 Ribeiro, D.A., Duarte, M.A., Matsumoto, M.A. et al. (2005). Biocompatibility in vitro tests of mineral trioxide aggregate and regular and white Portland cements. *J. Endod.* 31 (8): 605–607.

189 Ribeiro, D.A., Sugui, M.M., Matsumoto, M.A. et al. (2006). Genotoxicity and cytotoxicity of mineral trioxide aggregate and regular and white Portland cements on Chinese hamster ovary (CHO) cells in vitro. *Oral Surg. Oral Med. Oral Pathol. Oral Radiol. Endod.* 101 (2): 258–261.

190 Khalil, W.A. and Abunasef, S.K. (2015). Can mineral trioxide aggregate and nanoparticulate EndoSequence root repair material produce injurious effects to rat subcutaneous tissues? *J. Endod.* 41 (7): 1151–1156.

191 Dreger, L.A., Felippe, W.T., Reyes-Carmona, J.F. et al. (2012). Mineral trioxide aggregate and Portland cement promote biomineralization in vivo. *J. Endod.* 38 (3): 324–329.

192 Reyes-Carmona, J.F., Santos, A.S., Figueiredo, C.P. et al. (2010). Host-mineral trioxide aggregate inflammatory molecular signaling and biomineralization ability. *J. Endod.* 36 (8): 1347–1353.

193 Moretton, T.R., Brown, C.E. Jr., Legan, J.J., and Kafrawy, A.H. (2000). Tissue reactions after subcutaneous and intraosseous implantation of mineral trioxide aggregate and ethoxybenzoic acid cement. *J. Biomed. Mater. Res.* 52 (3): 528–533.

194 Sousa, C.J., Loyola, A.M., Versiani, M.A. et al. (2004). A comparative histological evaluation of the biocompatibility of materials used in apical surgery. *Int. Endod. J.* 37 (11): 738–748.

195 Torabinejad, M., Hong, C.U., Lee, S.J. et al. (1995). Investigation of mineral trioxide

aggregate for root-end filling in dogs. *J. Endod.* 21 (12): 603–608.

196 Silva, L.A.B., Pieroni, K.A.M.G., Nelson-Filho, P. et al. (2017). Furcation perforation: periradicular tissue response to biodentine as a repair material by histopathologic and indirect immunofluorescence analyses. *J. Endod.* 43 (7): 1137–1142.

197 Holland, R., Filho, J.A., de Souza, V. et al. (2001). Mineral trioxide aggregate repair of lateral root perforations. *J. Endod.* 27 (4): 281–284.

198 Holland, R., Bisco Ferreira, L., de Souza, V. et al. (2007). Reaction of the lateral periodontium of dogs' teeth to contaminated and noncontaminated perforations filled with mineral trioxide aggregate. *J. Endod.* 33 (10): 1192–1197.

199 Gomes Filho, J.E., Queiroz, Í.O., Watanabe, S. et al. (2016). Influence of diabetes mellitus on the mineralization ability of two endodontic materials. *Braz. Oral Res.* 30: S1806-83242016000100218.

200 Martins, C.M., Gomes-Filho, J.E., de Azevedo Queiroz, Í.O. et al. (2016). Hypertension undermines mineralization-inducing capacity of and tissue response to mineral trioxide aggregate endodontic cement. *J. Endod.* 42 (4): 604–609.

201 Cosme-Silva, L., Dal-Fabbro, R., Gonçalves, L.O. et al. (2019). Hypertension affects the biocompatibility and biomineralization of MTA, high-plasticity MTA, and Biodentine®. *Braz. Oral Res.* 33: e060.

202 Garcia, L.D.F.R., Huck, C., Magalhães, F.A.C. et al. (2017). Systemic effect of mineral aggregate-based cements: histopathological analysis in rats. *J. Appl. Oral Sci.* 25 (6): 620–630.

203 Khalil, W.A. and Eid, N.F. (2013). Biocompatibility of BioAggregate and mineral trioxide aggregate on the liver and kidney. *Int. Endod. J.* 46 (8): 730–737.

204 Demirkaya, K., Can Demirdöğen, B., Öncel Torun, Z. et al. (2016). In vivo evaluation of the effects of hydraulic calcium silicate dental cements on plasma and liver aluminium levels in rats. *Eur. J. Oral Sci.* 124 (1): 75–81.

205 Demirkaya, K., Demirdöğen, B.C., Torun, Z.Ö. et al. (2017). Brain aluminium accumulation and oxidative stress in the presence of calcium silicate dental cements. *Hum. Exp. Toxicol.* 36 (10): 1071–1080.

206 Simsek, N., Bulut, E.T., Ahmetoğlu, F., and Alan, H. (2016). Determination of trace elements in rat organs implanted with endodontic repair materials by ICP-MS. *J. Mater. Sci. Mater. Med.* 27 (3): 46.

207 Tanomaru-Filho, M., Andrade, A.S., Rodrigues, E.M. et al. (2017). Biocompatibility and mineralized nodule formation of Neo MTA Plus and an experimental tricalcium silicate cement containing tantalum oxide. *Int. Endod. J.* 50 (Suppl. 2): e31–e39.

208 Torabinejad, M., Hong, C.U., Pitt Ford, T.R., and Kettering, J.D. (1995). Antibacterial effects of some root end filling materials. *J. Endod.* 21 (8): 403–406.

209 Farrugia, C., Baca, P., Camilleri, J., and Arias Moliz, M.T. (2017). Antimicrobial activity of ProRoot MTA in contact with blood. *Sci. Rep.* 7: 41359.

210 Koutroulis, A., Batchelor, H., Kuehne, S.A. et al. (2019). Investigation of the effect of the water to powder ratio on hydraulic cement properties. *Dent. Mater.* 35 (8): 1146–1154.

211 Nekoofar, M.H., Haddad, D.C., Nolde, J., and Aseeley, Z. (2009). Water content of ampoule packaged with ProRoot MTA. *Int. Endod. J.* 42 (6): 549–551; author reply 552–553.

212 Shahi, S., Ghasemi, N., Rahimi, S. et al. (2015). The effect of different mixing methods on the pH and solubility of mineral trioxide aggregate and calcium-enriched mixture. *Iran Endod. J.* 10 (2): 140–143.

213 Saghiri, M.A., Garcia-Godoy, F., Gutmann, J.L. et al. (2014). Effects of various mixing techniques on physical properties of white mineral trioxide aggregate. *Dent. Traumatol.* 30 (3): 240–245.

214 Parashos, P., Phoon, A., and Sathorn, C. (2014). Effect of ultrasonication on physical properties of mineral trioxide aggregate. *Biomed. Res. Int.* 2014: 191984.

215 Nekoofar, M.H., Adusei, G., Sheykhrezae, M.S. et al. (2007). The effect of condensation pressure on selected physical properties of mineral trioxide aggregate. *Int. Endod. J.* 40 (6): 453–461.

216 Camilleri, J. (2011). Scanning electron microscopic evaluation of the material interface of adjacent layers of dental materials. *Dent. Mater.* 27 (9): 870–878.

217 Tsujimoto, M., Tsujimoto, Y., Ookubo, A. et al. (2013). Timing for composite resin placement on mineral trioxide aggregate. *J. Endod.* 39 (9): 1167–1170.

218 Kazemipoor, M., Azizi, N., and Farahat, F. (2018). Evaluation of microhardness of mineral trioxide aggregate after immediate placement of different coronal restorations: an in vitro study. *J. Dent. (Tehran).* 15 (2): 116–122.

219 Ballal, N.V., Sona, M., and Tay, F.R. (2017). Effects of smear layer removal agents on the physical properties and microstructure of mineral trioxide aggregate cement. *J. Dent.* 66: 32–36.

220 Lee, Y.L., Lin, F.H., Wang, W.H. et al. (2007). Effects of EDTA on the hydration mechanism of mineral trioxide aggregate. *J. Dent. Res.* 86 (6): 534–538.

221 Chu, J.H.R., Chia, K.Y., Qui, A.L. et al. (2020). The effects of sodium hypochlorite and ethylenediaminetetraacetic acid on the microhardness of Mineral Trioxide Aggregate and TotalFill Bioceramic Putty. *Aust. Endod. J.* 46 (1): 33–39.

222 Nekoofar, M.H., Oloomi, K., Sheykhrezae, M.S. et al. (2010). An evaluation of the effect of blood and human serum on the surface microhardness and surface microstructure of mineral trioxide aggregate. *Int. Endod. J.* 43 (10): 849–858.

223 Nekoofar, M.H., Stone, D.F., and Dummer, P.M. (2010). The effect of blood contamination on the compressive strength and surface microstructure of mineral trioxide aggregate. *Int. Endod. J.* 43 (9): 782–791.

224 Ramachandran, V.S. (1992). Interaction of admixtures in the cement–water system. In: *Application of Admixtures in Concrete*, 1e. Rilem Report no. 10 (eds. A.M.E. Paillere and F.N. Spon). London: CRC Press.

225 Storm, B., Eichmiller, F.C., Tordik, P.A., and Goodell, G.G. (2008). Setting expansion of gray and white mineral trioxide aggregate and Portland cement. *J. Endod.* 34 (1): 80–82.

226 Schembri Wismayer, P., Lung, C.Y., Rappa, F. et al. (2016). Assessment of the interaction of Portland cement-based materials with blood and tissue fluids using an animal model. *Sci. Rep.* 6: 34547.

227 Guimarães, B.M., Tartari, T., Marciano, M.A. et al. (2015). Color stability, radiopacity, and chemical characteristics of white mineral trioxide aggregate associated with 2 different vehicles in contact with blood. *J. Endod.* 41 (6): 947–952.

228 Sarkar, N.K., Caicedo, R., Ritwik, P. et al. (2005). Physicochemical basis of the biologic properties of mineral trioxide aggregate. *J. Endod.* 31: 97–100.

229 Tay, F.R., Pashley, D.H., Rueggeberg, F.A. et al. (2007). Calcium phosphate phase transformation produced by the interaction of the Portland cement component of white mineral trioxide aggregate with a phosphate-containing fluid. *J. Endod.* 33: 1347–1351.

230 Bozeman, T.B., Lemon, R.R., and Eleazer, P.D. (2006). Elemental analysis of crystal precipitate from gray and white MTA. *J. Endod.* 32 (5): 425–428.

231 Han, L. and Okiji, T. (2013). Bioactivity evaluation of three calcium silicate-based endodontic materials. *Int. Endod. J.* 46 (9): 808–814.

232 Reyes-Carmona, J.F., Felippe, M.S., and Felippe, W.T. (2010). The biomineralization ability of mineral trioxide aggregate and Portland cement on dentin enhances the push-out strength. *J. Endod.* 36 (2): 286–291.

233 Bohner, M. and Lemaitre, J. (2009). Can bioactivity be tested in vitro with SBF solution? *Biomaterials* 30: 2175–2179.

234 Ghoddusi, J., Sanaan, A., and Shahrami, F. (2007). Clinical and radiographic evaluation of root perforation repair using MTA. *N. Y. State Dent. J.* 73 (3): 46–49.

235 Saunders, W.P. (2008). A prospective clinical study of periradicular surgery using mineral trioxide aggregate as a root-end filling. *J. Endod.* 34 (6): 660–665.

236 Christiansen, R., Kirkevang, L.L., Hørsted-Bindslev, P., and Wenzel, A. (2009). Randomized clinical trial of root-end resection followed by root-end filling with mineral trioxide aggregate or smoothing of the orthograde gutta-percha root filling--1-year follow-up. *Int. Endod. J.* 42 (2): 105–114.

237 Kruse, C., Spin-Neto, R., Christiansen, R. et al. (2016). Periapical bone healing after apicectomy with and without retrograde root filling with mineral trioxide aggregate: a 6-year follow-up of a randomized controlled trial. *J. Endod.* 42 (4): 533–537.

238 Camilleri, J. (2011). Characterization and hydration kinetics of tricalcium silicate cement for use as a dental biomaterial. *Dent. Mater.* 27 (8): 836–844.

239 Schembri-Wismayer, P. and Camilleri, J. (2017). Why biphasic? Assessment of the effect on cell proliferation and expression. *J. Endod.* 43 (5): 751–759.

240 Charland, T., Hartwell, G.R., Hirschberg, C., and Patel, R. (2013). An evaluation of setting time of mineral trioxide aggregate and EndoSequence root repair material in the presence of human blood and minimal essential media. *J. Endod.* 39 (8): 1071–1072.

241 Guo, Y.J., Du, T.F., Li, H.B. et al. (2016). Physical properties and hydration behavior of a fast-setting bioceramic endodontic material. *BMC Oral Health.* 16: 23.

242 Lee, G.W., Yoon, J.H., Jang, J.H. et al. (2019). Effects of newly-developed retrograde filling material on osteoblastic differentiation in vitro. *Dent. Mater. J.* 38 (4): 528–533.

243 Walsh, R.M., Woodmansey, K.F., Glickman, G.N., and He, J. (2014). Evaluation of compressive strength of hydraulic silicate-based root-end filling materials. *J. Endod.* 40 (7): 969–972.

244 Kohli, M.R., Yamaguchi, M., Setzer, F.C., and Karabucak, B. (2015). Spectrophotometric analysis of coronal tooth discoloration induced by various bioceramic cements and other endodontic materials. *J. Endod.* 41 (11): 1862–1866.

245 Shokouhinejad, N., Nekoofar, M.H., Pirmoazen, S. et al. (2016). Evaluation and comparison of occurrence of tooth discoloration after the application of various calcium silicate-based cements: an ex vivo study. *J. Endod.* 42 (1): 140–144.

246 Damas, B.A., Wheater, M.A., Bringas, J.S., and Hoen, M.M. (2011). Cytotoxicity comparison of mineral trioxide aggregates and EndoSequence bioceramic root repair materials. *J. Endod.* 37 (3): 372–375.

247 Coaguila-Llerena, H., Vaisberg, A., and Velásquez-Huamán, Z. (2016). In vitro cytotoxicity evaluation of three root-end filling materials in human periodontal ligament fibroblasts. *Braz. Dent. J.* 27 (2): 187–191.

248 Edrees, H.Y., Abu Zeid, S.T.H., Atta, H.M., and AlQriqri, M.A. (2019). Induction of osteogenic differentiation of mesenchymal stem cells by bioceramic root repair material. *Materials (Basel)* 12 (14): E2311.

249 Chen, I., Karabucak, B., Wang, C. et al. (2015). Healing after root-end microsurgery by using mineral trioxide aggregate and a new calcium silicate-based bioceramic material as root-end filling materials in dogs. *J. Endod.* 41 (3): 389–399.

250 Damlar, I., Ozcan, E., Yula, E. et al. (2014). Antimicrobial effects of several calcium silicate-based root-end filling materials. *Dent. Mater. J.* 33 (4): 453–457.

251 Lovato, K.F. and Sedgley, C.M. (2011). Antibacterial activity of endosequence root repair material and proroot MTA against clinical isolates of Enterococcus faecalis. *J. Endod.* 37 (11): 1542–1546.

252 Moinzadeh, A.T., Aznar Portoles, C., Schembri Wismayer, P., and Camilleri, J. (2016). Bioactivity potential of EndoSequence BC RRM putty. *J. Endod.* 42 (4): 615–621.

253 Alsubait, S.A. (2017). Effect of sodium hypochlorite on push-out bond strength of four calcium silicate-based endodontic materials when used for repairing perforations on human dentin: an in vitro evaluation. *J. Contemp. Dent. Pract.* 18 (4): 289–294.

254 Kadić, S., Baraba, A., Miletić, I. et al. (2018). Push-out bond strength of three different calcium silicate-based root-end filling materials after ultrasonic retrograde cavity preparation. *Clin. Oral Investig.* 22 (3): 1559–1565.

255 Zhou, W., Zheng, Q., Tan, X. et al. (2017). Comparison of mineral trioxide aggregate and iRoot BP plus root repair material as root-end filling materials in endodontic microsurgery: a prospective randomized controlled study. *J. Endod.* 43 (1): 1–6.

256 Safi, C., Kohli, M.R., Kratchman, S.I. et al. (2019). Outcome of endodontic microsurgery using mineral trioxide aggregate or root repair material as root-end filling material: a randomized controlled trial with cone-beam computed tomographic evaluation. *J. Endod.* 45 (7): 831–839.

257 Shinbori, N., Grama, A.M., Patel, Y. et al. (2015). Clinical outcome of endodontic microsurgery that uses EndoSequence BC root repair material as the root-end filling material. *J. Endod.* 41 (5): 607–612.

8

Materials and Clinical Techniques for Endodontic Therapy of Deciduous Teeth

Nastaran Meschi, Mostafa EzEldeen, Gertrude Van Gorp, and Paul Lambrechts

Department of Oral Health Sciences, KU Leuven & Dentistry, University Hospitals Leuven, Leuven, Belgium

---

TABLE OF CONTENTS

8.1 Introduction

The necessity of guiding the primary dentition in order to reduce or eliminate functional disorders in the permanent teeth underlines the importance of paediatric dentistry. Morphological differences from the permanent dentition, such as a thinner enamel and wider pulp chamber, render deciduous teeth more prone to pulpal inflammation in cases of carious lesions and traumatic dental injuries. The treatment and preservation of diseased primary teeth aim to fulfil the following objectives: (i) enhancement of aesthetics and mastication; (ii) preservation of arch space, since premature loss of primary teeth may cause aberration of the arch length, resulting in mesial drift of the permanent teeth and consequent malocclusion; (iii) prevention of abnormal tongue habits and promotion of proper speech; and (iv) prevention of the psychological effects associated with tooth loss [1]. The ultimate goal is to preserve the deciduous teeth until the point of physiological exfoliation. An arsenal of treatment modalities has been developed to this end. Compliance of children and their parents or guardians, field isolation, magnification, a tight coronal seal, and biocompatible, nonallergenic, and easily applicable biomaterials are all indispensable in paediatric endodontics. The paediatric clinician requires not only knowledge of endodontic filling materials and a well-considered assessment of the treatment protocol, but also well-developed clinical and behavioural skills.

Endodontic Materials in Clinical Practice, First Edition. Edited by Josette Camilleri.
© 2021 John Wiley & Sons Ltd. Published 2021 by John Wiley & Sons Ltd.

This chapter summarizes the properties and clinical applications of the current most applied endodontic filling materials used in deciduous teeth. Clinical cases with long-term follow-up will highlight their technical applicability and outcomes.

8.2 The Primary Dentine–Pulp Complex

The pulp of a primary tooth is histologically similar to that of a permanent one [2]. However, the mesenchymal stem cells available in deciduous teeth – the stem cells of human exfoliated deciduous teeth (SHED) – can differentiate amongst others into neural cells and odontoblasts. Additionally, SHED have the highest multipotency and proliferative capacity of all adult mesenchymal cells investigated to date [3]. This is of paramount importance, as any external factor affecting the dentine will subsequently affect the pulp. Even if the primary dentine–pulp complex response to external stimuli is similar to that of the permanent dentition (namely a reduction in the number of odontoblasts and increase in the number of inflammatory cells), the high proliferative potential of SHED will favour healing of the injury. On one hand, the main factor affecting the dental pulp is bacterial infection via trauma, caries, or microleakage at the restorative material margins [2]. On the other, the toxicity of dental restorative materials is deleterious for the pulp as well. The remaining dentine thickness (RDT) acts as a buffer for the pulp, defines the depth of bacterial penetration, and hence defines the degree of pulpal inflammation. When decay is extended for more than 50% of dentine thickness, more extensive pulpal inflammation is noted for proximal as compared to occlusal carious lesions with similar depth [4]. However, the pulpal diagnosis for primary teeth is less reliable than that for mature permanent teeth, as young patients are less responsive on pulp vitality assessment than adults [5]. Pulp vitality assessment involves

pain history and clinical and radiographic examination. For carious lesions implying a deep cavity preparation (RDT < 0.5 mm), the treatment indication depends on the clinical and radiographic assessment. Clinically asymptomatic primary teeth with no lesion periapically or on the furcation level have in general solely coronally inflamed vital pulps and can be saved by indirect pulp treatment or pulpotomy – vital pulp therapy (VPT) techniques (Figure 8.1) [6]. Direct pulp capping of an exposed pulp due to a deep carious lesion is contraindicated in deciduous teeth [7]. If deep carious lesions evoke clinical or radiographic signs, then pulpectomy or extraction is more appropriate, depending on the stage of root resorption (Figure 8.1).

8.3 Pulp Treatments in Deciduous Teeth

8.3.1 Vital Pulp Therapy

8.3.1.1 Incomplete Caries Removal
If a deciduous tooth with a deep carious lesion (RDT < 0.5 mm) is clinically asymptomatic and no bone loss (periapical and on furcation level) is visible radiographically, attempts can be made to keep the pulp vital (Figure 8.1). The International Caries Consensus Collaboration (ICCC) recommends treating deep cavities either biologically by means of selective caries removal to the deepest soft dentine or using the Hall technique, in order to avoid pulp exposure [8]. Direct pulp capping due to a small pulp exposure after complete caries excavation in deciduous teeth has less reliable results than pulpotomy and is thus contraindicated [7]. The Hall technique involves no caries excavation; instead, a stainless-steel crown is emplaced to stop the carious process [9]. In case of selective caries removal, indirect pulp treatment can be performed by means of stepwise excavation (two sessions) or incomplete caries removal (one session). In both treatment modalities, caries is removed on the coronal cavity walls until

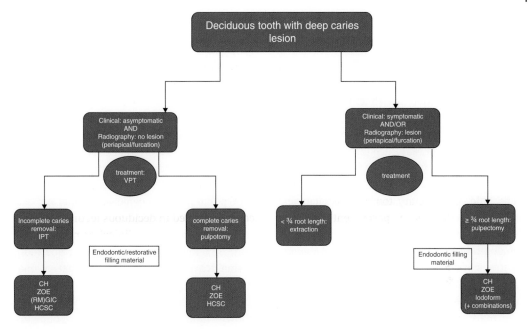

Figure 8.1 Treatment decision tree for deciduous teeth with deep carious lesions, with recommended endodontic/restorative filling material.

hard dentine is reached, in order to allow a good adhesion with the restorative material. Furthermore, the soft dentine on the pulpal floor is left untouched. In cases of stepwise excavation, 8–12 weeks after the first session, the temporary filling is removed and the carious lesion on the pulpal floor is reentered until firm dentine is reached. This reduces the chance of pulp exposure, but working in two sessions requires more compliance from the patient [10]. Field isolation is always recommended unless it is not accepted by the young patient. Magnification by means of loupes or an operating microscope is advisable. In deprived communities, or where there is anxiety over drilling, atraumatic restorative treatment (ART) can be performed [11]. This involves caries removal by means of manual instruments, often without local anaesthetics.

As bacterial infection is a critical aetiological factor in pulp necrosis, the restorative methods and materials applied in VPT must reduce or eliminate bacteria. In order to obtain an optimal adhesion with the restorative material, dentine conditioning is advisable.

Cleaning of the debris produced during caries removal is possible via application of ethylenediaminetetraacetic acid (EDTA), phosphoric acid, or polyacrylic acid. Due to the chelation of calcium promoted by EDTA and the surface etching caused by all acids, growth factors embedded in the dentine (e.g. transforming growth factor beta-1 (TGF-β1) and vascular endothelial growth factor (VEGF)) are released [12, 13], triggering odontoblasts to form tertiary dentine.

Controversy exists over the disinfection of the cavity. The ICCC states that there is no evidence to support the use of cavity disinfectants, as the application of etching agents such as 37% phosphoric acid is enough to remove the smear layer and reduce the number of bacteria left in the prepared cavity [8]. Nevertheless, etching of the soft dentine in deep carious lesions is not advisable. This thin demineralized dentine layer is not an adequate buffer for the pulp against the acidity of etching agents and the toxicity of restorative materials. Hence, a biocompatible buffer should be placed underneath the restorative material, or else the restorative material itself should be biocompatible.

8.3.1.2 Complete Caries Removal

Pulpotomy is the most common treatment for cariously exposed pulps in clinically symptom-free primary molars. Radiographically, no internal or external root resorption, furcation, or periapical radiolucency should be visible (Figure 8.1) [1, 6, 14]. Magnification by means of loupes or an operating microscope is advisable. After administration of local anaesthetic and rubber dam isolation, all caries is removed with a high-speed access bur (round end cutting tapered diamond bur) and copious water spray. After lowering the cusps (to remove all undercuts and provide optimal access to the pulp chamber), the entire roof of the pulp chamber is cut away with another high-speed access bur (round end cutting tapered diamond bur) to avoid carrying bacteria from the carious lesion to the pulp chamber. Copious water spray is used. Coronal pulp is then removed with a #6 or #8 round bur on a slow-speed handpiece or with a spoon excavator. The pulp chamber is thoroughly washed with sodium hypochlorite 2.5% to remove all debris and dried by aspiration (without air) and application of sterile paper points #130 or #140. Haemorrhage is controlled by use of thick paper points #130 or #140 or a sterile cotton pellet placed against the stumps of the pulp at the openings of the root canals (Figure 8.2).

Pulpotomy can be classified into three main approaches, depending on the material used: (i) preservation of the radicular pulp in a healthy state (by use of ferric sulphate (FS)); (ii) fixation of the radicular pulp by rendering it inert (by use of formocresol (FC); also known as Sweet's technique [15]); and (iii) encouragement of tissue regeneration and healing at the site of radicular pulp amputation (by use of biocompatible materials) [1, 14, 16].

FS is increasingly used, due to its haemostatic effect, ease of use, low cost, and good long-term success [14, 17]. It shows a clinical success rate ranging between 78 and 100% and a radiographic success rate between 74 and 100% [14, 16, 18, 19]. Moreover, the success of FS pulpotomy is dependent on the type of cement (pulpotomy base) used to fill the pulp chamber.

Historically, FC was the material of choice as a pulpotomy base in primary molars. It had a clinical success rate ranging between 83 and 100% and a radiographic success rate between 77 and 100% [14, 18]. However, studies have shown that it is mutagenic, genotoxic, and carcinogenic [20–23]. FC is a solution of cresol 35% and formaldehyde 19% in a vehicle of glycerine 15% and water (Buckley's formocresol). Formaldehyde is classified by the International Agency for Research on Cancer (IARC), part of the World Health Organization (WHO), as a known human carcinogen [24]. Following reports of wide systemic distribution of the medicament after application [1, 14], it has been replaced by other materials.

A biocompatible material is placed at the site of radicular pulp amputation in order to encourage tissue regeneration and healing [1, 14, 16]. Afterwards, the tooth is restored by means of a glass ionomer cement (GIC) or composite restoration or else by a stainless-steel crown, depending on the restorability of the tooth structure and the caries risk. However, no guidelines exist concerning the restorability of deciduous teeth post-pulpotomy. Hence, the restorative decision making remains at the clinician's discretion. If the pulp is hyperaemic and haemostasis cannot be obtained, then pulpectomy or extraction is indicated (Figure 8.1).

VPT requires periodic clinical and radiographic assessment of the treated tooth. The assessment generally should be performed every six months as part of the patient's periodic oral examinations. Radiographic evaluation of primary tooth pulpotomies should occur at least annually. Bitewing radiographs obtained as part of a patient's periodic examinations may suffice. However, if they do not display the inter-radicular area, a periapical radiograph will be necessary [25].

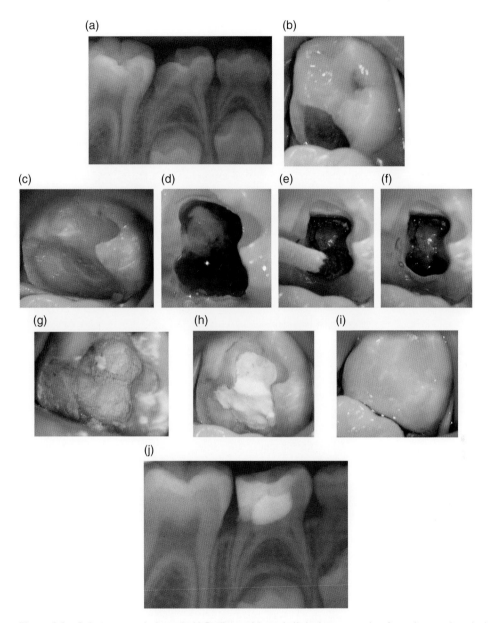

Figure 8.2 Pulpotomy technique. (a, b) Radiographic and clinical presentation for a deep carious lesion on the distal surface of the mandibular second primary molar. (c) Caries removal. (d)–(f) Coronal pulp amputation and control of bleeding. (g) Placement of hydraulic tricalcium silicate cement (Portland cement). (h) Subsequent placement of a layer of zinc phosphate cement. (i) Restoration by means of a composite resin filling. (j) Radiograph directly after treatment. *Source:* Josette Camilleri, Courtesy to Gertrude Van Gorp.

8.3.1.3 Restorative Materials for VPT of Deciduous Teeth

To prevent leakage of unreacted monomers from resin-based materials towards the pulp and enhance pulpal healing, a protective liner or biocompatible material is recommended in deep cavities (indirect pulp treatment) or on the radicular pulp (pulpotomy) [26]. Table 8.1 compares the advantages and disadvantages of several such filling materials. After placement

Table 8.1 Advantages and disadvantages of various filling materials for the endodontic treatment of deciduous teeth.

Endodontic filling material	Advantages	Disadvantages
CH[a–c]	Antimicrobial Inexpensive Induction of reactionary dentine Injectable Radiopaque	Caustic to pulp Induction of internal resorption
ZOE[a–c]	Antimicrobial Low pulpal toxicity Inexpensive Radiopaque Injectable	Lower success rates compared to MTA Difficult retreatment Resorbs slower than root Reduces adhesive bond strength
(RM) GIC[a]	Chemical bond to enamel and dentine Continuous fluoride release Fast set (RM) Biocompatible (conventional GIC) Easy to apply	Hydrophobic (conventional GIC) Slow set (conventional GIC) Toxic to pulp (RM)

Iodoform

	Advantages	Disadvantages
Iodoform[c]	Injectable Retreatable	Intracanal resorption
+ CH[c]	Antimicrobial Resorbs when extruded Resorbs faster than root (not for + ZO)	
+ ZO[c]	Radiopaque Moderate price	Slower resorption

HCSC

	Advantages		Disadvantages	
Portland cement[a,b]	Moderate price No discolouration		Slow set Low radiopacity	
MTA[a,b]	Most investigated Radiopaque	Biocompatible Bioactive Hydrophilic Antimicrobial	Grey/black Discolouration Expensive Slow set	Difficult to apply unretreatable[c]
Cem-Cement[a,b]	Moderate price Moderate colour stability Radiopaque		Slow set	
Biodentine[a,b]	Moderately fast set Moderate colour stability		Expensive Low radiopacity	

[a] For indirect pulp capping.
[b] For pulpotomy.
[c] For pulpectomy.

(a)　　　(b)　　　(c)　　　(d)　　　(e)

(f)　　　　　(g)

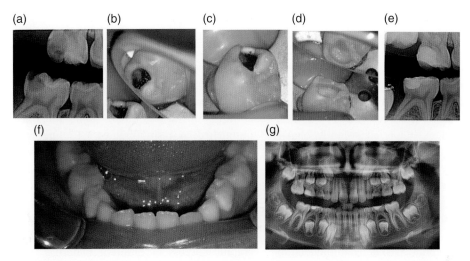

Figure 8.3 Indirect pulp treatment in two deciduous molars of a healthy 5.5-year-old boy without history of spontaneous pain. (Note: Before the age of three, removal of a throat cyst under general anaesthesia involved the administration of a lot of antibiotics.) (a) Bitewing radiograph of grossly decayed right lower and upper second primary molars. Notice a very small visible remaining dentine layer. (b, c) Clinical view (after local anaesthesia and rubber dam isolation) of the right mandibular second molar with a deep carious lesion. (d) Selective removal of soft carious dentine without pulp exposure and with clean cavity walls. The remaining 'firm' dentine in the depth of the lesion and the peripheral areas are cleaned with EDTA to enable a good restorative seal. No protective layer is placed. (e) Postoperative bitewing radiograph of the restored (composite filling) right lower and upper second primary molars, serving as a baseline for comparisons with future radiographs to determine treatment success. (f) Three-year follow-up showing stable restorations in teeth 85 and 75 (also indirect pulp treatment in the same period). Note the well-erupted first permanent molars. (g) Panoramic view on four-year follow-up, showing teeth 54, 75, and 85 with long-term stability of the restorations and healthy periapical tissues due to the hermetic seal, a critical condition in the success of an indirect pulp treatment. Note: Full coronal-coverage restoration with stainless-steel crowns is preferred, certainly in case of hypomineralization. *Source:* Josette Camilleri, Courtesy to Gertrude Van Gorp.

of the cavity liner or pulpotomy base cement, the rest of the cavity must be sealed with a well-bonded composite restoration or well-sealed steel crown to prevent any microleakage. Tight sealing of the cavity against bacterial microleakage seems to be the most important success factor in indirect pulp treatment, not the material or technique applied (Figure 8.3) [27].

8.3.1.3.1 Calcium Hydroxide
The first materials applied in pulp capping were dentine chips and pastes, including calcium hydroxide (CH) [28, 29]. Historically, CH played an important role in the evolution of VPT. It is antimicrobial and has the ability to extract growth factors from mineralized dentine, which induce reactionary dentine deposition [30]. However, it is caustic to the pulp due to its

alkaline pH [29]. In indirect pulp treatment, CH is generally used as a liner. A comparison of the clinical and microbiological effects of CH and gutta-percha when applied in indirect pulp treatment (incomplete caries excavation) in primary teeth after four to seven months found bacterial counts had decreased significantly in both groups [31]. However, the dentine turned hard after treatment in 85% of cases in the CH group, as compared with 68.4% in the gutta-percha one. These results were consistent with a randomized controlled clinical trial in which wax was applied in the control group instead of gutta-percha [32]. Nevertheless, inconsistent conclusions are drawn from reviews; the most evidence exists for the application of CH liners in indirect pulp therapy in primary teeth [33], but CH shows a higher probability of failure when compared with resin-modified glass ionomers and adhesive systems [34].

When used in pulpotomy, CH is applied in a thicker layer. It shows a clinical success rate ranging between 77 and 87% and a radiographic success rate between 66 and 77% [1, 14, 16]. Nevertheless, it has consistently higher rates of internal resorption [1, 14, 16, 17], reducing the chances of preserving the tooth until physiological exfoliation.

8.3.1.3.2 Zinc Oxide-Eugenol Due to its low pulpal toxicity and antibacterial properties, zinc oxide-eugenol (ZOE) is recommended in caries-free deep cavities [35]. ZOE prevents bacterial penetration towards the pulp in indirect pulp treatment [35]. Hence, the partially decalcified dentine remineralizes and the normal tissue pH is regained [36]. However, in pulpotomy studies, a higher success rate was reported following the use of FS/mineral trioxide aggregate (MTA) in comparison to FS/ZOE or FS/zinc oxide (eugenol-free) [19].

8.3.1.3.3 Glass Ionomer Cement (Indirect Pulp Treatment Only) Conventional or auto-cure GICs consist primarily of alumina, silica, and polyalkenoic acid and are self-curing restorative materials. GIC is known for its chemomechanical adhesion with dentine and enamel. It is the only restorative material that forms a chemical bond to tooth structures. Additionally, the newly developed chlorhexidine-containing GIC seems to reduce the level of bacteria in the soft carious dentine [37, 38]. However, all GICs lack the physical properties required for use in load-bearing areas [39].

Resin-modified GICs were developed to overcome the disadvantages of conventional GIC. They have a fast set due to polymerization after placement. Furthermore, the resin protects the GIC from dehydration and improves its physicomechanical properties. Resin-modified GICs do not require a dentine bonding agent. Nevertheless, because they contain hydrophilic resin monomers, they are not as biocompatible as conventional GIC [40].

An observational study of indirect pulp treatment in deeply decayed primary molars applied 2% chlorhexidine gluconate disinfectant after removal of infected dentine. Affected dentine on the pulpal floor remained untouched. A resin-modified GIC liner was placed and the teeth were restored with composite or stainless-steel crowns. After 12 months, the treatment was successful in 97% of the teeth. However, appropriate case selection was emphasized [41]. Furthermore, in a systematic review, the clinical and radiographic success of different materials (CH, adhesive systems, resin-modified GIC, and placebo) applied in indirect pulp treatment in primary teeth was questioned. Follow-up was conducted at between 24 and 48 months, and the authors concluded that the material type did not significantly affect the risk of treatment failure and that none of the mentioned materials was superior when used in indirect pulp treatment in primary teeth [34].

8.3.1.3.4 Hydraulic Calcium Silicate Cement The quest for new materials offering optimal clinical performance is never-ending in the field of dental science. One novel category is the hydraulic calcium silicate cements (HCSCs), which are known for their biocompatibility and bioactivity potential. Several HCSCs introduced and investigated since the early 1990s are discussed in this section (see also Table 8.1).

MTA is mixture of Portland cement and bismuth oxide. It generally comprises tricalcium silicate, dicalcium silicate, tricalcium aluminate, aluminoferrite (in the grey version), gypsum, and bismuth oxide [42]. Bismuth oxide powder is added (17–18 wt%) to make the aggregate radiopaque. The MTA paste is obtained by mixing three parts of powder with one part of water, producing a putty-like consistency. Mixing can be done on paper or on a glass slab using a plastic or metal spatula. This mix is then placed in the desired location using a large amalgam carrier or spatula and condensed lightly with a moistened cotton pellet [43, 44].

MTA has a pH of 10.2 immediately after mixing, increasing to 12.5 after three hours of setting – similar to that of CH [44]. The mixing time should be less than 4 minutes, and the working time is 70 (±2.58) minutes [43]. Grey MTA has a setting time of about 2 hours and 45 minutes [44], whilst white MTA has one of 2 hours and 20 minutes [45]. It has been used in VPT as it shows excellent biocompatibility [14, 43, 45, 46], promoting tissue regeneration and mineralization ability [1, 14, 43, 46, 47]. *In vivo*, it has proved better than CH at stimulating reparative dentine formation and maintaining pulpal integrity. It also consistently demonstrates less inflammation, hyperaemia, and necrosis, as well as a thicker and less porous calcified bridge, compared to CH [43]. Clinically, it shows superior results in terms of tissue regeneration ability and long-term success rates, with a clinical success rate ranging between 94 and 100% and a radiographic success rate ranging between 93 and 100% [1, 6, 14, 16, 18, 19, 43, 48]. Drawbacks include its high price, the blue-greyish to black discolouration it induces due to its bismuth oxide [49, 50], and its long setting time, which necessitates an additional session for proper setting in order not to jeopardize its physicochemical characteristics [44]. Moreover, clinicians are aware of its poor handling properties: even if the manufacturer's instructions are strictly followed, mixing the water and powder components in order to obtain a putty consistency is challenging, as is obtaining proper transportation to the tooth and proper adaptation to the region where the MTA is required [51].

Portland cement is produced by grinding cement clinker to a fine powder together with gypsum. Like MTA, it is mainly composed of tricalcium silicate and dicalcium silicate [52, 53]. Both MTA and Portland cement release CH when hydrated, which increases their pH to 12 and makes them antimicrobial [47]. Both show similar compressive strengths,

dimensional changes, and setting times [47, 51, 54, 55], and both have similar regeneration and mineralization abilities and biocompatibilities, *in vitro* and *in vivo* (animal studies) [45, 47, 54, 56–59]. Furthermore, human dental pulp cells show calcified bridge formation following exposure to Portland cement [47, 58]. Hence, it has recently been suggested as an alternative and moderately inexpensive HCSC for use in VPT [47, 51].

One of the drawbacks of Portland cement is that it has a lower radiopacity (similar to dentine) than MTA due to its lack of bismuth oxide [47, 54, 60] (Figures 8.3 and 8.4). On the other hand, this gives it the favourable property of not discolouring the tooth [47, 51, 60]. Studies evaluating leachable elements from different types of MTAs and Portland cements showed high quantities of acid-extractable trace elements (arsenic, chromium), especially from grey MTA and grey Portland cement. However, the release was negligible in a physiological-like solution [54, 61, 62].

Clinical trials on indirect pulp treatment with follow-up intervals ranging from six months [63] to two years [64] show a superior performance of MTA in comparison with CH. For pulpotomy procedures, MTA has been the most clinically applied and investigated HCSC. The current most complete data come from a Cochrane systematic review by Smail-Faugeron et al. [65], who concluded based on 12 trials (n = 740) that MTA reduced both clinical and radiographic failures when compared with FC, with a statistically significant difference at 12 months clinically and at 6, 12, and 24 months radiographically. When the comparison was made between CH and MTA (4 trials, n = 150), MTA showed significantly fewer clinical failures at 12 and 24 months and radiographic failures at 6, 12, and 24 months. Hence, to date, MTA is the most efficacious and biocompatible pulpotomy base cement for primary teeth, despite its high cost.

In 2008, a novel endodontic biomaterial was introduced as 'calcium-enriched mixture' (CEM; BioniqueDent YektazistDandan, Iran

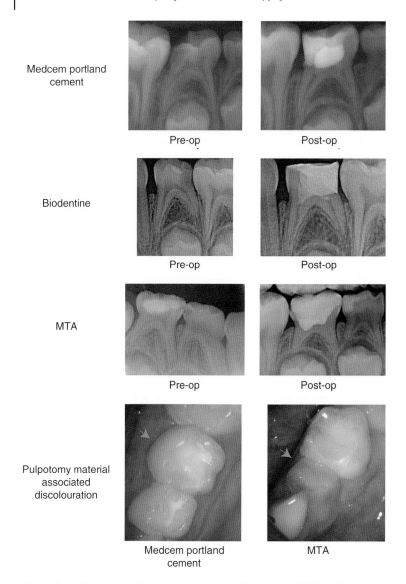

Figure 8.4 Pulpotomy of deciduous molars with various HCSCs: radiographic presentation (pre-op and one year post-op) and clinical image (one year post-op; green arrow = treated tooth). A difference in radiopacity is visible amongst the HCSCs (Portland cement < Biodentine < MTA). With regard to MTA-pulpotomy one year post-op, root canal obliteration is remarkable on the radiograph and greyish discolouration can be seen on the clinical image. *Source:* Josette Camilleri, Courtesy to Gertrude Van Gorp and Nastaran Meschi.

Polymer & Petrochemical Institute Tehran-Karaj, Iran; US Patent No. 20080206716) [66]. CEM is a newer-generation hydraulic cement with additives that enhance its material properties (Type 2 material). It consists mainly of calcium salts, calcium oxide, calcium silicate, and calcium phosphate compounds [67]. Like

MTA, it is delivered as a powder and a liquid, which are mixed manually just before application. No powder–liquid ratio is specified in the manufacturer's instructions, but they do mention that the amount of liquid may be varied depending on the required consistency of the cement (putty or creamy). This might jeopardize the material physical properties, since the addition of excess water increases the setting time and reduces the material strength [68–70]; however, it does not seem to affect the biological ones [71]. CEM sets in an aqueous environment and is as antibacterial as CH [72]. Its sealing ability, biocompatibility, pH, mixing time, and dimensional changes are comparable to those of white MTA [73, 74]. However, its initial setting time (50 minutes) and discolouration potential seem to be lower [66, 75] – and these are advantageous properties [66]. CEM is bismuth oxide-free. Also, it has the ability to maintain the pulp's integrity and to induce a calcified bridge [76]. Like MTA, it is based on the well-known tri- and dicalcium silicate phases [77]. Furthermore, its radiopacity results from the presence of barium sulphate. It is reported to be 2.2 mm Al – lower than that of white MTA (7.7 mm Al) [43, 67]. The minimum value required by the ISO standards is 3 mm Al [78].

Biodentine (Septodont, Saint Maur des Fosses, France) was introduced on the market in 2010. It is a newly formulated calcium silicate-based restorative cement indicated as a dentine replacement material [79, 80]. Hence, VPT is its most suitable clinical indication. Biodentine is available in a capsule containing the optimal ratio of powder (0.7 g) and a single-dose container of liquid (0.178 mg) [78, 81, 82]. It should be prepared by mixing with a Dental Mixer (Septodont, France) for 30 seconds at 4200 rpm [78, 81, 82]. The main component of the powder is a tricalcium silicate, plus calcium carbonate and zirconium oxide (the radiopacifier). It displays a radiopacity equivalent to 3.5 mm Al [78], which is less than that of white MTA (Figure 8.4). The liquid part is a solution of calcium chloride ($CaCl_2$) and a water-reducing agent [82]. The manufacturer reports a working time of 6 ($\pm$0.30) minutes and a setting time of 10 ($\pm$1.20) minutes, which is faster than either MTA, Portland cement, or CEM; this is due to the addition of $CaCl_2$ [78]. Biodentine releases CH during setting, which augments the pH significantly (to 12) and

makes it antimicrobial [83]. It reaches maximum hardness after one month and is colour-stable [84–86]. Due to its additives and low liquid–powder ratio, it is the strongest of the HCSCs [86].

An *in vitro* study investigating the effect of the overlying material on the final setting of Biodentine in primary molar pulpotomies showed no effect of ZOE, resin-modified GIC, or stainless-steel crowns cemented with GIC on the final set [87]. Hence, Biodentine can be immediately covered by a definitive restoration during pulpotomies. However, it may also be used as a temporary filling for up to six months with acceptable clinical performance (good anatomic form, marginal adaptation, and proximal contact). Moreover, it may be used as a dentine substitute for definitive dentinal treatment in restoration of posterior teeth [78, 88].

In a randomized clinical trial on indirect pulp therapy, 54 primary molars were equally divided into three groups: Biodentine, 2% chlorhexidine with resin-modified GIC, and CH [89]. The Biodentine group presented the highest (100%) clinical and radiographic success rates at 12-month follow-up.

In order to investigate the use of HCSCs in pulpotomy in a systematic way, clinical studies were retrieved from PubMed using the search terms 'pulpotomy AND primary tooth AND HCSC (PC/CEM/Biodentine™)'. The most recent studies (during the last decade) were selected, and are listed chronologically in Table 8.2. Those mentioning FC were excluded, because FC does not maintain the integrity of the pulp and is carcinogenic [20–23]. Based on the data obtained, the following conclusions can be drawn concerning the use of HCSCs in pulpotomy of deciduous teeth:

- The clinical and radiographic success rates of CEM, Portland cement, and Biodentine over an assessment period of 9–24 months are comparable/equivalent to the rates for MTA.
- The reparative dentine formation capacities of CEM, Portland cement, and Biodentine

Table 8.2 Clinical and radiographic (Rx) outcomes of pulpotomy studies conducted over the last decade (2009–2019) using Portland cement, CEM, and Biodentine, as retrieved from PubMed.

Year	Authors	Max. assessment period (months)	Number of teeth	Control material	Outcome Clinical	Outcome Rx
2019	Maroto et al. [90]	12	11	Portland cement	100% success	100% success. All reparative dentine formation
2019	Celik et al. [91]	24	44	MTA, Biodentine	Success: MTA 100% (2 PCO), Biodentine 89.4%	
2018	Nasseh et al. [92],	12	35	Biodentine	100% success	100% success. 25.7% PCO
2018	Caruso et al. [93]	18	400	CH, Biodentine	Success: CH 79.5%, Biodentine 89.5%	
2017	Shafie et al. [94]	7 days	90	MTA, CEM	MTA and CEM: 65.6% reported pain post-op	-
2017	Guven et al. [95]	24	116	ProRoot MTA, MTA-Plus, Biodentine, FS	Success: Biodentine 82.75%, MTA-Plus 86.2%, ProRoot MTA 93.1%, FS 75.9%	
2017	Bani et al. [96]	24	32	MTA, Biodentine	Success: MTA, Biodentine 96.8%	Success: Biodentine 93.6%, MTA 87.1%
2017	Carti et al. [97]	12	50	MTA, Biodentine	Success: MTA 96%, Biodentine 80%	Success: MTA 96%, Biodentine 60%
2016	Grewal et al. [98]	12	40	Biodentine, CH	Biodentine significantly better reparative dentine formation than CH	
2016	Togaru et al. [99]	12	90	MTA, Biodentine	Success: MTA, Biodentine 95.5%	
2016	Cuadros-Fernández et al. [100]	12	84	MTA, Biodentine	Success: MTA 92%, Biodentine 97%	Success: MTA 97%, Biodentine 95%
2015	Kusum et al. [101]	9	75	MTA, Biodentine, Propolis	Success: MTA 100%, Biodentine, Propolis 84%	Success: MTA 92%, Biodentine 80%, Propolis 72%
2014	Khorakian et al. [102]	24	102	CEM, ES/ZOE	Success: CEM, ES/ZOE 100%	Success: ES/ZOE 95.2%, CEM 90%
2013	Oliveira et al.[103]	24	45	CH, MTA, Portland cement	Success: Portland cement, MTA 100%	CH: many cases lost due to internal resorption
2011	Malekafzali et al. [104]	24	80	MTA, CEM	Success comparable for both groups, independent of time	
2009	Sakai et al. [105]	24	30	MTA, Portland cement	100% success	No statistical difference in reparative dentine formation. PCO: Portland cement 100%, MTA 57.14%

ES, electrosurgery; PCO, pulp canal obliteration.

are comparable/equivalent to the capacity of MTA.

- Since 2015, there has been an upgrowth of clinical trials including Biodentine in the test group.
- MTA, CEM, Portland cement, and Biodentine are superior to the traditional pulpotomy base cements/agents (CH and FS).
- Pulp canal obliteration is not seen as a failure (Figure 8.4).

A major drawback of MTA, Portland cement, and CEM is the need for temporization due to their slow setting times (see Table 8.1). Furthermore, ZOE delays setting, whilst GIC absorbs the water required for hydration [106]. Hence, these HCSCs cannot be layered immediately, necessitating a second visit necessary; this is especially inconvenient in paediatric dentistry.

8.3.2 Pulpectomy

8.3.2.1 Technique

Pulpectomy is a root canal procedure for pulp tissue that is irreversibly infected or necrotic due to caries or trauma and which shows limited preoperative radiological evidence of inter-radicular or periapical radiolucency. A successful pulpectomy retains a primary tooth in a symptom-free state until exfoliation [5].

Removal of the entire pulp tissue and obturation of the root canals with a suitable resorbable material is a challenging treatment approach, due to the complex anatomy and the programmed physiological resorption of the root canals in primary molars (Figure 8.5) [107]. The use of magnification (e.g. dental loupes, an operating microscope) is advisable [108]. After adequate local anaesthesia and rubber

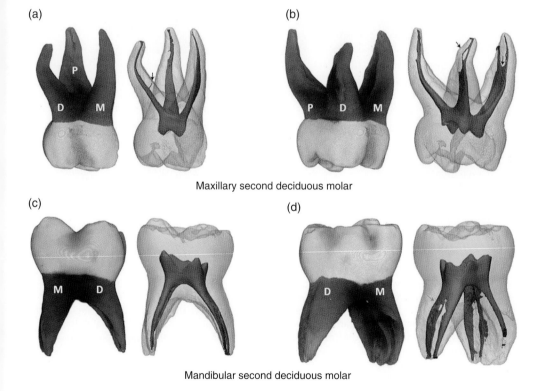

(a)

(b)

Maxillary second deciduous molar

(c)

(d)

Mandibular second deciduous molar

Figure 8.5 Primary molar root canal morphology from microcomputed tomography scans. (a) Morphology of a maxillary second primary molar with three roots: mesial (M), distal (D), and palatal (P). (b) 3D view showing the complex root canal configuration, including accessory canals (black arrows). (c) Morphology of a mandibular second primary molar with two roots: mesial and distal. (d) 3D view showing the complex root canal configuration, with three canals in the mesial root and two in the distal root, plus several accessory canals (blue arrows). *Source:* Josette Camilleri, Courtesy to Mostafa EzEldeen.

dam isolation, caries is removed with a high-speed access bur (round end cutting tapered diamond bur) and copious water spray (Figures 8.6 and 8.7). Once the cusps are lowered, the entire roof of the pulp chamber is cut away with another high-speed access bur (round end cutting tapered diamond bur) and copious water spray. Coronal pulp is removed with a #6 or #8 round bur on a slow-speed handpiece or with a sharp spoon excavator. The pulp chamber is then thoroughly washed with sodium hypochlorite 1% to remove all debris, necrotic pulp tissue, and dentine chips [109]. An appropriate enlargement (without undercuts) of the canal orifices using a small long-neck bur provides straight-line access to all the canals. Prior to chemomechanical instrumentation, the root canals are explored with slightly pre-curved size 0.08–0.10 K-files. The root canal working length is determined using an electronic apex locater and a shortened 2 mm of the apical foramen in order to prevent damage to the succeeding permanent tooth germ [110].

During chemomechanical preparation, the application of rotary NiTi files in primary molars significantly reduces the preparation time and improves the quality of obturation because of the more regular and uniform smooth root canal walls it provides [111]. A sufficient irrigation time is highly important for complete dissolution of pulp tissues

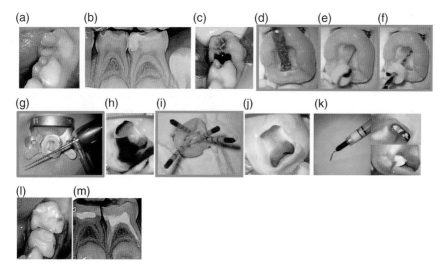

Figure 8.6 Pulpectomy of a left mandibular second molar with ZOE. Healthy five-year-old boy with a history of spontaneous pain and disturbing sleep after pulp capping performed by the referral dentist. (a) Tooth 75 presenting leakage of the coronal filling. (b) Preoperative radiograph showing secondary caries under the filling, continuous with the pulp chamber. No signs of internal resorption or inter-radicular or apical pathology. Mesial and distal caries present on tooth 74. (c) Tooth 75 isolated with a rubber dam following local anaesthesia. After access opening, excessive bleeding from the pulp chamber is indicative of irreversible pulpitis. (d) Removal of all carious tissue and access opening to expose the coronal pulp tissue in the pulp chamber with a high-speed access bur and copious water spray, finishing with round burs. (e) Exploration of the root canals with slightly pre-curved size 0.08–0.10 K-files (straight-line access to all the canals). (f) Preparation of the root canals with rotary NiTi files after working length determination with an electronic apex locater (shortened 2 mm of the apical foramen). (g) File clip of an electronic apex locator attached to the endodontic file to prevent overinstrumentation. After every instrumentation, the root canals should be gently irrigated with 1% sodium hypochlorite. (h) Haemostasis of tooth 75; a good haemostasis is difficult to obtain. (i) Drying of the root canals with sterile tapered paper points. (j) Tooth 75 before obturation. (k) Obturation of the root canals with ZOE delivered by a 0.80 flowable composite tip. (l) Pulp chamber filled with zinc phosphate cement and tooth restored with composite. (m) Postoperative radiograph showing adequate obturation of all root canals of tooth 75. Tooth 74 has received a pulpotomy with Portland cement. Green frames = preclinical images. *Source:* Josette Camilleri, Courtesy to Gertrude Van Gorp.

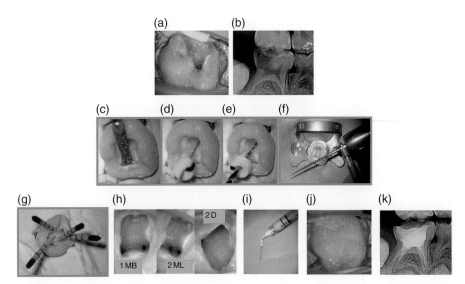

Figure 8.7 Pulpectomy of a right mandibular second molar with ZOE. Healthy five-year-old girl with a history of disturbing sleep and spontaneous pain. (a) Tooth 85 presenting a deep disto-occlusal carious lesion. (b) Preoperative radiograph showing a deep carious lesion reaching the pulp chamber. No signs of internal resorption or interradicular or apical pathology. (c) Removal of all carious tissue and access opening. (d) Exploration of the root canals with slightly pre-curved size 0.08–0.10 K-files (straight-line access to all the canals). (e) Preparation of the root canals with rotary NiTi files after working length determination with an electronic apex locater (2 mm short of working length). (f) File clip of an electronic apex locator attached to the endodontic file to prevent overinstrumentation. After application of a rotary file, the root canals should be gently irrigated with 1% sodium hypochlorite. (g) Drying of the root canals with sterile tapered paper points. (h) Orifices of five canals: three mesial (M) and two distal (D). (i) Obturation of the root canals with ZOE delivered by a 17 mm NaviTip (Ultradent Products, South Jordan, UT, USA). (j) Pulp chamber filled with zinc phosphate cement and tooth restored with composite. (k) Postoperative radiograph showing an adequate obturation of all root canals. Green frames = preclinical images. *Source:* Josette Camilleri, Courtesy to Gertrude Van Gorp.

and a proper debridement of the root canal system. A gentle but copious irrigation with 1% sodium hypochlorite [5] or saline [16] is recommended.

After irrigation, a sterile paper point is left in each canal for a few seconds to dry it out before obturation. There are numerous ways of delivering the obturation materials to the pulp chamber and canals, and no material or technique has been shown to be superior to all others [65, 112]. For example, NaviTips (Ultradent Products, South Jordan, UT, USA) can be used efficiently (Figure 8.7) [113], but the most important condition for success is a good coronal seal to prevent microleakage on placement of a permanent restoration [114]. This involves placing a GIC or reinforced ZOE directly on the floor of the pulp chamber in order to prevent coronal leakage. Prior to rubber dam

removal, the coronal part is restored with resin composite. A preformed metal crown is recommended in all endodontically treated primary teeth that are to be retained in the mouth in the long term [107, 115].

A postoperative radiograph is acquired immediately after root canal treatment to allow an evaluation of the obturation level and to provide future reference. Root canal fillings are categorized based on distance to the radiographic apex: underfilled (shorter than 2 mm), optimal (0–2 mm), or overfilled (over apex) [116]. Recall appointments for clinical and radiographic evaluation at 6, 12, and 18 months are recommended. However, the American Academy of Pediatric Dentistry (AAPD) leaves the type and frequency of follow-up radiographs of primary teeth pulpectomy to clinician discretion [25]. Clinical criteria for success are defined as being completely free of clinical signs and symptoms including pain, swelling, fistula, and sensitivity to percussion and having no pathologic mobility. The criteria for radiographic success include analysis of inter-radicular or periapical radiopacities (stabilization, regression), lack of pathologic external root resorption, and integrity of the periodontal ligament [117]. Failure of root canal treatment in primary molars may be evident from the development of new radiolucent defects or the enlargement of existing ones [118, 119].

8.3.2.2 Restorative Materials

Although an arsenal of root canal filling materials for permanent teeth exists, anatomical and developmental differences between permanent and deciduous teeth impose criteria that make most of them not applicable for deciduous teeth. The ideal root canal filling material for a primary tooth would be biocompatible with the periapical tissues and underlying tooth germ, resorbable at the same rate as the primary tooth root, easily applicable, colour-stable, inexpensive, easily resorbable when accidentally extruded beyond the root canal, antimicrobial, dimensionally stable, retreatable, and radiopaque [120]. Such a material has not yet been found, but the following are the most applied and investigated: CH, ZOE, iodoform, and the combination of iodoform with CH or ZOE (see Table 8.1) [120, 121].

8.3.2.2.1 Zinc Oxide-Eugenol
Since 1930, ZOE – in the United States, especially ZOE without setting accelerators – has been the most used root canal filling material in pulpectomy of primary teeth [120, 122]. As previously mentioned, it is inexpensive and has antimicrobial capacities (see Table 8.1). A drawback is that it resorbs at a slower rate than the roots of deciduous teeth [117, 123]; it can remain in the alveolar bone for months or even years, causing mild (irritation) to severe (necrosis) foreign-body reaction to the periapical tissues [124–126]. Furthermore, it has been described that ZOE negatively influences the

bond strength of adhesive systems to primary dentine [127]. Hence, alternatives have been developed and investigated, as discussed in the rest of this section.

8.3.2.2.2 Iodoform
Iodoform was introduced as a root canal filling material for primary teeth due to its antibacterial property, ability to be resorbed when placed in excess, and lack of undesirable effects on the periapical structures and underlying tooth germ [128–130]. It is also radiopaque, retreatable, and easily applicable by means of a sterile syringe and disposable plastic needles [131]. Its only drawback is that it can resorb inside the root canal [129]. Commercially, it is sold as KRI paste (Pharmachemie, Zurich, Switzerland), which is a mixture of iodoform (80.8%), camphor, parachlorophenol, and menthol [130].

Iodoform + CH CH is added to iodoform in a number of commercial products, including Metapex (Meta Biomed, Cheongju City, South Korea) (Figure 8.8) and Vitapex (New Dental Chemical Products, Tokyo, Japan), in order to combine their beneficial properties. Vitapex, also sold as Diapex (DiaDent Group International, Burnaby, BC, Canada) in the United States, is a combination of 30% CH, 40.4% iodoform, and 22.4% silicone oil. Its properties are similar to those of iodoform (Table 8.1) [121]. The outcome of its use in primary teeth with irreversible pulpitis is similar to that with ZOE pulpectomies, and more favourable than that with CH ones [132]. As the success rates of solely CH-containing root canal filling materials are significantly lower than those of ZOE or iodoform (-containing mixtures), they cannot be recommended as pulpectomy sealers for primary teeth [133]. Nevertheless, Vitapex does not show antibacterial effects against most pure cultures [134].

Iodoform + Zinc Oxide Iodoform has also been combined with zinc oxide (eugenol-free). Maisto's paste was introduced in 1967 and consists of zinc oxide, iodoform, parachlorophenol

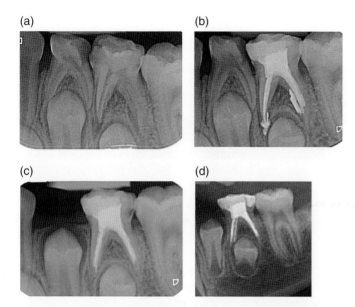

Figure 8.8 Pulpectomy of a left mandibular second molar with Metapex (Meta Biomed, Cheongju City, South Korea). Healthy nine-year-old boy with a history of swelling. (a) Preoperative radiograph showing a deep carious lesion with minor interradicular mesially and apical pathology on tooth 75, as well as a distal deep carious lesion reaching the pulp on tooth 74. (b) Postoperative radiograph of tooth 75, showing extrusion of Metapex into the interradicular area (tooth 74 was extracted). (c) Radiograph at 10-month follow-up showing resorption of the overfilled obturation material and healthy interradicular tissue, as well as a distal carious lesion, which was restored. (d) Radiograph at 15-month follow-up, showing no pathologies of tooth 75. *Source:* Courtesy to Gertrude Van Gorp.

camphor, lanolin, and thymol [121]. Studies report higher success rates with Maisto's paste than with ZOE alone [135, 136]. A similarly combined cement is Endoflas (Sanlor & CFA, Bogota, Colombia) (Figure 8.9), which consists of tri-iodmethane and iodine dibutilorthocresol (40.6%), zinc oxide (56.5%), CH (1.07%), and barium sulphate (1.63%), plus a liquid consisting of eugenol and paramonochlorophenol [121]. However, Endoflas does not seem to have a success rate as high as that of ZOE [129, 135]. A drawback of these pastes is that the presence of the zinc oxide slows their resorption [121].

Evaluation of Root Canal Filling Materials in Primary Teeth

A systematic review and meta-analysis comparing CH + iodoform pastes with ZOE found no statistically significant differences in the clinical and radiographic success rates at 6- and 12-month follow-up, but that ZOE was more successful at 18-month follow-up [122].

Another systematic review and meta-analysis of the Cochrane database found no significant difference between Metapex and ZOE at 6 and 12 months (two trials, 62 participants) or between Endoflas and ZOE at 6 months (two trials, 80 participants) [65]. It did find some low-quality evidence to suggest that ZOE might be better than Vitapex at 12 months (two trials, 161 participants) [65].

Based on these findings, the following conclusions and recommendations can be made concerning root canal filling materials for primary teeth:

- There is no conclusive evidence that any one root canal filling material or technique is superior to any other, which implies that the choice remains at the clinician's discretion [65].
- CH + iodoform pastes may be utilized for pulpectomy in primary teeth nearing exfoliation [122].
- ZOE may be utilized when exfoliation is not expected to occur soon [122].

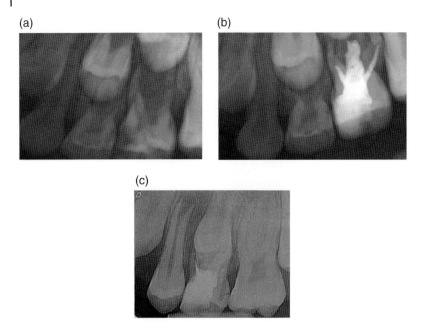

Figure 8.9 Pulpectomy of a left upper second molar with Endoflas (Sanlor & CFA, Bogota, Colombia). Healthy nine-year-old boy with a history of swelling. (a) Preoperative radiograph of tooth 65 showing a deep carious lesion mesially, and on the mesial radicular side an enlargement of the periodontal ligament. (b) Postoperative radiograph of tooth 65 showing an adequate filling of the distal roots and an underfilling of the palatal and mesial ones. (c) Radiograph at three-year follow-up showing resorption of the obturation material and a normal physiological root resorption of tooth 65, allowing maintenance of the arch length and integrity. A distal carious lesion was developed but not treated, as the tooth had to be extracted. *Source:* Courtesy to Gertrude Van Gorp.

- There is room for research to confirm whether ZOE is more effective than CH + iodoform pastes and for an exploration of other alternatives [65].

8.4 Conclusion

Considerable efforts have been made in the field of biomaterials and in dental science in order to give paediatric dentists and endodontists the tools they need to maintain deciduous teeth until physiological exfoliation. However, as paedo-endo is a challenging clinical domain in which precision and fast handling are requirements, we demand high standards of our biomaterials. The arsenal of endodontic obturation materials for paedo-endo shows some drawbacks that still need to be overcome, and a biomaterial with *all* of the following properties has yet to be developed: biocompatible, bioactive, good sealing ability, fast setting, colour-stable, radiopaque, user-friendly, inexpensive, antimicrobial, and adaptable to the overlying restorative material. Furthermore, there is a lack of long-term (at least 12 months) high-quality comparative studies and randomized controlled clinical trials in indirect pulp therapy, and in pulpectomy of deciduous teeth more specifically.

References

1 Camp, J.H. and Fuks, A.B. (2006). Pediatric endodontics: endodontic treatment for the primary and young permanent dentition. In: *Pathways of the Pulp*, 9e (eds. S. Cohen and K.M. Hargreaves), 822–882. Maryland Heights, MO: Mosby Elsevier.

2 Fuks, A.B., Hebling, J., and de Souza Costa, C.A. (2016). The primary pulp: developmental and biomedical background. In: *Pediatric Endodontics: Current Concepts in Pulp Therapy for Primary and Young Permanent Teeth* (eds. A.B. Fuks and B. Peretz), 7–22. Philadelphia, PA: Springer.

3 Martinez Saez, D., Sasaki, R.T., Neves, A.D., and da Silva, M.C. (2016). Stem cells from human exfoliated deciduous teeth: a growing literature. *Cells Tissues Organs* 202 (5–6): 269–280.

4 Kassa, D., Day, P., High, A., and Duggal, M. (2009). Histological comparison of pulpal inflammation in primary teeth with occlusal or proximal caries. *Int. J. Paediatr. Dent.* 19 (1): 26–33.

5 American Academy of Pediatric Dentistry (2014–2015). Reference Manual: Guideline on Pulp Therapy for Primary and Immature Permanent Teeth. Available from https://www.aapd.org/media/Policies_Guidelines/BP_PulpTherapy.pdf (accessed 10 August 2020).

6 Subramaniam, P., Konde, S., Mathew, S., and Sugnani, S. (2009). Mineral trioxide aggregate as pulp capping agent for primary teeth pulpotomy: 2 year follow up study. *J. Clin. Pediatr. Dent.* 33 (4): 311–314.

7 Fuks, A.B. (2013). Pulp therapy for the primary dentition. In: *Pediatric Dentistry: Infancy through Adolescence*, 5e (eds. J.R. Pinkham, P.S. Casamassimo, H.W. Fields Jr., et al.), 331–351. St Louis, MO: Elsevier Saunders Co.

8 Schwendicke, F., Frencken, J.E., Bjorndal, L. et al. (2016). Managing carious lesions: consensus recommendations on carious tissue removal. *Adv. Dent. Res.* 28 (2): 58–67.

9 Innes, N.P., Evans, D.J., and Stirrups, D.R. (2007). The Hall technique; a randomized controlled clinical trial of a novel method of managing carious primary molars in general dental practice: acceptability of the technique and outcomes at 23 months. *BMC Oral Health* 7: 18.

10 Coll, J.A. (2016). Indirect pulp treatment, direct pulp capping, and stepwise caries excavation. In: *Pediatric Endodontics: Current Concepts in Pulp Therapy for Primary and Young Permanent Teeth* (eds. A.B. Fuks and B. Peretz), 37–50. Philadelphia, PA: Springer.

11 Frencken, J.E. (2018). *The Art and Science of Minimal Intervention Dentistry and Atraumatic Restorative Treatment.* Orleton: Stephen Hancocks.

12 Mathieu, S., Jeanneau, C., Sheibat-Othman, N. et al. (2013). Usefulness of controlled release of growth factors in investigating the early events of dentin–pulp regeneration. *J. Endod.* 39 (2): 228–235.

13 Galler, K.M., Widbiller, M., Buchalla, W. et al. (2016). EDTA conditioning of dentine promotes adhesion, migration and differentiation of dental pulp stem cells. *Int. Endod. J.* 49 (6): 581–590.

14 Fuks, A.B. (2008). Vital pulp therapy with new materials for primary teeth: new directions and treatment perspectives. *J. Endod.* 34 (7 Suppl): S18–S24.

15 Sweet, C.A. (1930). Procedure for treatment of exposed and pulpless deciduous teeth. *J. Am. Dent. Assoc.* 17: 1150–1153.

16 Rodd, H.D., Waterhouse, P.J., Fuks, A.B. et al. (2006). Pulp therapy for primary molars. *Int. J. Paediatr. Dent.* 16 (Suppl. 1): 15–23.

17 Huth, K.C., Hajek-Al-Khatar, N., Wolf, P. et al. (2012). Long-term effectiveness of four pulpotomy techniques: 3-year randomised controlled trial. *Clin. Oral Investig.* 16 (4): 1243–1250.

18 Simancas-Pallares, M.A., Diaz-Caballero, A.J., and Luna-Ricardo, L.M. (2010). Mineral trioxide aggregate in primary teeth pulpotomy. A systematic literature review. *Med. Oral Patol. Oral Cir. Bucal* 15 (6): e942–e946.

19 Doyle, T.L., Casas, M.J., Kenny, D.J., and Judd, P.L. (2010). Mineral trioxide aggregate produces superior outcomes in vital primary molar pulpotomy. *Pediatr. Dent.* 32 (1): 41–47.

20 Pashley, E.L., Myers, D.R., Pashley, D.H., and Whitford, G.M. (1980). Systemic distribution

of 14C-formaldehyde from formocresol-treated pulpotomy sites. *J. Dent. Res.* 59 (3): 602–608.

21 Myers, D.R., Shoaf, H.K., Dirksen, T.R. et al. (1978). Distribution of 14C-formaldehyde after pulpotomy with formocresol. *J. Am. Dent. Assoc.* 96 (5): 805–813.

22 Ko, H., Jeong, Y., and Kim, M. (2017). Cytotoxicities and genotoxicities of cements based on calcium silicate and of dental formocresol. *Mutat. Res.* 815: 28–34.

23 Ranly, D.M. (1985). Assessment of the systemic distribution and toxicity of formaldehyde following pulpotomy treatment: part one. *ASDC J. Dent. Child.* 52 (6): 431–434.

24 World Health Organization IARC Monographs on the Evaluation of Carcinogenic Risks to Humans. Available from https://publications.iarc.fr/Book-And-Report-Series/Iarc-Monographs-On-The-Identification-Of-Carcinogenic-Hazards-To-Humans#:~:text=The%20IARC%20Monographs%20on%20the,the%20weight%20of%20the%20evidence (accessed 10 August 2020).

25 American Academy of Pediatric Dentistry Review Council on Clinical Affairs (2014). Pulp Therapy for Primary and Immature Permanent Teeth. Available from https://www.aapd.org/media/Policies_Guidelines/BP_PulpTherapy.pdf (accessed 10 August 2020).

26 de Souza Costa, C.A., do Nascimento, A.B., and Teixeira, H.M. (2002). Response of human pulps following acid conditioning and application of a bonding agent in deep cavities. *Dent. Mater.* 18 (7): 543–551.

27 Kuhn, E., Chibinski, A.C., Reis, A., and Wambier, D.S. (2014). The role of glass ionomer cement on the remineralization of infected dentin: an in vivo study. *Pediatr. Dent.* 36 (4): E118–E124.

28 Glass, R.L. and Zander, H.A. (1949). Pulp healing. *J. Dent. Res.* 28 (2): 97–107.

29 Zander, H.A. (1939). Reaction of the pulp to calcium hydroxide. *J. Dent. Res.* 18: 373–379.

30 Graham, L., Cooper, P.R., Cassidy, N. et al. (2006). The effect of calcium hydroxide on solubilisation of bio-active dentine matrix components. *Biomaterials* 27 (14): 2865–2873.

31 Pinto, A.S., de Araujo, F.B., Franzon, R. et al. (2006). Clinical and microbiological effect of calcium hydroxide protection in indirect pulp capping in primary teeth. *Am. J. Dent.* 19 (6): 382–386.

32 Bressani, A.E., Mariath, A.A., Haas, A.N. et al. (2013). Incomplete caries removal and indirect pulp capping in primary molars: a randomized controlled trial. *Am. J. Dent.* 26 (4): 196–200.

33 Boutsiouki, C., Frankenberger, R., and Kramer, N. (2018). Relative effectiveness of direct and indirect pulp capping in the primary dentition. *Eur. Arch. Paediatr. Dent.* 19 (5): 297–309.

34 Santos, P.S.D., Pedrotti, D., Braga, M.M. et al. (2017). Materials used for indirect pulp treatment in primary teeth: a mixed treatment comparisons meta-analysis. *Braz. Oral Res.* 31: e101.

35 Murray, P.E., Hafez, A.A., Smith, A.J., and Cox, C.F. (2002). Bacterial microleakage and pulp inflammation associated with various restorative materials. *Dent. Mater.* 18 (6): 470–478.

36 Goodis, H.E., Marshall, S., Tay, F.R., and Marshall, G.W. Jr. (2012). Repair of pulpal injury with dental materials. In: *Seltzer and Bender's Dental Pulp* (eds. K.M. Hargreaves, H.E. Goodis and F.R. Tay), 301–322. New Malden: Quintessence.

37 Frencken, J.E., Imazato, S., Toi, C. et al. (2007). Antibacterial effect of chlorhexidine-containing glass ionomer cement in vivo: a pilot study. *Caries Res.* 41 (2): 102–107.

38 Turkun, L.S., Turkun, M., Ertugrul, F. et al. (2008). Long-term antibacterial effects and physical properties of a chlorhexidine-containing glass ionomer cement. *J. Esthetic Restorat. Dent.* 20 (1): 29–44; disc. 5.

39 Mount, G.J., Tyas, M.J., Ferracane, J.L. et al. (2009). A revised classification for direct

tooth-colored restorative materials. *Quintessence Int.* 40 (8): 691–697.

40 Nicholson, J.W. and Czarnecka, B. (2008). The biocompatibility of resin-modified glass-ionomer cements for dentistry. *Dent. Mater.* 24 (12): 1702–1708.

41 Rosenberg, L., Atar, M., Daronch, M. et al. (2013). Observational: prospective study of indirect pulp treatment in primary molars using resin-modified glass ionomer and 2% chlorhexidine gluconate: a 12-month follow-up. *Pediatr. Dent.* 35 (1): 13–17.

42 Torabinejad, M. and Moaddel, H. (2015). Substances and method for replacing natural tooth material. US patent 20150157538.

43 Rao, A., Rao, A., and Shenoy, R. (2009). Mineral trioxide aggregate – a review. *J. Clin. Pediatr. Dent.* 34 (1): 1–7.

44 Torabinejad, M., Hong, C.U., McDonald, F., and Pitt Ford, T.R. (1995). Physical and chemical properties of a new root-end filling material. *J. Endod.* 21 (7): 349–353.

45 Camilleri, J., Montesin, F.E., Brady, K. et al. (2005). The constitution of mineral trioxide aggregate. *Dent. Mater.* 21 (4): 297–303.

46 Camilleri, J. and Pitt Ford, T.R. (2006). Mineral trioxide aggregate: a review of the constituents and biological properties of the material. *Int. Endod. J.* 39 (10): 747–754.

47 Steffen, R. and van Waes, H. (2009). Understanding mineral trioxide aggregate/ Portland-cement: a review of literature and background factors. *Eur. Arch. Paediatr. Dent.* 10 (2): 93–97.

48 Cardoso-Silva, C., Barberia, E., Maroto, M., and Garcia-Godoy, F. (2011). Clinical study of mineral trioxide aggregate in primary molars. Comparison between grey and white MTA – a long term follow-up (84 months). *J. Dent.* 39 (2): 187–193.

49 Marciano, M.A., Duarte, M.A., and Camilleri, J. (2015). Dental discoloration caused by bismuth oxide in MTA in the presence of sodium hypochlorite. *Clin. Oral Investig.* 19 (9): 2201–2209.

50 Camilleri, J. (2014). Color stability of white mineral trioxide aggregate in contact with

hypochlorite solution. *J. Endod.* 40 (3): 436–440.

51 Islam, I., Chng, H.K., and Yap, A.U. (2006). Comparison of the physical and mechanical properties of MTA and Portland cement. *J. Endod.* 32 (3): 193–197.

52 Niu, L.N., Jiao, K., Wang, T.D. et al. (2014). A review of the bioactivity of hydraulic calcium silicate cements. *J. Dent.* 42 (5): 517–533.

53 Prati, C. and Gandolfi, M.G. (2015). Calcium silicate bioactive cements: biological perspectives and clinical applications. *Dent. Mater.* 31 (4): 351–370.

54 Camilleri, J., Montesin, F.E., Curtis, R.V., and Ford, T.R. (2006). Characterization of Portland cement for use as a dental restorative material. *Dent. Mater.* 22 (6): 569–575.

55 Storm, B., Eichmiller, F.C., Tordik, P.A., and Goodell, G.G. (2008). Setting expansion of gray and white mineral trioxide aggregate and Portland cement. *J. Endod.* 34 (1): 80–82.

56 Ribeiro, D.A., Duarte, M.A., Matsumoto, M.A. et al. (2005). Biocompatibility in vitro tests of mineral trioxide aggregate and regular and white Portland cements. *J. Endod.* 31 (8): 605–607.

57 Holland, R., de Souza, V., Nery, M.J. et al. (2001). Reaction of rat connective tissue to implanted dentin tube filled with mineral trioxide aggregate, Portland cement or calcium hydroxide. *Braz. Dent. J.* 12 (1): 3–8.

58 Barbosa, A.V., Sampaio, G.C., Gomes, F.A. et al. (2009). Short-term analysis of human dental pulps after direct capping with Portland cement. *Open Dent. J.* 3: 31–35.

59 Camilleri, J., Kralj, P., Veber, M., and Sinagra, E. (2012). Characterization and analyses of acid-extractable and leached trace elements in dental cements. *Int. Endod. J.* 45 (8): 737–743.

60 Islam, I., Chng, H.K., and Yap, A.U. (2006). X-ray diffraction analysis of mineral trioxide aggregate and Portland cement. *Int. Endod. J.* 39 (3): 220–225.

61 Duarte, M.A., De Oliveira Demarchi, A.C., Yamashita, J.C. et al. (2005). Arsenic release provided by MTA and Portland cement. *Oral Surg. Oral Med. Oral Pathol. Oral Radiol. Endod.* 99 (5): 648–650.

62 Monteiro Bramante, C., Demarchi, A.C., de Moraes, I.G. et al. (2008). Presence of arsenic in different types of MTA and white and gray Portland cement. *Oral Surg. Oral Med. Oral Pathol. Oral Radiol. Endod.* 106 (6): 909–913.

63 George, V., Janardhanan, S.K., Varma, B. et al. (2015). Clinical and radiographic evaluation of indirect pulp treatment with MTA and calcium hydroxide in primary teeth (in-vivo study). *J. Indian Soc. Pedod. Prev. Dent.* 33 (2): 104–110.

64 Hilton, T.J., Ferracane, J.L., and Mancl, L. (2013). Comparison of CaOH with MTA for direct pulp capping: a PBRN randomized clinical trial. *J. Dent. Res.* 92 (7 Suppl): 16s–22s.

65 Smail-Faugeron, V., Glenny, A.M., Courson, F. et al. (2018). Pulp treatment for extensive decay in primary teeth. *Cochrane Database Syst. Rev.* 5: CD003220.

66 Asgary, S., Shahabi, S., Jafarzadeh, T. et al. (2008). The properties of a new endodontic material. *J. Endod.* 34 (8): 990–993.

67 Asgary, S. (2007). Endodontic filling material. US patent 20080206716.

68 Cutajar, A., Mallia, B., Abela, S., and Camilleri, J. (2011). Replacement of radiopacifier in mineral trioxide aggregate; characterization and determination of physical properties. *Dent. Mater.* 27 (9): 879–891.

69 Koutroulis, A., Batchelor, H., Kuehne, S.A. et al. (2019). Investigation of the effect of the water to powder ratio on hydraulic cement properties. *Dent. Mater.* 35 (8): 1146–1154.

70 Fridland, M. and Rosado, R. (2005). MTA solubility: a long term study. *J. Endod.* 31 (5): 376–379.

71 Shahravan, A., Jalali, S.P., Torabi, M. et al. (2011). A histological study of pulp reaction to various water/powder ratios of white mineral trioxide aggregate as pulp-capping

material in human teeth: a double-blinded, randomized controlled trial. *Int. Endod. J.* 44 (11): 1029–1033.

72 Asgary, S. and Kamrani, F.A. (2008). Antibacterial effects of five different root canal sealing materials. *J. Oral Sci.* 50 (4): 469–474.

73 Asgary, S., Eghbal, M.J., and Parirokh, M. (2008). Sealing ability of a novel endodontic cement as a root-end filling material. *J. Biomed. Mater. Res. A* 87 (3): 706–709.

74 Asgary, S., Eghbal, M.J., and Ehsani, S. (2010). Periradicular regeneration after endodontic surgery with calcium-enriched mixture cement in dogs. *J. Endod.* 36 (5): 837–841.

75 Eghbal, M.J., Torabzadeh, H., Bagheban, A.A. et al. (2016). Color stability of mineral trioxide aggregate and calcium enriched mixture cement. *J. Investig. Clin. Dent.* 7 (4): 341–346.

76 Mehrdad, L., Malekafzali, B., Shekarchi, F. et al. (2013). Histological and CBCT evaluation of a pulpotomised primary molar using calcium enriched mixture cement. *Eur. Arch. Paediatr. Dent.* 14 (3): 191–194.

77 Primus, C.M. (2014). Products and distinctions. In: *Mineral Trioxide Aggregate in Dentistry* (ed. J. Camilleri), 151–172. Heidelberg: Springer.

78 Septodont (2010). Biodentine Active Biosilicate Technology: Scientific File.

79 Camilleri, J. (2013). Investigation of Biodentine as dentine replacement material. *J. Dent.* 41 (7): 600–610.

80 Koubi, G., Colon, P., Franquin, J.-C. et al. (2013). Clinical evaluation of the performance and safety of a new dentine substitute, Biodentine, in the restoration of posterior teeth – a prospective study. *Clin. Oral Investig.* 17 (1): 243–249.

81 Laurent, P., Camps, J., De Meo, M. et al. (2008). Induction of specific cell responses to a Ca(3)SiO(5)-based posterior restorative material. *Dent. Mater.* 24 (11): 1486–1494.

82 Goldberg, M., Pradelle-Plasse, N., Tran, X.V. et al. (2009). Emerging trends in (bio) material research. In: *Biocompatibility or Cytotoxic Effects of Dental Composites* (ed. M. Goldberg). Moreton In Marsh: Coxmoor.

83 Koutroulis, A., Kuehne, S.A., Cooper, P.R., and Camilleri, J. (2019). The role of calcium ion release on biocompatibility and antimicrobial properties of hydraulic cements. *Sci. Rep.* 9 (1): 19019.

84 Yoldas, S.E., Bani, M., Atabek, D., and Bodur, H. (2016). Comparison of the potential discoloration effect of bioaggregate, Biodentine, and white mineral trioxide aggregate on bovine teeth: in vitro research. *J. Endod.* 42 (12): 1815–1818.

85 Valles, M., Mercade, M., Duran-Sindreu, F. et al. (2013). Influence of light and oxygen on the color stability of five calcium silicate-based materials. *J. Endod.* 39 (4): 525–528.

86 Grech, L., Mallia, B., and Camilleri, J. (2013). Investigation of the physical properties of tricalcium silicate cement-based root-end filling materials. *Dent. Mater.* 29 (2): e20–e28.

87 Pham, C.L., Kratunova, E., Marion, I. et al. (2019). Effect of overlying material on final setting of Biodentine (R) in primary molar pulpotomies. *Pediatr. Dent.* 41 (2): 140–145.

88 Weissrock, G., Franquin, P., Colon, P., and Koubi, G. (2009). A clinical study of a new Ca_3SiO_5-based material indicated as a dentine substitute. *Journee Scientifique du CNEOC Brest* 45: 74–101.

89 Boddeda, K.R., Rani, C.R., Vanga, N.R., and Chandrabhatla, S.K. (2019). Comparative evaluation of Biodentine, 2% chlorhexidine with RMGIC and calcium hydroxide as indirect pulp capping materials in primary molars: an in vivo study. *J. Indian Soc. Pedod. Prev. Dent.* 37 (1): 60–66.

90 Maroto, M., Barreiro, S., and Barberia, E. (2019). Portland cement as pulp dressing agent in pulpotomy treatment of primary molars: a 12-month clinical study. *Eur. J. Paediatr. Dent.* 20 (1): 23–26.

91 Celik, B.N., Mutluay, M.S., Arikan, V., and Sari, S. (2019). The evaluation of MTA and Biodentine as a pulpotomy materials for carious exposures in primary teeth. *Clin. Oral Investig.* 23 (2): 661–666.

92 Nasseh, H.N., El Noueiri, B., Pilipili, C., and Ayoub, F. (2018). Evaluation of Biodentine pulpotomies in deciduous molars with physiological root resorption (stage 3). *Int. J. Clin. Pediatr. Dent.* 11 (5): 393–394.

93 Caruso, S., Dinoi, T., Marzo, G. et al. (2018). Clinical and radiographic evaluation of Biodentine versus calcium hydroxide in primary teeth pulpotomies: a retrospective study. *BMC Oral Health* 18 (1): 54.

94 Shafie, L., Barghi, H., Parirokh, M. et al. (2017). Postoperative pain following pulpotomy of primary molars with two biomaterials: a randomized split mouth clinical trial. *Iranian Endod. J.* 12 (1): 10–14.

95 Guven, Y., Aksakal, S.D., Avcu, N. et al. (2017). Success rates of pulpotomies in primary molars using calcium silicate-based materials: a randomized control trial. *Biomed. Res. Int.* 2017: 4059703.

96 Bani, M., Aktas, N., Cinar, C., and Odabas, M.E. (2017). The clinical and radiographic success of primary molar pulpotomy using Biodentine and mineral trioxide aggregate: a 24-month randomized clinical trial. *Pediatr. Dent.* 39 (4): 284–288.

97 Carti, O. and Oznurhan, F. (2017). Evaluation and comparison of mineral trioxide aggregate and Biodentine in primary tooth pulpotomy: clinical and radiographic study. *Niger. J. Clin. Pract.* 20 (12): 1604–1609.

98 Grewal, N., Salhan, R., Kaur, N., and Patel, H.B. (2016). Comparative evaluation of calcium silicate-based dentin substitute (Biodentine(R)) and calcium hydroxide (pulpdent) in the formation of reactive dentin bridge in regenerative pulpotomy of vital primary teeth: triple blind, randomized clinical trial. *Contemp. Clin. Dent.* 7 (4): 457–463.

99 Togaru, H., Muppa, R., Srinivas, N. et al. (2016). Clinical and radiographic evaluation

of success of two commercially available pulpotomy agents in primary teeth: an in vivo study. *J. Contemp. Dent. Pract.* 17 (7): 557–563.

100 Cuadros-Fernandez, C., Lorente Rodriguez, A.I., Saez-Martinez, S. et al. (2016). Short-term treatment outcome of pulpotomies in primary molars using mineral trioxide aggregate and Biodentine: a randomized clinical trial. *Clin. Oral Investig.* 20 (7): 1639–1645.

101 Kusum, B., Rakesh, K., and Richa, K. (2015). Clinical and radiographical evaluation of mineral trioxide aggregate, Biodentine and propolis as pulpotomy medicaments in primary teeth. *Restor. Dent. Endod.* 40 (4): 276–285.

102 Khorakian, F., Mazhari, F., Asgary, S. et al. (2014). Two-year outcomes of electrosurgery and calcium-enriched mixture pulpotomy in primary teeth: a randomised clinical trial. *Eur. Arch. Paediatr. Dent.* 15 (4): 223–228.

103 Oliveira, T.M., Moretti, A.B., Sakai, V.T. et al. (2013). Clinical, radiographic and histologic analysis of the effects of pulp capping materials used in pulpotomies of human primary teeth. *Eur. Arch. Paediatr. Dent.* 14 (2): 65–71.

104 Malekafzali, B., Shekarchi, F., and Asgary, S. (2011). Treatment outcomes of pulpotomy in primary molars using two endodontic biomaterials. A 2-year randomised clinical trial. *Eur. J. Paediatr. Dent.* 12 (3): 189–193.

105 Sakai, V.T., Moretti, A.B., Oliveira, T.M. et al. (2009). Pulpotomy of human primary molars with MTA and Portland cement: a randomised controlled trial. *Br. Dent. J.* 207 (3): E5; disc. 128–129.

106 Camilleri, J. (2011). Scanning electron microscopic evaluation of the material interface of adjacent layers of dental materials. *Dent. Mater.* 27 (9): 870–878.

107 Ahmed, H.M. (2014). Pulpectomy procedures in primary molar teeth. *Eur. J. Gen. Dent.* 3 (1): 3–10.

108 Ahmed, H.M. (2013). Anatomical challenges, electronic working length determination and current developments in root canal preparation of primary molar teeth. *Int. Endod. J.* 46 (11): 1011–1022.

109 Zehnder, M. (2006). Root canal irrigants. *J. Endod.* 32 (5): 389–398.

110 Ahmad, I.A. and Pani, S.C. (2015). Accuracy of electronic apex locators in primary teeth: a meta-analysis. *Int. Endod. J.* 48 (3): 298–307.

111 Govindaraju, L., Jeevanandan, G., and Subramanian, E.M.G. (2017). Comparison of quality of obturation and instrumentation time using hand files and two rotary file systems in primary molars: a single-blinded randomized controlled trial. *Eur. J. Dent.* 11 (3): 376–379.

112 Mahajan, N. and Bansal, A. (2015). Various obturation methods used in deciduous teeth. *Int. J. Med. Dent. Sci.* 4 (1): 708–713.

113 Khubchandani, M., Baliga, M.S., Rawlani, S.S. et al. (2017). Comparative evaluation of different obturation techniques in primary molars: an in vivo study. *Eur. J. Gen. Dent.* 6 (1): 42–47.

114 Moskovitz, M., Sammara, E., and Holan, G. (2005). Success rate of root canal treatment in primary molars. *J. Dent.* 33 (1): 41–47.

115 Kher, M.S. and Rao, A. (2019). Pulp therapy in primary teeth. In: *Contemporary Treatment Techniques in Pediatric Dentistry* (eds. M.S. Kher and A. Rao), 75–98. Cham: Springer Nature Switzerland AG.

116 Nakornchai, S., Banditsing, P., and Visetratana, N. (2010). Clinical evaluation of 3Mix and Vitapex as treatment options for pulpally involved primary molars. *Int. J. Paediatr. Dent.* 20 (3): 214–221.

117 Mortazavi, M. and Mesbahi, M. (2004). Comparison of zinc oxide and eugenol, and Vitapex for root canal treatment of necrotic primary teeth. *Int. J. Paediatr. Dent.* 14 (6): 417–424.

118 Moskovitz, M., Yahav, D., Tickotsky, N., and Holan, G. (2010). Long-term follow up of root canal treated primary molars. *Int. J. Paediatr. Dent.* 20 (3): 207–213.

119 Chen, X., Liu, X., and Zhong, J. (2017). Clinical and radiographic evaluation of pulpectomy in primary teeth: a 18-months clinical randomized controlled trial. *Head Face Med.* 13 (1): 12.

120 Fuks, A.B., Guelmann, M., and Kupietzky, A. (2012). Current developments in pulp therapy for primary teeth. *Endod. Top.* 23: 50–72.

121 Moskovitz, M. and Tickotsky, N. (2016). Pulpectomy and root canal treatment (RCT) in primary teeth: techniques and materials. In: *Pediatric Endodontics: Current Concepts in Pulp Therapy for Primary and Young Permanent Teeth* (eds. A.B. Fuks and B. Peretz), 71–102. Cham: Springer International.

122 Najjar, R.S., Alamoudi, N.M., El-Housseiny, A.A. et al. (2019). A comparison of calcium hydroxide/iodoform paste and zinc oxide eugenol as root filling materials for pulpectomy in primary teeth: a systematic review and meta-analysis. *Clin. Exp. Dent. Res.* 5 (3): 294–310.

123 Ozalp, N., Saroglu, I., and Sonmez, H. (2005). Evaluation of various root canal filling materials in primary molar pulpectomies: an in vivo study. *Am. J. Dent.* 18 (6): 347–350.

124 Sadrian, R. and Coll, J.A. (1993). A long-term followup on the retention rate of zinc oxide eugenol filler after primary tooth pulpectomy. *Pediatr. Dent.* 15 (4): 249–253.

125 Barker, B.C. and Lockett, B.C. (1971). Endodontic experiments with resorbable paste. *Aust. Dent. J.* 16 (6): 364–372.

126 Hendry, J.A., Jeansonne, B.G., Dummett, C.O. Jr., and Burrell, W. (1982). Comparison of calcium hydroxide and zinc oxide and eugenol pulpectomies in primary teeth of dogs. *Oral Surg. Oral Med. Oral Pathol.* 54 (4): 445–451.

127 Pires, C.W., Lenzi, T.L., Soares, F.Z.M., and Rocha, R.O. (2018). Zinc oxide eugenol paste jeopardises the adhesive bonding to primary dentine. *Eur. Arch. Paediatr. Dent.* 19 (3): 163–169.

128 Estrela, C., Estrela, C.R., Hollanda, A.C. et al. (2006). Influence of iodoform on antimicrobial potential of calcium hydroxide. *J. Appl. Oral Sci. Rev. FOB* 14 (1): 33–37.

129 Nurko, C., Ranly, D.M., Garcia-Godoy, F., and Lakshmyya, K.N. (2000). Resorption of a calcium hydroxide/iodoform paste (Vitapex) in root canal therapy for primary teeth: a case report. *Pediatr. Dent.* 22 (6): 517–520.

130 Holan, G. and Fuks, A.B. (1993). A comparison of pulpectomies using ZOE and KRI paste in primary molars: a retrospective study. *Pediatr. Dent.* 15 (6): 403–407.

131 Nurko, C. and Garcia-Godoy, F. (1999). Evaluation of a calcium hydroxide/iodoform paste (Vitapex) in root canal therapy for primary teeth. *J. Clin. Pediatr. Dent.* 23 (4): 289–294.

132 Barcelos, R., Santos, M.P., Primo, L.G. et al. (2011). ZOE paste pulpectomies outcome in primary teeth: a systematic review. *J. Clin. Pediatr. Dent.* 35 (3): 241–248.

133 Subramaniam, P. and Gilhotra, K. (2011). Endoflas, zinc oxide eugenol and metapex as root canal filling materials in primary molars – a comparative clinical study. *J. Clin. Pediatr. Dent.* 35 (4): 365–369.

134 Tchaou, W.S., Turng, B.F., Minah, G.E., and Coll, J.A. (1996). Inhibition of pure cultures of oral bacteria by root canal filling materials. *Pediatr. Dent.* 18 (7): 444–449.

135 Mass, E. and Zilberman, U.L. (1989). Endodontic treatment of infected primary teeth, using Maisto's paste. *ASDC J. Dent. Child.* 56 (2): 117–120.

136 Reddy, V.V. (1996). Clinical and radiological evaluation of zinc oxide-eugenol and Maisto's paste as obturating materials in infected primary teeth – nine months study. *J. Indian Soc. Pedod. Prev. Dent.* 14 (2): 39–44.

9

Adhesion to Intraradicular and Coronal Dentine

Possibilities and Challenges

Mutlu Özcan[1], Claudia Angela Maziero Volpato[2], and Luiz Fernando D'Altoé[3]

[1] *Division of Dental Biomaterials, Center for Dental and Oral Medicine, Clinic for Reconstructive Dentistry, University of Zürich, Zürich, Switzerland*
[2] *Department of Dentistry, Federal University of Santa Catarina (UFSC), Florianópolis, Santa Catarina, Brazil*
[3] *Department of Dentistry, University of the Extreme South of Santa Catarina (UNESC), Criciúma, Santa Catarina, Brazil*

TABLE OF CONTENTS

9.1   Introduction

Human dentine is chemically composed of minerals in the form of apatite crystals (about 70 vol%), organic matrix (20 vol%), and water (10 vol%). The volumetric percentage between these components varies according to tooth size, shape, location on the arch, and age-related changes or dental diseases [1]. Various morphological structures of dentine, such as dentinal tubules, incremental growth lines (Von Ebner and Owen), Tomes granular layer, and intratubular, intertubular, and interglobular dentine, have already been identified as demonstrating histological differentiations within the dentinal structure [2].

The dentinal tubules, filled with glycoprotein, give dentine a high permeability [3, 4]. The mixture of collagen fibres, noncollagenous proteins, and glycosaminoglycans (GAGs) provides a matrix capable of absorbing a large amount of water, which explains the natural humidity of this substrate [2]. Most collagen fibres in the organic matrix are classified as Type I collagens, having a diameter of 50–100 nm, and are distributed obliquely or perpendicularly around the dentinal tubules. The number of collagen fibres decreases from superficial to deep dentine due to the fact that the latter has larger dentinal tubules [5].

Root dentine is characterized by the presence of dentinal tubules starting from the pulp and moving to the interface with the cementum (Figure 9.1) [6]. The tubules contain cytoplasmic extensions of the odontoblasts and are filled with glycoprotein solution containing approximately 12% water. Compared to the coronal dentine, root dentine has a smaller amount

Endodontic Materials in Clinical Practice, First Edition. Edited by Josette Camilleri.

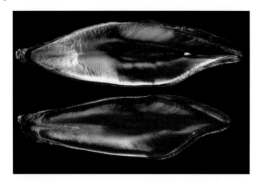

Figure 9.1 Image made with polarized light, showing the presence of dentinal tubules. *Source:* Mutlu Özcan, Claudia Angela Maziero Volpato, Luiz Fernando D'Altoé.

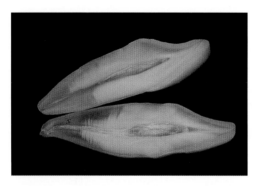

Figure 9.2 Detail of root dentine, showing its translucent appearance in the apical portion. *Source:* Mutlu Özcan, Claudia Angela Maziero Volpato, Luiz Fernando D'Altoé.

of intertubular dentine and a smaller number, density, and diameter of dentinal tubules [1]. In root dentine, the number of dentinal tubules decreases towards the apical region, where the dentin is quite irregular, translucent, and may be devoid of tubules entirely (Figure 9.2) [7]. When dentinal tubules are present in this region, they are usually sclerotic and obliterated with minerals that resemble those of the peritubular dentine [8]. In addition, unlike in human enamel, which is made up of approximately 97% minerals, 2% water, and 1% organic matrix [9], a very humid environment is found throughout root dentine [3]. The complexity of the anatomical structure of root dentine complicates durable adhesion of resin-based materials in this region.

9.2 Adhesion to Human Dentine

The adhesion of restorative or capping materials to human dentine has been a matter of controversy in the dental literature [10, 11]. The wide variation in dentinal structure in the same tooth makes dentine a very complex substrate in this regard [12]. However, the differences between coronal and root dentine are not a barrier to dentin adhesion [8]. Bonding techniques are typically very sensitive to humidity, being influenced by substrate type, adhesive system, and application technique. Thus, standardization of procedures and care during clinical steps are fundamental to the success of the adhesive protocol.

The longevity of the adhesive interface is directly related to the quality of the hybrid layer [13], comprising the bond between the polymer present in the adhesive resin and the collagen present in dentine. When acid etching is performed in dentine, demineralization, collagen fibre exposure, and light opening of dentinal tubules have been observed [14, 15]. The primer applied to the demineralized dentine then maintains the collagen structure and may increase the free surface energy. In addition, after promoting evaporation of water and solvent, the primer binds to the adhesive resin, causing it to penetrate capillary into the dentinal tubules [16]. A decreasing number, density, and diameter of the dentinal tubules in different root areas can lead to a significant reduction in the thickness of the hybrid layer from cervical to apical [14].

Conventional bonding can be employed to restore vital and nonvital teeth [17]. In conventional bonding systems, also known as total-etch adhesive systems, dental tissues are conditioned with phosphoric acid, followed by the application of adhesive resin in two (primer and adhesive present in the same solution) or three (primer and adhesive applied separately) clinical steps. When the acid is applied to the enamel, demineralization of this substrate creates microporosities, which will then be filled

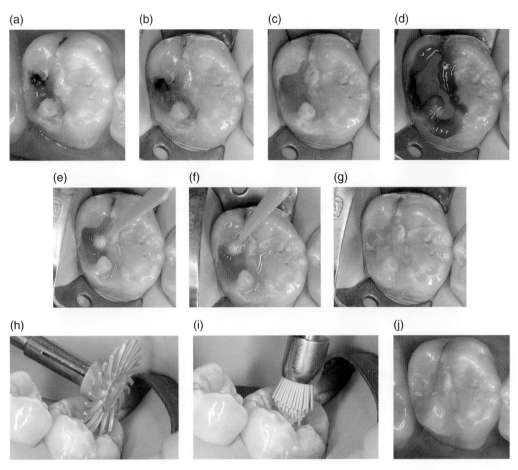

Figure 9.3 (a) Occlusal cavity with irregularities that disturb the chewing function of the patient. *Source:* Mutlu Özcan, Claudia Angela Maziero Volpato, Luiz Fernando D'Altoé. (b) Initial appearance after absolute isolation. *Source:* Mutlu Özcan, Claudia Angela Maziero Volpato, Luiz Fernando D'Altoé. (c) Completed cavity after removal of decayed tissue. Note the presence of enamel and dentine. *Source:* Mutlu Özcan, Claudia Angela Maziero Volpato, Luiz Fernando D'Altoé. (d) Selective acid conditioning of enamel with 35% phosphoric acid (Ultra-Etch; Ultradent, South Jordan, UT, USA). *Source:* Mutlu Özcan, Claudia Angela Maziero Volpato, Luiz Fernando D'Altoé. (e) Application of the acidic primer for 20 seconds (Clearfil SE Bond; Kuraray Noritake Dental, Tokyo, Japan). *Source:* Mutlu Özcan, Claudia Angela Maziero Volpato, Luiz Fernando D'Altoé. (f) Application and polymerization of the adhesive system (Clearfil SE Bond) for 10 seconds following evaporation of the primer solvent. *Source:* Mutlu Özcan, Claudia Angela Maziero Volpato, Luiz Fernando D'Altoé. (g) View of the restoration after stratification of the resin composite (Z350 XT; 3M ESPE, St Paul, MN, USA). *Source:* Mutlu Özcan, Claudia Angela Maziero Volpato, Luiz Fernando D'Altoé. (h) Polishing with a spiral diamond disc (Sof-Lex; 3M ESPE). *Source:* Mutlu Özcan, Claudia Angela Maziero Volpato, Luiz Fernando D'Altoé. (i) Final polishing with a silicon carbide brush (Occlubrush; Kerr Dental, Brea, CA, USA). *Source:* Mutlu Özcan, Claudia Angela Maziero Volpato, Luiz Fernando D'Altoé. (j) Occlusal view of the restoration completed after one week. *Source:* Mutlu Özcan, Claudia Angela Maziero Volpato, Luiz Fernando D'Altoé.

by the hydrophobic resin monomers present in the adhesive, helping in the micromechanical retention of the restoration. On dentine, phosphoric acid removes the smear layer, exposing collagen fibres, which will be infiltrated by resinous monomers to form the hybrid layer [18].

Commercially available self-etching systems can be classified according to the number of operative steps into 'two-step' and 'all-in-one' systems; this classification affects the adhesion quality to dentine (Figure 9.3). In self-etching adhesives, primers can partially demineralize the underlying dentine whilst simultaneously providing monomers to fill the created microporosities. In 'two-step' systems, washing the surface after acid etching is unnecessary and thus maintenance of the interfibrillary spaces by humidity is not required as demineralization products and acid etching residues are incorporated and polymerized with the adhesive resin to the dentine [4, 19]. These agents may have acid-functionalized monomers in their composition, such as 10-methacryloyloxydecyl dihydrogen phosphate (10-MDP), which favour dentine surface demineralization due to the maintenance of a local pH between 1.5 and 3.0, at which range acid groups bind to the hydroxyapatite, forming suitable adhesion between the methacrylate network and the dentine [19]. In single-step adhesives, the three basic components (acid, primer, and adhesive resin) are combined where dentine substrate hybridization is achieved in a single clinical step [20, 21].

Regardless of the adhesive system employed, studies agree on the need for micromechanical enticement resulting from the bond between the adhesive resin and the collagen present in the dentinal tubules, which is primarily responsible for the quality of the adhesive interface [4, 22]. The stronger the bond, the better the marginal sealing, the less the microleakage, and the longer the survival of the restorations. However, according to some studies, there is no direct and significant correlation between bond strength and marginal sealing [23]. Microleakage has been suggested as the major factor responsible for the degradation of the adhesive interface over time, despite the previously achieved bond-strength results [24–26]. When water can penetrate existing spaces, usually as a result of incomplete penetration of the resin into demineralized dentine, the bond strength may decrease, marginal discolouration and secondary caries may occur, and postoperative sensitivity may increase [25, 27]. Likewise, with regard to the longevity of the filling in the intraradicular system, the quality of adhesion on the coronal dentine is essential.

9.3 Adhesion to Root Dentine in Vital Teeth

Vital teeth with cervical lesions and deep cavities exhibit root dentine exposure, most often associated with dentine sensitivity [4, 15]. According to the hydrodynamic theory, when enamel is lost and dentine is exposed, a change in dentine fluid velocity can stimulate pain receptors found in the most inner portions of the tubules or predentine, causing sensitivity [3, 4].

In shallow cavities, dentine has a smaller amount of dentinal tubules (20.000 mm^2), with an average diameter of 0.6 µm, and a predominance of intertubular dentine (96% of the area), which is rich in collagen. Already in deep cavities, the amount of tubules is about 45.000 mm^2, with an average diameter of 2.4 µm, and there is a small amount of intertubular dentine (12% of the area) [28]. This is fundamental to undertaking restoration with proper sealing on these substrates. In addition, it is important to highlight the fact that different dentine substrate patterns can be found in a single tooth, making it impossible to obtain a homogeneous hybrid layer over the entire length of cavity preparations. Variations in the presence of caries (infected, contaminated, sclerosed, reactive, or repair tertiary dentine), tubular orientation (transverse, longitudinal, or oblique section), and depth (superficial, middle, or deep) also present a compromised dentine on which to bond [19, 29].

During cavity preparation for direct or indirect restorations, dentine is covered by a layer containing remnants of dental structure, saliva, and bacteria. This layer, known as the smear layer, blocks the entry of adhesive resin to dentinal tubules and decreases dentinal permeability by up to 86% [30]. However, it can be easily removed by conditioning with 30–40% phosphoric acid for 15–20 seconds [6]. Acid etching of the dentine surface removes the smear layer and enables the bonding of resin-based materials to demineralized dentine, allowing sealing by adhesive resin and helping prevent postoperative hypersensitivity and recurrent caries [25].

In the bonding procedure, the humidity of the dentine should be maintained, since the mesh of collagen fibres separated by 15–20 nm-wide spaces is supported by the presence of water [31]. If the dentine surface is excessively dry, collagen fibres without mineral support can collapse, closing the microscopic spaces created during conditioning, which are critical for the longevity of the adhesion. On the other hand, excess moisture on the dentinal surface impairs the bond strength and sealing of dentinal tubules [25].

One other important aspect in this regard is the polymerization contraction that occurs during the making of direct restorations using resin composite. When resin-based materials polymerize, the monomer molecules join together to form intertwining chains and the mass is reduced by about 2–7%. The strength of polymerization shrinkage often exceeds the bond strength of dentine adhesives to dentine, which may result in failures due to dental surfaces yielding to weaker adhesion [21, 32].

9.4 Pulp Protection Materials and Their Effect on Adhesion to Dentine

The preservation of pulp vitality depends on a number of clinical factors. The use of pulp-capping biomaterials on deep dentine can also preserve vitality, as the success of vital pulp treatment is dependent on the choice of materials when remaining dentine thickness is less than 0.5 mm [33]. Adequate management of the pulp tissues is necessary [34], followed by placement of an adequate pulp-protection material. Compounds such as calcium hydroxide (CH) have been used for over a century, but the most recent guidelines [35] suggest the use of glass ionomer cement (GIC) or of hydraulic calcium silicate cements (HCSCs), such as mineral trioxide aggregate (MTA) or Biodentine

(Septodont, Saint Maur des Fosses, France), placed over disinfected dentine.

CH is a biocompatible material [36] with antimicrobial properties [37] that stimulates the formation of sclerotic dentine [38]. When it is first applied to the exposed pulp, superficial necrosis occurs [39], which induces a slight irritation that stimulates the pulp to repair, forming a bridge of sclerotic dentine through cell differentiation [38], extracellular matrix (ECM) secretion, and subsequent mineralization [39]. However, CH cement does not have good adhesive properties [40] and is subject to dissolution over time [36], leading to the formation of dead spaces [40] and microleakage [41].

GICs are materials that involve a significant acid–base reaction as part of their setting, where the acid is a water-soluble polymer and the base is a special glass [42]. They are considered self-etching cements, since they bond chemically to dentine through ion exchange at the tooth–material interface [43]. They also have an insulating effect in relation to thermal changes in the oral environment [44], acting as antibacterial agents [45] and presenting low levels of marginal infiltration [46]. However, their bond strength is considered low, with values ranging from 2.6 to 9.6 MPa for enamel and from 1.1 to 4.1 MPa for dentine [47].

MTA was the first HCSC available for clinical use and is composed of tricalcium and dicalcium silicate. It is recommended for pulp capping, pulpotomy, and treatment of immature teeth with nonvital pulps or open apices, due to its biocompatibility [48] and potential bioactivity [49, 50]. However, it has some critical shortcomings, namely its prolonged setting time [51], high solubility during setting [51], potential for discolouration [52, 53], and difficulty in handling [54, 55]. Its bond strength is influenced by its long setting time and its surface following acid conditioning [56].

The reaction of HCSCs with water leads to the formation of calcium silicate hydrate and CH [57]; the CH interacts with tissue fluids, resulting in bioactivity [49, 50]. Although several formulations are available on the market, Biodentine is the most optimized and specifically developed for pulp-related procedures. Biodentine powder contains tricalcium silicate, zirconium oxide, and calcium carbonate, and its liquid is composed of water plus calcium chloride and a hydrosoluble polymer [54, 58, 59]. It has good sealing ability [60], relatively short setting time [54], high alkalinity [61], and good biocompatibility and bioactive potential [62, 63].

More recently, additives such as calcium phosphate [64], silicon oxide [65], and resin components [66] have been added to HCSCs, with the aim of improving biological activity [67], strengthening the material [65], and providing the ability to command cure the material in a way that avoids problems with bonding composite resin to the underlying substrate [68]. Commercial examples of these cements are TotalFill (FKG Dentaire, La Chaux-de-Fonds, Switzerland), BioAggregate (Verio Dental, Vancouver, BC, Canada), and TheraCal LC (Bisco, Schaumburg, IL, USA), respectively. The solubility of TheraCal LC is reported to be less than that of MTA and CH [69], but the addition of resin induces important changes in its hydration properties [59].

The quality of the adhesion between pulp-capping materials and resin composites is critical for optimal stress distribution at the interface, reduction of microleakage, and the general success and longevity of direct restorations. Resin composite is frequently the material of choice for placement over pulp-capping materials because of the low loads applied on them, reducing the possibility of dislocation. Thus, acid etching has been employed on these materials, followed by the application of adhesive resin systems. However, studies demonstrate that acid etching results in the formation of porosities in the glass ionomer and in the destruction of part of the microstructure of Biodentine, reducing the adhesive strength [70, 71]. Primers that contain acetone or alcohol may affect the properties of CH, resulting in

high erosion and lower compressive strength values [72]. Water-based adhesive resin systems may result in lower bond strength due to incomplete polymerization of monomers and the high water content of HCSCs, which can interfere with the polymerization of self-etching adhesive resins [73]. Although some authors recommend that materials such as MTA and Biodentine be covered with other materials, such as GIC [56], studies show that a weak bond occurs, leading to their displacement [74]. Thus, from a bonding perspective, the use of resin-based materials such as Theracal LC as pulp-capping biomaterials is still the best strategy, due to their greater resistance to the effects of acid conditioning and adhesive procedures [69]. However, the European Society of Endodontology (ESE) guidelines do not recommend the use of such materials [35]. The implications of the effects of resins on dental pulp are further discussed in Chapter 2.

9.5 Adhesion to Root Dentine in Nonvital Teeth

In nonvital teeth, structural changes that occur as a result of access to the pulp chamber, endodontic instrumentation, or intraradicular preparation to receive intraradicular posts leave the root dentine exposed, necessitating its restoration [75]. These clinical procedures may alter the mechanical properties of the teeth, whilst modifying the viable dentine surface for adhesion [76]. In addition, these teeth will have less water and an increased risk of root fracture [75].

Restoration of endodontically treated teeth is usually performed with prefabricated or custom-made intraradicular posts. Most prefabricated posts consist of unidirectional fibres (glass, carbon, quartz, or polyethylene) embedded in a highly cross-linked resin matrix, which might be an epoxy resin, a methacrylate matrix, or a proprietary resin [77]. These posts present acceptable biomechanical behaviour with high flexural strength and a modulus of elasticity similar to that of dentine and favourable aesthetics [78]. They are usually luted within the intraradicular preparation, using resin-based luting cement to fix them and to fill the space between them and the root canal walls. Their surface conditioning prior to adhesive resin cementation depends on the micromorphology of the post surface, the matrix composition that surrounds the fibres, and the resin-based luting cement [79]. Thus, manufacturer's recommendations must be strictly followed.

Some techniques that may be used to maintain the dental structure and reduce intraradicular wear caused by post preparation are suggested in the literature [80, 81]. Here, the core is made inside the pulp chamber and retained in the root canal. In 1980, Nayyar et al. [80] suggested the removal of obturated gutta-percha to a depth of 2–4 mm from the canal orifice and restoration with amalgam, in what is known as the 'coronoradicular restoration technique'. More recently, other core build-up materials have been used for root reconstruction, including GIC, composite resins, and bioactive materials, with or without prefabricated posts [81]. For the success of such techniques, it is essential that the material presents adequate strength, exhibits a high level of resistance to bacterial leakage, and is dimensionally stable in the presence of oral fluids. In addition, the tooth must have sufficient coronary structure to promote adhesion [80].

The success of adhesive resin cementation of posts to root dentine depends on mastery of the technique employed (materials and adhesive resin technique) and knowledge of the features of devitalized dentine (dentine tissue morphology and geometric characteristics of the root canal space) [82]. Necrotic teeth have bacterial toxins and pulp-tissue remnants in direct contact with the intraradicular dentine. In addition, during instrumentation of canal walls with endodontic files, a significant amount of smear layer is produced [83]. Whilst the first layer is about 1–2 μm thick and consists of organic matter and dentine particles, the second extends into the dentinal tubules to about 10 μm, forming smear plugs [84]. The composition of these layers varies according to the dentine substrate, endodontic instrument, and irrigation method employed [9].

The smear layer may contain dentine debris, remnants of plasticized gutta-percha, saliva, toxins, bacteria, irrigant, and obturator cement products, as well as organic content due to the presence of viable or necrotic pulp tissue [85]. The diversity of these contaminants prevents chemical interactions and penetration of adhesive resins into root dentine, as the smear layer acts as a physical barrier [86]. This layer should thus be carefully removed in order to optimize the adhesive potential of root dentine, by the use of irrigation solutions employed during and after endodontic instrumentation [87]. Sodium hypochlorite (NaOCl) has been shown to be quite effective in this regard [88], as compared to ethylenediaminetetraacetic acid (EDTA) [87] and chlorhexidine gluconate (CHX) [89].

NaOCl has antibacterial properties, dissolves dentine collagen, and aids in the removal of organic debris formed during instrumentation and intraradicular preparation [90]. However, its use may inhibit polymerization of resin-based luting cement due to its strong oxidizing property [91]. After rinsing with NaOCl, an oxygen-rich layer is formed on the dentine surface, resulting in inhibition of resin polymerization, reduction of adhesion, and consequent increase of microleakage [91]. In order to compensate for these limitations, studies have indicated the use of NaOCl solutions associated with chelating agents, such as EDTA at about 17% concentration, as a good strategy for removal of the smear layer and achieve adhesion between resin-based materials and intra-radicular dentine [92]. However, the use of EDTA for longer than one minute may lead to excessive dentine demineralization [93].

CHX has the ability to reduce the proteolytic activity of dentine, inhibiting matrix metalloproteinases (MMPs). These enzymes can degrade proteins in the ECM, including denatured collagen [94], and may thus degrade the unprotected collagen left after incomplete infiltration of resin monomers into the conditioned dentine; this could be related to the progressive degradation of the hybrid layer [95]. The use of CHX thus prevents the self-degradation of exposed collagen fibrils, contributing to the bond strength of resin-based materials with dentine [96]. However, its inhibitory effect seems to be related to its dose and the product concentration; therefore, the relationship between CHX concentration and the long-term stability of dentine adhesion is not yet clear [97].

Eugenol present in endodontic sealers has the ability to partially or totally inhibit polymerization of resin composite materials. Lower bond-strength values were reported when zinc oxide-eugenol (ZOE)-based root canal sealers were used for endodontic obturation [98]. In the clinical stage, it is important that the canal walls are mechanically cleaned by endodontic instruments and that alcohol or detergent is rubbed against them to remove any eugenol. Acid etching also assists in eugenol removal, so long as the root walls have been precleaned and no coarse cement residues are still present [99]. Studies have suggested that hydroxide- and resin-based sealers may be an interesting alternative to eugenol-based cements [99, 100]. However, sealers containing CH are difficult to remove from the edges of dentine, reducing the adhesion capacity of resin cement and leading to low bond-strength values [100, 101]. The epoxy resin-based sealer AH Plus (Dentsply Sirona, Bensheim, Germany) offers reduced viscosity and improved fluidity properties. A recent study showed it had superior bond strength compared to other endodontic sealers: EndoSequence BC (Brasseler, Savannah, GA, USA), Sealapex (SyBronendo, Orange, CA, USA), Sealer Plus (MK Life, Porto Alegre, Brazil), and Endofill (Dentsply Sirona) [102]. The authors thus recommended the use of endodontic sealers based on epoxy resin when intraradicular posts are cemented with composite resin [102].

Figure 9.4 (a) Extensive restorations on teeth 14 and 15 with adhesive failure and loss of dental tissue. *Source:* Mutlu Özcan, Claudia Angela Maziero Volpato, Luiz Fernando D'Altoé. (b) Absolute isolation of Mutlu Özcan, Claudia Angela Maziero Volpato, Luiz Fernando D'Altoé the area. *Source:* Mutlu Özcan, Claudia Angela Maziero Volpato, Luiz Fernando D'Altoé. (c) Occlusal view after removal of old resin composite. *Source:* Mutlu Özcan, Claudia Angela Maziero Volpato, Luiz Fernando D'Altoé. (d) View of the cavities after caries and old restoration removal. *Source:* Mutlu Özcan, Claudia Angela Maziero Volpato, Luiz Fernando D'Altoé. (e) Root canal opening filled with resin-modified GIC (Ionoseal; Voco, Cuxhaven, Germany), followed by selective conditioning of the enamel with 35% phosphoric acid (Ultra-Etch; Ultradent, South Jordan, UT, USA). *Source:* Mutlu Özcan, Claudia Angela Maziero Volpato, Luiz Fernando D'Altoé. (f) Primer application (Clearfil SE Bond; Kuraray Noritake Dental, Tokyo, Japan). *Source:* Mutlu Özcan, Claudia Angela Maziero Volpato, Luiz Fernando D'Altoé. (g) Adhesive resin application (Clearfil SE Bond). *Source:* Mutlu Özcan, Claudia Angela Maziero Volpato, Luiz Fernando D'Altoé. (h) Resin composite insertion using incremental technique. *Source:* Mutlu Özcan, Claudia Angela Maziero Volpato, Luiz Fernando D'Altoé. (i) Cavity filling with resin composite (Filtek One Bulk Fill; 3M ESPE, St Paul, MN, USA). *Source:* Mutlu Özcan, Claudia Angela Maziero Volpato, Luiz Fernando D'Altoé. (j) Ultrasonic tip used for guttapercha removal. *Source:* Mutlu Özcan, Claudia Angela Maziero Volpato, Luiz Fernando D'Altoé. (k) Matrix system (Supermat; Kerr Dental, Brea, CA, USA), adapted prior to the adhesion procedure. *Source:* Mutlu Özcan, Claudia Angela Maziero Volpato, Luiz Fernando D'Altoé. (l) Application of self-etching adhesive resin bonding (ED Primer II; Kuraray Noritake Dental). *Source:* Mutlu Özcan, Claudia Angela Maziero Volpato, Luiz Fernando D'Altoé. (m) Removal of excess adhesive with absorbent paper cones. *Source:* Mutlu Özcan, Claudia Angela Maziero Volpato, Luiz Fernando D'Altoé. (n) View immediately after adhesive resin cementation of the two fibreglass posts (Whitepost; FGM, Joinville, Brazil) with resin-based luting cement (Panavia F; Kuraray Noritake Dental). *Source:* Mutlu Özcan, Claudia Angela Maziero Volpato, Luiz Fernando D'Altoé. (o) Final view of the resin composite filling (Filtek One Bulk Fill) for subsequent preparation for indirect restorations. *Source:* Mutlu Özcan, Claudia Angela Maziero Volpato, Luiz Fernando D'Altoé.

In intraradicular preparations, almost all dentine walls have an opposite wall, which creates a cavity with very unfavourable geometry for adhesion [29]. This is due to the high configuration factor (C-factor), which allows for plastic deformation of the resin-based luting cement during its polymerization [103]. In association with this, the presence of an intraradicular post creates more adhesive interfaces, whilst in the dental root – where bending forces and tensional torsion are present – the repetitive stress generated during function can lead to microcracks

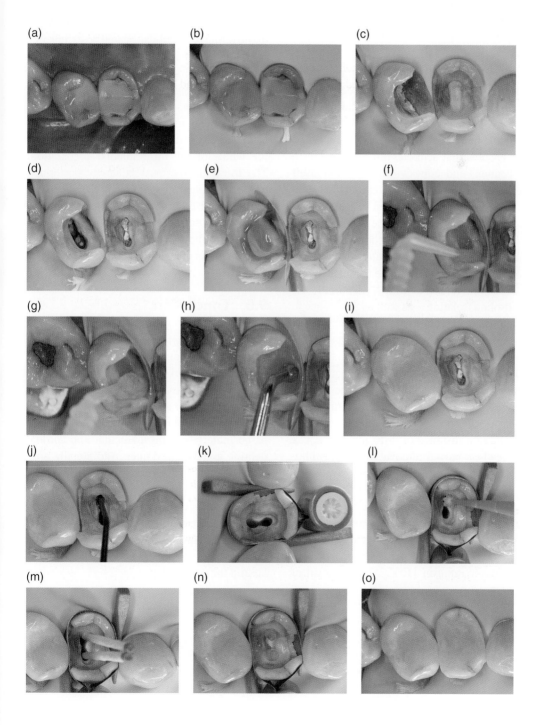

and adhesive interface failures [75]. The limited light access to the photo-polymerization device should also be considered, as it indicates the use of photo-transmitter posts [104]. Light can pass through these posts, but it is not sufficient to ensure proper polymerization of adhesive cement in the most apical portion [105], reinforcing the need for a dual-setting resin-based luting cement [106].

In adhesive restorative procedures for nonvital teeth, the same clinical care should be taken as for vital ones [11, 15]. This includes the routine use of absolute isolation. Adhesive techniques are sensitive to humidity, making a dry operative field a priority [86]. Isolation of the area ensures that acid etching, adhesive resin application, and adhesive cementation itself are performed in a very safe clinical environment. The success of adhesion to root dentine is directly proportional to the quality of the hybrid layer, and the key to obtaining an adequate hybrid layer is infiltration of the adhesive resin bonding agent in the complete depth of the demineralized dentine [8]. Thus, the use of absolute isolation – as well as adherence to all adhesive cementation steps – will certainly have a positive impact on the success of the adhesive protocol.

The acid etching of intraradicular preparations can be accomplished by the use of 38–43% phosphoric acid, with the purpose of removing the smear layer and demineralizing dentine to a distance of 2–10 μm [107]. The acid leads to partial removal of the peritubular dentine, opening of the dentinal tubules, and exposure of the scaffold collagen, creating a suitable surface to receive the adhesive resin and resin-based luting cement [108]. Liquid-viscosity phosphoric acids are preferred to gel formulas for more effective smear-layer removal [109]. After removal of the acid using abundant water rinse, the dentine substrate should not be excessively dried, so that demineralized dentine dehydration does not occur.

The adhesive resin should be applied with a disposable micro-applicator, and excess adhesive should be removed with absorbent paper tips. Dual-polymerized adhesive cement, used in the luting of the prefabricated posts, ensures complete polymerization in the most apical portion of the intraradicular preparation and increases the degree of conversion of monomers to polymers and the working time [106]. Current versions of self-mixing adhesive cements have slim tips that can easily access the whole of the intraradicular preparation. The intraradicular post is slowly positioned within the preparation, allowing excess cement to drain and be properly removed. The post-core is then built up incrementally with resin composite, allowing the steps needed to make the prosthesis to be undertaken (Figure 9.4).

9.6 Conclusion

The nature of root dentine, with low tubular density and a moist environment, makes it a very complex substrate for bonding procedures. Despite these limitations, the same clinical care taken for adhesive procedures in vital teeth should be practised when bonding resin-based materials to intraradicular and coronal dentine in devitalized ones. Additionally, adequate absolute isolation, cleaning, and preparation of the dentine substrate, selection of suitable adhesive resin and adhesive cements, and adherence to the adhesive protocol are all critical in ensuring the success and longevity of adhesive interfaces at both the intraradicular and the coronal levels.

References

1 Marshall, G.W. Jr., Marshall, S.J., Kinney, J.H., and Balooch, M. (1997). The dentin substrate: structure and properties related to bonding. *J. Dent.* 25: 441–458.

2 Dai, X.F., Ten Cate, A.R., and Limeback, H. (1991). The extent and distribution intratubular collagen fibrils in human dentine. *Arch. Oral Biol.* 36: 775–778.

3 Pashley, D.H. and Carvalho, R.M. (1997). Dentine permeability and dentine adhesion. *J. Dent.* 25: 355–372.

4 Pashley, D.H., Pashley, E.L., Carvalho, R.M., and Tay, F.R. (2002). The effects of dentin permeability on restorative dentistry. *Dent. Clin. N. Am.* 46: 211–245.

5 Pashley, D.H., Ciucchi, B., Sano, H., and Horner, J.A. (1993). Permeability of dentin to adhesive agents. *Quintessence Int.* 24: 618–631.

6 Perdigão, J., Moore, K.C., and Swift, E.J. Jr. (1992). A scanning electron microscopy study of human dentin and its interaction with third-generation dentin bonding systems. *Acta Microsc.* 1: 193–203.

7 Mjör, I.A., Smith, M.R., Ferrari, M., and Mannocci, F. (2001). The structure of dentine in the apical region of human teeth. *Int. Endod. J.* 34: 346–353.

8 Ferrari, M., Mannocci, F., Vichi, A. et al. (2000). Bonding to root canal: structural characteristics of the substrate. *Am. J. Dent.* 13: 255–260.

9 Weatherell, J.A., Robinson, C., and Hallsworth, A.S. (1974). Variations in the chemical composition of human enamel. *J. Dent. Res.* 53: 180–192.

10 Takahashi, A., Inoue, S., Kawamoto, C. et al. (2002). In vivo long-term durability of the bond to dentin using two adhesive systems. *J. Adhes. Dent.* 4: 151–159.

11 Hashimoto, M., De Munck, J., Ito, S. et al. (2004). In vitro effect of nanoleakage expression on resin-dentin bond strengths analyzed by microtensile bond test, SEM/EDX and TEM. *Biomaterials* 25: 5565–5574.

12 Breschi, L., Mazzoni, A., Ruggeri, A. Jr. et al. (2008). Dental adhesion review: aging and stability of the bonded interface. *Dent. Mater.* 24: 90–101.

13 Yoshiyama, M., Carvalho, R.M., Sano, H. et al. (1996). Regional bond strengths of resins to human root dentine. *J. Dent.* 24: 435–442.

14 Toledano, M., Osorio, R., Ceballos, L. et al. (2003). Microtensile bond strength of several adhesive systems to different dentin depths. *Am. J. Dent.* 16: 292–298.

15 Ferrari, M. and Tay, F.R. (2003). Technique sensitivity in bonding to vital, acid-etched dentin. *Oper. Dent.* 28: 3–8.

16 De Munck, J., Van Landuyt, K.L., Peumans, M. et al. (2005). A critical review of the durability of adhesion to tooth tissue: methods and results. *J. Dent. Res.* 84: 118–132.

17 Freedman, G. and Leinfelder, K. (2002). Seventh-generation adhesive systems. *Dent. Today* 11: 106–111.

18 Nakabayashi, N., Nakamura, M., and Yasuda, N. (1991). Hybrid layer as a dentin-bonding mechanism. *J. Esthet. Dent.* 4: 133–138.

19 Tay, F.R. and Pashley, D.H. (2001). Aggressiveness of contemporary self-etching systems. I: Depth of penetration beyond dentin smear layers. *Dent. Mater.* 17: 296–308.

20 Van Meerbeek, B., De Munck, J., Yoshida, Y. et al. (2003). Buonocore memorial lecture. Adhesion to enamel and dentin: current status and future challenges. *Oper. Dent.* 28: 215–235.

21 Ito, S., Tay, F.R., Hashimoto, M. et al. (2005). Effects of multiple coatings of two all-in-one adhesives on dentin bonding. *J. Adhes. Dent.* 7: 133–141.

22 Baseggio, W., Consolmagno, E.C., de Carvalho, F.L. et al. (2009). Effect of deproteinization and tubular occlusion on microtensile bond strength and marginal microleakage of resin composite restorations. *J. Appl. Oral Sci.* 17: 462–466.

23 Heintze, S.D., Forjanic, M., and Roulet, F.J. (2007). Automated margin analysis of contemporary adhesive systems in vitro: evaluation of discriminatory variables. *J. Adhes. Dent.* 9: 359–369.

24 Pereira, P.N., Okuda, M., Nakajima, M. et al. (2001). Relationship between bond strengths

and nanoleakage: evaluation of a new assessment method. *Am. J. Dent.* 14: 100–104.

25 Pioch, T., Staehle, H.J., Wurst, M. et al. (2002). The nanoleakage phenomenon: influence of moist vs dry bonding. *J. Adhes. Dent.* 4: 23–30.

26 Zhao, S.J., Zhang, L., Tang, L.H., and Chen, J.H. (2010). Nanoleakage and microtensile bond strength at the adhesive–dentin interface after different etching times. *Am. J. Dent.* 23: 335–340.

27 Pioch, T., Staehle, H.J., Duschner, H., and García-Godoy, F. (2001). Nanoleakage at the composite–dentin interface: a review. *Am. J. Dent.* 14: 252–258.

28 Leloup, G., D'Hoore, W., Bouter, D. et al. (2001). Meta-analytical review of factors involved in dentin adherence. *J. Dent. Res.* 80: 1605–1614.

29 Tay, F.R. and Pashley, D.H. (2002). Dental adhesives of the future. *J. Adhes. Dent.* 4: 91–103.

30 Pashley, D.H., Michelich, V., and Kehl, T. (1981). Dentin permeability: effects of smear layer removal. *J. Prosthet. Dent.* 46: 531–537.

31 Van Meerbeek, B., Yoshida, Y., Lambrechts, P. et al. (1998). A TEM study of two water-based adhesive systems bonded to dry and wet dentin. *J. Dent. Res.* 77: 50–59.

32 Singh, T.V., Patil, J.P., Raju, R.C. et al. (2015). Comparison of effect of C-factor on bond to human dentin using different composite resin materials. *J. Clin. Diagn. Res.* 9: 88–91.

33 Murray, P.E., About, I., Lumley, P.J. et al. (2002). Cavity remaining dentin thickness and pulpal activity. *Am. J. Dent.* 15: 41–46.

34 Ricucci, D., Siqueira, J.F. Jr., Li, Y., and Tay, F.R. (2019). Vital pulp therapy: histopathology and histobacteriology-based guidelines to treat teeth with deep caries and pulp exposure. *J. Dent.* 86: 41–52.

35 Duncan, H.F., Galler, K.M., Tomson, P.L. et al. (2019). European Society of Endodontology position statement: management of deep caries and the exposed pulp. *Int. Endod. J.* 52: 923–934.

36 Hilton, T.J., Ferracane, J.L., and Mancl, L. (2013). Comparison of CaOH with MTA for direct pulp capping: a PBRN randomized clinical trial. *J. Dent. Res.* 92: 16s–22s.

37 Stuart, K., Miller, C., Brown, C. Jr., and Newton, C. (1991). The comparative antimicrobial effect of calcium hydroxide. *Oral Surg. Oral Med. Oral Pathol. Oral Radiol. Endod.* 72: 101–104.

38 Graham, L., Cooper, P.R., Cassidy, N. et al. (2006). The effect of calcium hydroxide on solubilization of bio-active dentine matrix components. *Biomaterials* 27: 2865–2873.

39 Schroder, U. (1985). Effects of calcium hydroxide-containing pulp capping agents on pulp cell migration, proliferation, and differentiation. *J. Dent. Res.* 64: 541–548.

40 Taira, Y., Shinkai, K., Suzuki, M. et al. (2011). Direct pulp capping effect with experimentally developed adhesive resin systems containing reparative dentin-promoting agents on rat pulp: mixed amounts of additives and their effect on wound healing. *Odontology* 99: 135–147.

41 Cox, C.F. and Suzuki, S. (1994). Re-evaluating pulp protection: calcium hydroxide liners vs. cohesive hybridization. *J. Am. Dent. Assoc.* 125: 823–831.

42 Nicholson, J.W. and Croll, T.P. (1997). Glass ionomers in restorative dentistry. *Quintessence Int.* 28: 705–714.

43 Wilson, A.D., Crisp, S., and Ferner, A.J. (1976). Reactions in glass ionomer cements: IV. Effect of chelating comonomers on setting behavior. *J. Dent. Res.* 55: 490–495.

44 Mount, G.J. (1998). Clinical performance of glass-ionomers. *Biomaterials* 19: 573–579.

45 Coogan, M.M. and Creaven, P.J. (1993). Antimicrobial effects of dental cements. *Int. Endod. J.* 26: 355–361.

46 Ermis, R.B. (2002). Two-year clinical evaluation of four polyacid-modified resin composites and a resin-modified glass-ionomer cement in class V lesions. *Quintessence Int.* 33: 542–548.

47 Perondi, P.R., Oliveira, P.H.C., Cassoni, A. et al. (2014). Ultimate tensile strength and microhardness of glass ionomer materials. *Braz. Dent. Sci.* 17: 16–22.

48 Camilleri, J., Montesin, F.E., Papaioannou, S. et al. (2004). Biocompatibility of two commercial forms of mineral trioxide aggregate. *Int. Endod. J.* 37: 699–704.

49 Tay, F.R., Pashley, D.H., Rueggeberg, F.A. et al. (2007). Calcium phosphate phase transformation produced by the interaction of the Portland cement component of white mineral trioxide aggregate with a phosphate-containing fluid. *J Endod.* 33: 1347–1351.

50 Sarkar, N.K., Caicedo, R., Ritwik, P. et al. (2005). Physicochemical basis of the biologic properties of mineral trioxide aggregate. *J. Endod.* 31: 97–100.

51 Torabinejad, M., Hong, C.U., McDonald, F., and Pitt Ford, T.R. (1995). Physical and chemical properties of a new root-end filling material. *J. Endod.* 21: 349–353.

52 Camilleri, J. (2014). Color stability of white mineral trioxide aggregate in contact with hypochlorite solution. *J. Endod.* 40: 436–440.

53 Valles, M., Mercade, M., Duran-Sindren, F. et al. (2013). Influence of light and oxygen on the color stability of five calcium silicate-based materials. *J. Endod.* 39: 525–528.

54 Grech, L., Mallia, B., and Camilleri, J. (2013). Investigation of the physical properties of tricalcium silicate cement-based root-end filling materials. *Dent. Mater.* 29: 20–28.

55 Shin, J.H., Jang, J.H., Park, S.H., and Kim, E. (2014). Effect of mineral trioxide aggregate surface treatments on morphology and bond strength to composite resin. *J. Endod.* 40: 1210–1216.

56 Oskoee, S.S., Bahari, M., Kimyai, S. et al. (2014). Shear bond strength of calcium enriched mixture cement and mineral trioxide aggregate to composite resin with two different adhesive systems. *J. Dent. (Tehran).* 11: 665–671.

57 Camilleri, J. (2015). Mineral trioxide aggregate: present and future developments. *Endod. Top.* 32: 31–46.

58 Active Biosilicate Technology™, Septodont (2010). Biodentine™ scientific file. Saint-Maur-des-Fosse's Cedex, France: R&D Department.

59 Camilleri, J. (2014). Hydration characteristics of Biodentine and Theracal used as pulp capping materials. *Dent. Mater.* 30: 709–715.

60 Ravichandra, P.V., Vemisetty, H., Deepthi, K. et al. (2014). Comparative evaluation of marginal adaptation of biodentine and other commonly used root end filling materials – an in vitro study. *J. Clin. Diagn. Res.* 8: 243–245.

61 Kjellsen, K. and Justnes, H. (2004). Revisiting the microstructure of hydrated tricalcium silicate – a comparison to Portland cement. *Cem. Concr. Compos.* 26: 947–956.

62 Koubi, G., Colon, P., Franquin, J.C. et al. (2013). Clinical evaluation of the performance and safety of a new dentine substitute, Biodentine, in the restoration of posterior teeth – a prospective study. *Clin. Oral Investig.* 17: 243–249.

63 Daltoé, M.O., Paula-Silva, F.W., Faccioli, L.H. et al. (2016). Expression of mineralization markers during pulp response to Biodentine and mineral trioxide aggregate. *J. Endod.* 42: 596–603.

64 Zamparini, F., Siboni, F., Prati, C. et al. (2019). Properties of calcium silicate-monobasic calcium phosphate materials for endodontics containing tantalum pentoxide and zirconium oxide. *Clin. Oral Investig.* 23: 445–457.

65 Camilleri, J., Sorrentino, F., and Damidot, D. (2015). Characterization of un-hydrated and hydrated BioAggregate and MTA Angelus. *Clin. Oral Investig.* 19: 689–698.

66 Arias-Moliz, M.T., Farrugia, C., Lung, C.Y.K. et al. (2017). Antimicrobial and biological activity of leachate from light curable pulp capping materials. *J. Dent.* 64: 45–51.

67 Barrere, F., van Blitterswijk, C.A., and de Groot, K. (2006). Bone regeneration: molecular and cellular interactions with

calcium phosphate ceramics. *Int. J. Nanomedicine* 1: 317–332.

68 Kayahan, M.B., Nekoofar, M.H., McCann, A. et al. (2013). Effect of acid etching procedures on the compressive strength of 4 calcium silicate-based endodontic cements. *J. Endod.* 39: 1646–1648.

69 Poggio, C., Lombardini, M., Colombo, M. et al. (2015). Solubility and pH of direct pulp capping materials: a comparative study. *J. Appl. Biomater. Funct. Mater.* 13: e181–e185.

70 Panahandeh, N., Torabzadeh, H., Ghassemi, A. et al. (2015). Effect of bonding application time on bond strength of composite resin to glass ionomer cement. *J. Dent. (Tehran).* 12: 859–867.

71 Camilleri, J. (2013). Investigation of Biodentine as dentine replacement material. *J. Dent.* 41: 600–610.

72 El-Araby, A. and Al-Jabab, A. (2005). The influence of some dentin primers on calcium hydroxide lining cement. *J. Contemp. Dent. Pract.* 6: 1–9.

73 Bayrak, S., Tunç, E.S., Saroglu, I., and Egilmez, T. (2009). Shear bond strengths of different adhesive systems to white mineral trioxide aggregate. *Dent. Mater. J.* 28: 62–67.

74 Dawood, A.E., Manton, D.J., Parashos, P., and Wong, R.H. (2016). The effect of working time on the displacement of Biodentine™ beneath prefabricated stainless steel crown: a laboratory study. *J. Investig. Clin. Dent.* 7: 391–395.

75 Lin, L.M., Skribner, J.E., and Gaengler, P. (1992). Factors associated with endodontic treatment failures. *J. Endod.* 18: 625–627.

76 Gaston, B.A., West, L.A., Liewehr, F.R. et al. (2001). Evaluation of regional bond strength of resin cement to endodontic surfaces. *J. Endod.* 27: 321–324.

77 Zicari, F., De Munck, J., Scotti, R. et al. (2012). Factors affecting the cement–post interface. *Dent. Mater.* 28: 287–297.

78 Lassila, L.V., Tanner, J., Le Bell, A.M. et al. (2004). Flexural properties of fiber reinforced root canal posts. *Dent. Mater.* 20: 29–36.

79 Mazzitelli, C., Papacchini, F., Monticelli, F. et al. (2012). Effects of post surface treatments on the bond strength of self-adhesive cements. *Am. J. Dent.* 25: 159–164.

80 Nayyar, A., Walton, R.E., and Leonard, L.A. (1980). An amalgam coronal radicular dowel and core technique for endodontically treated posterior teeth. *J. Prosthet. Dent.* 43: 511–515.

81 Subash, D., Shoba, K., Aman, S. et al. (2017). Fracture resistance of endodontically treated teeth restored with biodentine, resin modified GIC and hybrid composite resin as a core material. *J. Clin. Diagn. Res.* 11: ZC68–ZC70.

82 Ekambaram, M., Yiu, C.K.Y., and Matinlinna, J.P. (2015). Bonding of adhesive resin to intraradicular dentine: a review of the literature. *Int. J. Adhes. Adhes.* 60: 92–103.

83 Serafino, C., Gallina, G., Cumbo, E., and Ferrari, M. (2004). Surface debris of canal walls after post space preparation in endodontically treated teeth: a scanning electron microscopic study. *Oral Surg. Oral Med. Oral Pathol. Oral Radiol. Endod.* 97: 381–387.

84 Mader, C.D., Baumgartner, J.C., and Peters, D.D. (1984). Scanning electron microscopic investigation of the smeared layer on root canal walls. *J. Endod.* 10: 477–483.

85 Violich, D.R. and Chansler, N.P. (2010). The smear layer in endodontics – a review. *J. Endod.* 43: 2–15.

86 Gulabivala, K., Patel, B., Evans, G., and Ng, Y. (2005). Effects of mechanical and chemical procedures on root canal surfaces. *Endod. Top.* 10: 103–122.

87 Breschi, L., Mazzoni, A., Dorigo, E.S., and Ferrari, M. (2009). Adhesion to intraradicular dentin: a review. *J. Adhes. Sci. Technol.* 23: 1053–1083.

88 Mayhew, J.T., Windchy, A.M., Goldsmith, L.J., and Getteman, L. (2000). Effect of root canal sealers and irrigation agents on retention of preformed posts luted with a resin cement. *J. Endod.* 26: 341–344.

89 Lindblad, R.M., Lassila, L.V., Salo, V. et al. Effect of chlorhexidine on initial adhesion of fiber-reinforced post to root canal. *J. Dent.* 38: 796–801.

90 Inoue, S., Murata, Y., Sano, H., and Kashiwada, T. (2002). Effect of NaOCl treatment on bond strength between indirect resin core-buildup and dentin. *Dent. Mater. J.* 21: 343–354.

91 Ozturk, B. and Ozer, F. (2004). Effect of NaOCl on bond strengths of bonding agents to pulp chamber lateral walls. *J. Endod.* 30: 362–365.

92 García-Godoy, F., Loushine, R.J., Itthagarun, A. et al. (2005). Application of biologically-oriented dentin bonding principles to the use of endodontic irrigants. *Am. J. Dent.* 18: 281–290.

93 Calt, S. and Serper, A. (2002). Time-dependent effects of EDTA on dentin structures. *J. Endod.* 28: 17–19.

94 Montagner, A.F., Sarkis-Onofre, R., Pereira-Cenci, T., and Cenci, M.S. (2014). MMP inhibitors on dentin stability: a systematic review and meta-analysis. *J. Dent. Res.* 93: 733–743.

95 Breschi, L., Mazzoni, A., Nato, F. et al. (2010). Chlorhexidine stabilizes the adhesive interface: a 2-year in vitro study. *Dent. Mater.* 26: 320–325.

96 Carrilho, M.R., Tay, F.R., Pashley, D.H. et al. (2005). Mechanical stability of resin–dentin bond components. *Dent. Mater.* 21: 232–241.

97 Collares, F.M., Rodrigues, S.B., Leitune, V.C. et al. (2013). Chlorhexidine application in adhesive procedures: a meta-regression analysis. *J. Adhes. Dent.* 15: 11–18.

98 Bohrer, T.C., Fontana, P.E., Wandscher, V.F. et al. (2018). Endodontic sealers affect the bond strength of fiber posts and the degree of conversion of two resin cements. *J. Adhes. Dent.* 20: 165–172.

99 Hagge, M.S., Wong, R.D., and Lindemuth, J.S. (2002). Retention strengths of five luting cements on prefabricated dowels after root canal obturation with a zinc oxide/eugenol sealer: 1. Dowel space preparation/cementation at one week after obturation. *J. Prosthodont.* 11: 168–175.

100 Skupien, J.A., Sarkis-Onofre, R., Cenci, M.S. et al. (2015). A systematic review of factors associated with the retention of glass fiber posts. *Braz. Oral Res.* 29: 1–8.

101 Demiryurek, E.O., Kulunk, S., Yuksel, G. et al. (2010). Effects of three canal sealers on bond strength of a fiber post. *J. Endod.* 36: 497–501.

102 Soares, I.M.V., Crozeta, B.M., Pereira, R.D. et al. (2020). Influence of endodontic sealers with different chemical compositions on bond strength of the resin cement/glass fiber post junction to root dentin. *Clin. Oral Investig.* https://doi.org/10.1007/s00784-020-03212-9.

103 Bouillaguet, S., Troesch, S., Wataha, J.C. et al. (2003). Microtensile bond strength between adhesive cements and root canal dentin. *Dent. Mater.* 19: 199–205.

104 Moazzami, S.M., Kazemi, R., Alami, M. et al. (2012). Light conduction capability of different light-transmitting FRC posts. *J. Dent. Mater. Tech.* 1: 40–46.

105 Goracci, C., Corciolani, G., Vichi, A., and Ferrari, M. (2008). Light-transmitting ability of marketed fiber posts. *J. Dent. Res.* 87: 1122–1126.

106 Wu, H., Hayashi, M., Okamura, K. et al. (2009). Effects of light penetration and smear layer removal on adhesion of post-cores to root canal dentin by self-etching adhesives. *Dent. Mater.* 25: 1484–1492.

107 Pashley, D.H., Zhang, Y., Agee, K.A. et al. (2000). Permeability of demineralized dentin to HEMA. *Dent. Mater.* 16: 7–14.

108 Nakabayashi, N., Kojima, K., and Masuhara, E. (1982). The promotion of adhesion by the infiltration of monomers into tooth substrates. *J. Biomed. Mater. Res.* 16: 265–273.

109 Scotti, N., Scansetti, M., Rota, R. et al. (2013). Active application of liquid etching agent improves adhesion of fibre posts to intraradicular dentine. *Int. Endod. J.* 46: 1039–1045.

Index

Endodontic Materials in Clinical Practice, First Edition. Edited by Josette Camilleri.
© 2021 John Wiley & Sons Ltd. Published 2021 by John Wiley & Sons Ltd.